Alex Brecher
Natalie Stein

The
BIG Book
on the
GASTRIC BYPASS

Everything You Need To Know To Lose Weight and Live Well with the Roux-en-Y Gastric Bypass Surgery

Thank you for reading **The Big Book on the Gastric Bypass: Everything You Need to Know to Lose Weight and Live Well with the Roux-en-Y Gastric Bypass Surgery**

We hope the book has been a valuable resource for you as you decide whether to get theRoux-en-Y Gastric Bypass Surgery.

Need another copy? You can order them online from:

- BariatricPal.com

- Amazon

- Barnes and Noble

You can get them in print and in electronic forms for e–readers including the Kindle, iPad, Nook, Kobo and Sony. They're great gifts for other bariatric patients as well as your friends and family who want to support you in your journey.

If you liked this book, you'll also love the companion books in this series.

The Big Book on the Lap-Band: Everything You Need to Know to Lose Weight and Live Well with the Adjustable Gastric Band!

And

The Big Book on the Gastric Sleeve: Everything You Need to Know to Lose Weight and Live Well with the Vertical Sleeve Gastrectomy

And coming soon…

Life after Weight Loss Surgery: Tips and Tricks for Losing Weight and Living Well

Look out for these and more weight loss surgery books from Alex Brecher and Natalie Stein to help you succeed in your weight loss journey

Acknowledgements

The authors would like to thank everyone who made this book possible. Surgeons, from Alex's own bariatric surgeon to the many other knowledgeable and talented surgeons he has worked with over the years, influenced this book's content. Many of these surgeons, as well as integrated health members who are similarly dedicated to the weight loss surgery community, also support BariatricPal.com with their membership and insights on the boards. The expertise and commitment of these healthcare professionals drive patient success with gastric bypass.

The authors' friends and family members have continuously supported the production of this book and the others in the series. The process has been much easier with their encouragement.

The staff of BariatricPal.com keeps the boards running smoothly each day. Their skills and dedication keep old members coming back and continue to recruit new members. The trust and popularity promoted by the BariatricPal.com staff allow for better service to the weight loss surgery community. The staff maintains an incredible degree of courtesy and respect on the boards so that no member feels excluded or uncomfortable. This book strives to maintain this welcoming atmosphere.

This book would not have been possible without the thousands of BariatricPal.com community members who continue to support the forums and provide inspiration to the authors. Member moderators deserve special recognition and thanks for their generous roles as community leaders and role models. Many additional members are also highly participative and very engaged in the boards. The authors are grateful to all BariatricPal.com users, who inspired this book.

In particular, the authors would like to thank all BariatricPal.com members who were kind enough to share their stories in this book. They embody the true giving spirit of BariatricPal.com, and their willingness to share their stories to benefit others is overwhelming. It was a pleasure to work with each of them, and the book would not have been the same without them. Many of these generous members had already shared parts of their stories in previously published pieces in the BariatricPal.com member newsletters.

Finally, heartfelt thanks to the book's editor, *Melissa Se*, and illustrator, *Gary Crump*. The illustrator's clear and beautiful drawings are designed to help readers visualize the descriptions in the text—and in this case, each drawing truly is worth a thousand words. The editor took the manuscript from its initial submission to an edited and formatted final form, directing the authors in their third book.

Thank you to each of you who has made this book possible and to all of its readers.

Contents

Acknowledgements.. v

List of Tables... xii

List of Figures... xiii

Note From the Authors.. xv

Prologue xix

1. Obesity—A Costly Epidemic... 1
   The Rising Obesity Epidemic 2
   Obesity — An Expensive Affair Indeed... 3
   Health Risks of Obesity 6
   Obesity Threatens Quality Of Life 13
   Take Control – You Are Worth It!.. 27

2. Options for Losing Weight: Diets, Exercise, Weight Loss Drugs, and Surgery 37
   Losing Weight Is Tough 38
   Why Dieting Alone Can't Help 38
   Why Exercise Won't Help You Lose Weight... 42
   What You Need To Know About Weight Loss Drugs............................. 43
   Get the Lowdown on Weight Loss Surgery 45

3. All About The Roux-En-Y Gastric Bypass (RYGB) 63
   What Is Roux-En-Y Gastric Bypass, How It Works, and the Surgical Procedure............. 65
   Overview of the Roux-en-Y Gastric Bypass (RYGB)............................. 67
   The Roux-en-Y Gastric Bypass Operation 68
   More Roux-en-Y Gastric Bypass Facts.. 72

4. RYGB & It's Potential Benefits 77

    How Much Weight Do People Lose After Gastric Bypass? 80

    Weight Loss Depends On You! 81

    Beyond Weight Loss: More Potential Benefits of RYGB 84

    Other Improvements in Your Physical Health after the RYGB 86

    Additional Benefits from RYGB: Better Quality of Life 87

5. Roux-en-Y Gastric Bypass: Risks and Considerations 97

    Risks of the Roux-en-Y Gastric Bypass 98

    Possible Complications 100

    Reducing Your Risk of Complicaions 104

6. Considering Roux-En-Y Gastric Bypass? ....What You Need To Know 111

    Eligibility Criteria for Roux-En-Y Gastric Bypass 112

    Gastric Bypass and Pregnancy 114

    Roux-en-Y Gastric Bypass as a Revisional Surgery 115

    What about RYGB and Adolescents? 116

    A Brief Overview: Review of RYGB's Effects 119

7. Planning for the Gastric Bypass 125

    Doing More Research on RYGB 126

    Possible Sources of Information 127

    Online Communities 128

    Choosing a Surgeon 131

    A Few More Considerations 138

8. Roux-En-Y Gastric Bypass Costs, Insurance
    and More 145

    Cost of the RYGB 146

    Insurance 148

    Paying Out-of-Pocket and Financing Options 155

    Medical Tourism: Going to Another Country for the RYGB 157

    Considerations with Medical Tourism 162

9. Pre-Surgery Tips 171

    How to Prepare For Your Pre-Op Appointment 172

    Likely Medical Tests 176

    Psychological Evaluation 178

    Working with a Dietitian 182

The Pre-Surgery Liquid Diet..187

Pre-Surgery Exercise Program...189

10. Final Preparation for RYGB..197

Preparing Ahead Of Time...198

Ways to Make Post-Op Recovery Easier...201

Packing for the Hospital...202

Getting Help...206

Last-Minute Checks...207

11. Your Time at the Hospital After Surgery...213

Healthy Recovery in the Hospital..216

Your First Few Days at Home...220

Pain Medications & Alternative Pain Management Strategies................220

Returning To Normal Activities and Work..226

12. Aftercare: Your Post-Surgery Care Program.......................................231

Post-Op Care: Surgeon Appointments and Medical Tests......................233

Post-Op Care for Medical Tourism RYGB Patients 233

Food Lists to Menu Planning..235

Post-operative Psychological Challenges 238

Setting Goals and Troubleshooting..239

Staying Positive Post-Surgery! 244

13. Post-Surgery Diet: From Liquid Diet to Solid Foods 251

Why You Need to Follow the Post-Surgery Diet..252

Phase 1 – Liquid Diet..256

Liquids to Avoid...260

Phase 2 – Pureed Diet...266

Foods on a Pureed Foods Diet...267

Phase 3 – Soft Foods Diet 273

Foods from Phases 1 and 2 While in Phase 3 274

Handy Food Lists 276

14. RYGB Diet 101...283

Overview of Phase 4 – The Solid Foods Diet..284

Food Lists for the Solid Diet 286

Help with Meal Planning on the RYGB Diet..293

Strategies for Reducing Hunger...296

Guidelines for Success on the Gastric Bypass Diet..................................297

15. The RYGB Diet & Nutrition 305

    Calories and Weight Loss 306

    Protein as an Energy Source 310

    Not All Fats Are Equal 313

    Caloric Carbohydrates and Dietary Fiber 316

    An Overview of the Micronutrients 318

    Condiments on the RYGB Diet 327

    Calories, Alcohol, and Your Weight 331

    The Nutrition Facts Panel: One of Your New Best Friends 332

16. Physical Activity to Control Weight Loss 339

    Physical Activity Burns Calories to Help
    You Control Your Weight 340

    The Psychosocial Benefits of Physical Activity 345

    Aerobic Exercise: What it is and How Much to Do 350

    Strength or Resistance Training:
    What It Is and How Much to Do 353

    Restrictions after the RYGB 356

    Getting Active after the Roux-en-Y Gastric Bypass 357

    Sticking to the Exercise Program: Problems and Solutions 366

17. The First Year After RYGB Is Filled With Changes 383

    Physical Changes – Weight Loss and Other Effects 384

    Changes in Your Social Life 386

    Improvements in Chronic Conditions 387

    Side Effects after Gastric Bypass 388

    Weight Milestones & Non-Scale Victories 392

    What to Expect: Overcoming Challenges 394

    Do Not Let Plateaus Derail Your Diet 395

18. The Benefits of a Strong Support System 405

    Building Your Support System 406

    How You Can Support Yourself 406

    Family and Friends for Support 407

    A Supportive Work Environment 410

    Support from Your Healthcare Team 412

    Online Support 413

19. Bariatricpal .Com and Other Online Resources..417

    Benefits of Online Resources 418

    Introduction to BariatricPal.com 420

    A Brief Tour of BariatricPal.com 421

    BariatricPal.com Grows with You..422

    Other Features on BariatricPal.com 422

    Other Online Resources 427

Epilogue 431

Glossary of Terms 433

List of Figures

Figure 1: The Digestive System 51

Figure 2: Nutrient Malabsorption to Help in Weight Loss after RYGB..66

Figure 3 : Standard Nutrition Label 333

List of Tables

Table 1: Relationship between obesity rates and medical costs 5

Table 2: Interpreting Blood Sugar Tests 9

Table 3: Cut-off values for diagnosing type 2 diabetes from an oral glucose tolerance test 9

Table 4: Blood Pressure Range 11

Table 5: BMI Table 19

Table 6: Common approaches to dieting 40

Table 7: Sample of foods and calorie counts 43

Table 8: Weight loss drugs (FDA approved) 44

Table 9: Examples of medications that may help you lose weight (not FDA approved) 45

Table 10: Weight loss surgery-Myths Vs. Reality 46

Table 11: Summary of types of weight loss surgery 58

Table 12: Comparing RYGB to other weight loss options 106

Table 13: Review of RYGB's Effects 120

Table 14: Checklist of factors to consider when thinking about the sleeve 122

Table 15: Foods on a Liquid Diet 188

Table 16: Standard guidelines for a clear liquid diet 201

Table 17: Liquids You Can and Cannot Have 256

Table 18: Summary of what you can and cannot have on a full liquid diet 259

Table 19: Sample meal plans during phase 1 of the RYGB diet 262

Table 20: Sample daily menu for your post-surgery clear liquid diet 265

Table 21: Sample menu for a day on the full liquid diet 266

Table 22: Foods Allowed/Not Allowed in Phase2 270

Table 23: Sample Menus for Phase 2 – Pureed Foods Diet 272

Table 24: Sample Menus for Phase 3 – Semi-Solid or Soft Foods Diet 276

Table 25: Monitoring Your Diet and Yourself 279

Table 26: Estimate Time to Lose Weight 285

Table 27: Sample Meal Patterns for Phase 4 294

Table 28: Basic Meal Plan (to help keep up you protein intake and provide a balanced diet) 296

Table 29: Create Your Own Menu – Template1 301

Table 30: Create Your Own Menu – Template 2 302

Table 31: Calories & Weight Change 306

Table 32: High-protein foods 311

Table 33: Medium-protein foods 312

Table 34: Low-protein foods 313

Table 35: Different types of fat & the general recommendations for healthy intake 314

Table 36: Vitamin/Mineral and Requirement 323

Table 37: Sample day on the RYGB diet with a few condiments 328

Table 38: Condiment Substitutions to Try 329

Table 39: Maintain a detailed diet record 336

Table 40: Calories burned doing different activities at different weights 341

Table 41: Sample Plan for Starting a Workout Plan 361

Table 42: Four-week exercise log 373

Table 43: Cravings 397

Note From the Authors

From Alex:

When I began my weight loss journey in 2003, I had no idea that it would lead to all of this. I only wanted a way to lose weight and get myself together. I had been fighting obesity my entire life, and I was desperate for a long-term solution that did not involve starving myself, being obsessed with food, and regaining weight every time I stopped dieting. At 5 feet 7 inches tall, I hit a high of 255 pounds during college. I was able to successfully lose some weight, even a lot of weight, when I dieted, but the weight always came back when I stopped dieting.

I began seriously considering weight loss surgery because of a friend of mine. Since getting the laparoscopic adjustable gastric band (lap-band), he had been losing weight and was looking better than I had ever seen him. After doing a small bit of research, I decided that the lap-band could be my own ticket to controlling my eating and my weight. I got the band in 2003 and assumed that I could easily figure out what I needed to know by searching the Internet when I had questions. I had thought there would be unlimited sites talking about the lap-band and providing social support, information, and encouragement to all of the lap-band patients like me who were so dedicated to losing weight but needed a helping hand.

Boy, was I wrong! There were not that many resources available, and the ones that were there were not that useful. They did not have the information I needed or they did not have a friendly, welcoming vibe that made me want to go back. I wanted a place to go to communicate with other lap-band patients. I wanted to learn from them and to be able to ask my questions and receive advice and suggestions from people who had already been exactly where I was. That is why I started LapBandTalk.com almost immediately after my surgery in 2003. I want all of the lap-band patients out there, and the people who are considering the lap-band as a tool to fight obesity, to have a place to go for the assistance and answers they need, starting from before surgery and for as long as they want to continue the lap-band lifestyle and stay healthy.

LapBandTalk.com took off beyond anything I had ever imagined, and I realized that patients who were interested in or had gotten other weight loss surgery procedures had similar needs. I started RNYTalk.com for Roux-en-Y gastric bypass patients as well as additional boards for other bariatric procedures. These boards, at one time under the larger umbrella name of WLS Boards (Weight Loss Surgery Boards), are now assembled as BariatricPal.com.

BariatricPal.com includes hundreds of thousands of members. Some are successfully maintaining their goal weights or are losing weight, and they attribute part of their weight loss to weight loss surgery. Other members are preparing for surgery or are trying to decide whether weight loss surgery may be right for them. I am proud of our weight loss surgery community and believe it serves a vital purpose in promoting patient success. The site is the first choice for many weight loss surgery patients, including many who use it daily for information, encouragement, and a sense of community.

BariatricPal.com continues to grow and evolve to meet the needs of weight loss surgery patients everywhere. The fully functional smartphone apps for iPhones and Androids and the app for the Kindle make the site accessible at all times from anywhere that you have access to the Internet. I try to be highly sensitive to members' needs and respond to them. Whether it is getting feedback from members, discussing latest trends in other weight loss surgery with surgeons, or attending the annual conference of the American Society for Metabolic and Bariatric Surgery across the country from my home, I do what I can to continually meet your needs.

Consistent with my goal of providing help to all weight loss surgery patients, I am particularly proud of the fact that full membership to BariatricPal.com is free. Not one member is paying a dime to use the site, and I have no plans to change this. Members get unlimited access to all of the services that BariatricPal.com offers, such as the discussion forums, apps, surgeon directory, ability to upload photos, personal blogs, chat rooms, and newsletters. You can read more about the site throughout the book and especially in the final chapter of this book.

Today, the situation on the Internet has dramatically improved from when I got my lap-band procedure done in 2003. You have several hundred, if not thousands, of options for getting information and for meeting people to talk online or arrange to meet in person. Despite this, BariatricPal.com remains one of the premier sites. It is the largest, so you are sure to find people who are or were in your situation. It is non-biased, and my staff and I are very careful to keep it friendly.

So why did I feel the need for this book? It is true that you can find almost all of this information when you read the fine print online and get materials from your surgeon and hospital. But do you really want to? This book has all of the information in one place, so it is more convenient. Plus, it is organized according to what stage you are at in your weight loss journey. It goes from deciding about whether to get the gastric bypass, through the surgery, all the way to living the RYGB lifestyle. It is available as an e-book so it is easy to access, and you can print it out a chapter at a time if you want to stick it in your purse or pocket and read it a bit at a time.

For me, weight loss surgery has been everything that I had hoped for. I have lost 100 pounds and kept it off for years. I am happier than I ever was. I am active and have energy, and food does not dictate my thoughts and life. I cannot be more grateful than I am toward the lap-band as a tool for weight loss, and I hope to support others who are considering weight loss surgery or who already have it to make lasting weight loss a possibility.

That is the purpose of this book. I hope you find that it is an excellent resource and guide for your own journey.

Alex Brecher

Alex Brecher
Founder
BariatricPal.com

Note from Natalie:

I was proud to play a role in helping Alex with this book. I have been increasingly involved in BariatricPal.com, and working with Alex on the monthly newsletters and other behind-the-scenes work. Writing books for the weight loss community seemed to be a fantastic way to continue to reach out and provide a trustworthy and complete source of information. This book, focused on the Roux-en-Y gastric bypass, joins the Big Book series' other two books on the adjustable gastric band (lap-band) and vertical sleeve gastrectomy (gastric sleeve).

As a nutritionist, I am often overwhelmed by the consequences of obesity. The physical effects, including type 2 diabetes, heart disease, arthritis, and sleep apnea, are only part of it. If you suffer from obesity or know someone who does, you know that the psychological battles, low self-esteem and social stigma, discrimination, and judgment are just as significant. They are part of daily life for obese individuals.

I am just as overwhelmed by how difficult it is to beat obesity. Fast food is on every corner, every family and social event revolves around eating, junk food is cheap and delicious, we use cars to take us everywhere, and our lives are often too busy to exercise or cook healthy meals. Nobody can make the best health decisions all the time.

Fighting obesity is tough, and giving up can seem easier. However, giving up can be devastating. For many people, weight loss surgery has been the only successful treatment for obesity in their whole lives, or at least in decades. If you are among the people who have tried every diet under the sun without success and you are ready to make a permanent and dramatic lifestyle change, you might be a good candidate for the gastric bypass.

We wanted to put everything together in a single book to make it easier for you find information. Unfortunately, some RYGB patients do not do all of the background research that they should before deciding to get the surgery. It is heartbreaking to hear from weight loss surgery patients who jumped into the surgery without having realistic expectations about weight loss or lifestyle changes. Just as sad is when weight loss surgery patients think they are doing everything right but are not losing the weight they wanted because they do not have the correct information about what to eat and how to make healthy lifestyle changes.

By the time Alex asked me if I would work with him on this book, I was already starting to "meet" (in a virtual sense—online!) a large number of wonderful members through my experiences working with and writing for BariatricPal.com. Community members impressed me in several ways. I admire their dedication to their weight loss despite the hardships they faced. I respect that each of them has a personal story that brought them to BariatricPal.com, and I appreciate the common ground that all RYGB patients share.

Most of all, what struck me about so many of the BariatricPal.com members that I talked to, and continues to amaze me, is their generosity. They express gratitude for BariatricPal.com and members who have helped them along the way and would like nothing more than to give back to the weight loss surgery community. They love to help others that are beginning their RYGB journeys just like they were helped.

You will see bits and pieces of some of their stories throughout this book. This is just a small sample of the warm and caring people that I have met so far. I am sincerely grateful to those of you who have been kind enough to share your stories for this book. I know that you will touch thousands of lives.

I hope, in some small way, that this book is inspirational and informative for anyone interested in the Roux-en-Y gastric bypass and living a healthy lifestyle.

Natalie Stein

Natalie Stein, MS, MPH
Author

Prologue

Are you sick and tired of struggling with obesity? If you have been obese for years and have tried every weight loss diet without lasting success, weight loss surgery may be the right choice for you. *The Big Book on the Gastric Bypass: Everything You Need to Lose Weight and Live Well with the Roux-en-Y Gastric Bypass* is your complete guide to the Roux-en-Y gastric bypass.

Like so many other patients that have struggled with obesity for many years, you may find that the gastric bypass is the tool you need to eat well and finally lose weight for good. The Big Book guides you through each step of the journey, from deciding to get RYGB, finding a surgeon, and paying for surgery to recovering from surgery, following the bypass diet, and losing weight and keeping it off for life.

The Big Book on the Gastric Bypass: Everything You Need to Lose Weight and Live Well with the Roux-en-Y Gastric Bypass treats you with the respect you deserve and provides facts and analysis in simple language. It discusses everything related to obesity, weight loss, the gastric bypass, and the weight loss surgery diet so that you can make the best decisions for yourself. The book further helps you by being a source of advice and motivation. It contains stories from real-life bypass patients, told in their words. When you are ready to learn all about losing weight and living well with the Roux-en-Y gastric bypass, grab your copy of the book and get reading!

Chapter 1: Obesity – A Widespread Disease

This chapter talks about the obesity epidemic and provides a reminder of the dangers of obesity. It contributes to type 2 diabetes, heart disease, stroke, sleep apnea, and osteoarthritis. It can make you depressed, and you might already be familiar with the social stigma, such as people looking down on you, that comes with obesity. Still, one-third of Americans are obese, and another third are overweight. Our lifestyles and surroundings make losing weight difficult. Each day we face fast food, junk food, not enough opportunities for exercise, and too much time sitting around. How much is obesity affecting you?

Chapter 2: Options For Losing Weight: Diets, Exercise, Weight Loss Drugs, and Surgery

Why is weight loss so difficult when it sounds so simple? Eat less and exercise more, and you should lose weight, right? It is not so easy though. This chapter takes a look at your options for losing weight and why they do not work for most people.

- Diets do not usually work in the long term if you do not make them true lifestyle changes; you will gain the weight right back if you try extreme diets such as low-carb diets or diets that only let you eat boxed meals or shakes.
- Exercise programs are healthy, but they do not usually burn off enough calories to motivate you to continue them.
- Weight loss drugs can be dangerous and are not necessarily effective.

Weight loss surgery, or bariatric surgery, is an alternative option for losing weight and keeping it off. The major types in the United States are:

- Vertical sleeve gastrectomy
- Roux-en-Y gastric bypass
- Sleeve plication (or curvature plication)
- Laparoscopic adjustable gastric band (brand name: Lap-Band)

This chapter discusses each of these approaches to weight loss so you can consider more seriously whether weight loss surgery, possibly the gastric bypass, may be the right choice for you.

Chapter 3: All About The Roux-En-Y Gastric Bypass (RYGB)

You may be considered the gastric bypass as an obesity treatment, but do you know exactly what it is and how it works? This chapter describes the gastric bypass procedure and how it can help you lose weight if you follow the bypass diet. During surgery, the surgeon forms a small pouch out of your stomach and closes off the rest of your stomach so that it cannot be used. The bottom of the small stomach pouch gets attached to a spot toward the middle or bottom of the small intestine so that food bypasses the upper part of the small intestine where nutrient absorption usually takes place.

As explained in the chapter, the surgery is usually laparoscopic, or minimally invasive, but it can be open. After surgery, when you swallow, food travels down your throat, into the small stomach pouch, and to the middle or lower end of your small intestine. The small stomach pouch helps you feel full faster so you are less likely to eat as much. The bypass portion of the gastric bypass helps reduce nutrient absorption so that you do not get as many calories. The Roux-en-Y gastric bypass is intended to be permanent, and you need to follow the bypass diet for life.

Chapter 4: RYGB & It's Potential Benefits

The stomach pouch that you have after RYGB is much smaller than your original stomach. It can hold only about 15 percent of the amount of food that your original stomach could hold. You are likely to eat less and lose weight when you have the gastric bypass because of the smaller amount of food that you can eat. Also, you can lose some weight because will not be absorbing as many calories from your food. Finally, the RYGB changes some of your hormones so that you do not feel as hungry. This chapter talks about how much weight you can expect to lose with the RYGB if you follow the bypass lifestyle. It also explains some of the other benefits of losing weight with the bypass, such as feeling better and getting off of some of your medications.

Chapter 5: Roux-En-Y Gastric Bypass: Risks And Considerations

Any surgical procedure has risks, and this chapter presents them to you so that you can make an informed decision about whether you think the Roux-en-Y gastric bypass is worthwhile for you. Infections and bleeding can occur. Other serious complications include a staple line leak and an obstruction. Rarely, some complications can require a second surgery. Pain is usually severe as you recover from surgery. Nausea, vomiting, and gastrointestinal discomfort are possible but are often preventable if you follow your surgeon's diet and other instructions carefully. You will also likely experience dumping syndrome after RYGB. Chapter 5 makes sure that you are going into the procedure with all the information you need.

Chapter 6: Considering Roux-En-Y Gastric Bypass – What You Need To Know

Now that you know how the Roux-en-Y gastric bypass procedure, how it can help you lose weight, and what the risks are, it is time to start thinking about whether you are a good candidate to get RYGB. Chapter 6 introduces the eligibility criteria for obese patients who want the gastric bypass, as well as exclusion criteria—contraindications (medical conditions) that may prevent you from getting it. The chapter also talks about some special conditions, such as pregnancy, revisional weight loss surgery patients, and adolescents. By the end of this chapter, you will have a much better idea about whether RYGB is for you.

Chapter 7: Planning For the Gastric Bypass

After deciding to get the bypass, it is time to plan your surgery. This chapter suggests sources for expanding your knowledge about the surgery. Selecting a surgeon is an important step in your journey, and we give you tips on finding a surgeon who is qualified and a good fit for your personality. We also introduce the other members of the healthcare team, such as a mental health professional and dietitian. These health professionals will be working with you for years. Finally, the chapter discusses some characteristics to look for when you are deciding where to get your surgery done. While it is not as cozy as a smaller clinic, a bariatric center in a large hospital has many advantages.

Chapter 8: Roux-En-Y Gastric Bypass Costs, Insurance, and More

Financing your surgery can be challenging, but you have multiple options. This chapter walks you through finding out whether your insurance coverage includes RYGB and the steps of getting your pre-approval letter. Finance plans can help you cover the surgery if you do not have health insurance coverage and you cannot afford to pay the entire cost in cash. Since some other nations often offer Roux-en-Y gastric bypass at lower overall costs than in the U.S., each year thousands of patients go to Mexico or other countries for their procedures. This chapter provides advice and tips for medical tourism.

Chapter 9: Pre-Surgery Tips

Surgery day is approaching. You have chosen a surgeon and figured out financing, and you are getting excited! What is next? Relax, take a deep breath, and dig into Chapter 9! As you prepare for surgery, you will meet with your surgeon for medical tests and to discuss your concerns. You will get a psychological evaluation, and a dietitian may work with you on a pre-surgery diet as well as some plans for your post-surgery gastric bypass diet.

Chapter 10: Final Preparation for RYGB

Chapter 10 goes over some of the pre-surgery details, such as getting time off work and making sure your kitchen is well stocked. The chapter provides lists of what to take to the hospital and what to leave at home. If you are going abroad for your Roux-en-Y gastric bypass, do not miss the checklist of important things to take care of as surgery approaches! This chapter has you covered through checking into the hospital and going in for your procedure.

Chapter 11: Your Time At The Hospital After Surgery

Congratulations! You are now an RYGB patient! Taking precautions during this important period in your gastric bypass journey can make your weight loss easier and faster down the road. Chapter 11 talks about what to expect during the rest of your time in the hospital. We also give some advice for speeding your recovery when you get home. During this period, you will gradually return to your normal activities and to work.

Chapter 12: Aftercare: Your Post-Surgery Care Program

Since the gastric bypass is a lifelong procedure, your post-op care goes from the end of surgery through the rest of your life. The more seriously you take your post-surgery care, the more likely you are to avoid complications and have weight loss success with the bypass. Your post-op, or aftercare, program usually includes:

- Your post-surgery surgeon appointments
- Medical tests that you may have

- Other healthcare appointments in your post-surgery care program
- Support group meetings and other sources of support
- Staying positive and persistent during this time

Chapter 13: Post-Surgery Diet: From Liquid Diet to Solid Foods

Food is central to weight loss and health, but you cannot jump right into your long-term RYGB diet right after surgery. The first four to six weeks after surgery are for focusing on recovery, not on weight loss. Eating the right foods now can help you prevent complications later. Chapter 13 goes through your diet during the first several weeks after surgery. During this time, stick carefully to the allowed foods and get into the habit of measuring portions. Drink plenty of water throughout the day but not at meals. This chapter has food lists for each phase plus suggested meal plans and other tips to get you through these first several weeks. Chapter 13 covers the first three out of these four phases of your post-surgery diet progression:

- Liquid diet
- Pureed diet
- Soft foods diet
- Regular RYGB diet

Chapter 14: RYGB Diet 101

You get to start the solid foods diet after you successfully complete the semi-solid phase. The solid foods phase is designed to be your long-term diet; it will help you lose weight and maintain your weight for as long as you choose to follow it. This chapter will let you stick to your RYGB diet with confidence. You will see lists of foods and their serving sizes for each food group plus suggested meal plans and tips for following the Roux-en-Y gastric bypass diet. We will teach you how to make your own meal plans so you can eat the foods you prefer and change up your diet to prevent boredom.

Chapter 15: The RYGB Diet & Nutrition

You can eat most foods on the gastric bypass diet, but you will do best if you focus on high-protein and nutrient-dense foods. We will show you how! This chapter tells you about water, protein, carbohydrates, fats, vitamins, and minerals—all the nutrients you need to stay healthy! High-protein and nutrient-dense choices are critical for preventing deficiencies, so we will tell you what you need to know. You will also get to learn about nutrition labels so you choose healthy foods. It will become natural if you practice it constantly!

Chapter 16: Physical Activity to Control Weight Loss

Physical activity, or exercise, helps you burn calories and control your weight, and this chapter has a list of common activities and the calories you can burn doing them. Regular exercise has other benefits too. It reduces your risk for the obesity-related chronic diseases discussed in Chapter 1, and improves your mood. You can start, after getting your surgeon's approval, with light exercise, such as slow walking or water aerobics. Then progress as you are comfortable. In the chapter, you can find recommendations for amount and types of exercise and ways to fit it in when you are short on time. Of course, sticking to an exercise program is even harder than starting one—and there are tons of tips in the chapter so that you are able to stick to your program—and enjoy it! Chapter 16 talks about:

- Why exercise is good for your weight and health
- Recommended amounts of exercise
- How a complete beginner can safely and gradually start a physical activity program when you still have a lot of weight to lose
- How to make your program more advanced as you progress
- How to stick to your exercise program for the long term

Chapter 17: The First Year After RYGB Is Filled With Changes

The changes during the first year can be overwhelming—unless you are prepared for them! Chapter 16 gives you a nice overview of the changes to expect—keeping in mind, of course, that each individual's gastric bypass experience is slightly different. During the first year on the RYGB diet, you can expect significant weight loss and changes in your body. You will probably feel better about yourself and notice that others treat you differently as you lose weight. This chapter helps you recognize symptoms of complications so you know whether to call your surgeon. Chapter 16 also provides tips on staying motivated. Cosmetic surgery to remove extra skin is something that you may want to consider as you lose weight, and the chapter outlines the most common options.

Chapter 18: The Benefits of a Strong Support System

The previous chapter discussed some of the changes to expect after your Roux-en-Y gastric bypass. With so many changes, you will need a lot of support. Chapter 18 helps you build a fail-proof support system. This chapter will talk about the sources of support that may be available to you. These include:

- Yourself
- Your family and friends
- Members of your medical team
- Other bariatric surgery patients from your support group meetings and online communities

Chapter 19: Bariatricpal.Com and Other Online Resources

There is always more to learn. You can read The Big Book on the Gastric Bypass: Everything You Need to Lose Weight and Live Well with the Roux-en-Y Gastric Bypass, call your surgeon, and talk to all of the members of your support groups, and you will never know every detail about the gastric bypass that you will be wondering about eventually. That is where online resources come in; there is a nearly infinite array of sites that can answer your questions. BariatricPal.com is an online community with more than 200,000 members, many of whom have been in your shoes and can provide advice from personal experience. Members are encouraging, too, so you can feel comfortable there. Membership is free and features include regular newsletters, a profile page with space for your photos and a blog, a surgeon directory with member ratings and reviews, and a live chat room.

Ready to get started? Read on…

1

Obesity—A
Costly Epidemic

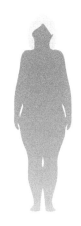

You can choose not to be obese.

Do you want to hear that again?

You can choose not to be obese.

Obesity may not *seem* like a choice. Why would anyone *choose* to suffer the health consequences and feel the embarrassment of being obese? If you could, wouldn't you *choose* to be a normal weight? You would be more energetic, healthier, able to fit into fashionable clothes, and someone who gets involved in everything.

But you have been struggling with your weight for years and possibly for your whole life. You have tried every diet on the planet; none has worked for more than a few weeks or months. You have health problems or worry about developing them. The United States and entire world are getting fatter. Of course, you cannot *choose* not to be obese. Or can you?

"What's the point? Why even bother to try?"

With everything appearing to be stacked against you, you might wonder why you fight obesity so hard. We know why. Deep down, you still have a glimmer of hope. One day, you might figure out a permanent solution to your weight. *Is the roux-en-Y gastric bypass surgery the solution for you?* It could very well be. Thousands of patients worldwide have succeeded in losing weight after getting the gastric bypass. Many of them can tell you that it changed their lives and can change yours.

This entire book is dedicated to the gastric bypass—what it is, how it can help you lose weight, how you get it, and what happens afterward. We will get to all of that. For now, let's start at the beginning—with obesity. This chapter will cover the following topics:

- The obesity epidemic in the U.S
- Harmful effects of obesity
- Causes of obesity in society
- Your own causes of obesity
- Your motivation for losing weight
- Defining obesity with the BMI

The Rising Obesity Epidemic

The dictionary defines an "epidemic" as a disease "affecting a disproportionately large number of individuals within a population."[1] This definition qualifies obesity as an epidemic in the United States and most nations worldwide.

An Epidemic Is a Disease

Obesity is a disease because it makes us sick. As this chapter will explain, obesity causes chronic illnesses, such as type 2 diabetes and heart disease. It can lead to painful conditions, such as osteoarthritis, and mental illness, such as depression. After tobacco use, obesity is the second leading underlying cause of death in the U.S.

An Epidemic Is Widespread

The Centers for Disease Control and Prevention report that more than one out of every three American adults is obese.[2] Another third of the adult population is overweight, which means that they are at risk for becoming obese. This leaves less than one-third of the entire American adult population at a "normal" weight. In fact, obesity is so widespread in the U.S. that there are more obese people than so-called "normal-weight" people!

Obesity is not just an American problem. More than 500 million people worldwide are obese; 1.4 billion are overweight or obese.[3] In fact, the World Health Organization lists obesity and overweight as one of the top risk factors for death in the world.[4]

Obesity—An Expensive Affair Indeed

Obesity is expensive. Even worse, the costs of obesity are growing as fast as the rates of obesity. In 1998 less than 20% of adults in the U.S. were obese; that year, total medical costs related to obesity were $78.5 billion in medical costs.[5] By 2008 the rate of obesity was significantly higher; more than one-third of Americans were obese. Medical costs related to obesity were $147 billion.[6] And in 2010 medical costs due to obesity hit $190 billion. To put that number in perspective, nearly one-tenth of all medical spending in the U.S. is the result of obesity.

Who Pays for Obesity?

Medicare and Medicaid Pay Some of the Cost of Obesity

Medicare and Medicaid pay about half of the medical costs caused by obesity. Medicare is a health insurance program run by the national government. It covers:

- Adults over age 65
- People with disabilities
- People with end-stage renal disease (or chronic kidney failure)
- Low-income individuals that may not be able to afford another health insurance plan or health care

Medicaid is the health insurance program for low-income adults and children and individuals with disabilities. It is a federal program, but each state has the ability to modify the program.

Medicare is funded by the U.S. federal government, and Medicaid is funded by both the federal government and by individual state governments. Because about half of obesity-related medical costs are paid for by Medicare and Medicaid, everyone's tax dollars are paying for nearly $100 billion per year of the medical costs of obesity. To put it another way, the total costs of these healthcare insurance programs for the needy would be 10% less if obesity did not exist.

Who Else Pays for Obesity?

If Medicare and Medicaid pay for about half of the nation's obesity bill, who covers the rest? The payers are individuals, like you, and private healthcare insurance companies. Compared to an employee who is at a healthy weight, someone who is mildly obese (we will get to the exact definitions in a minute) can cost an employer-sponsored insurance plan about an extra $1,850 per year. A more obese individual can cost a healthcare coverage plan about $3,086 extra per year, while a very obese person can cost an extra $5,530 per year compared to someone who is not obese.

Why Is Obesity So Expensive?

You may be wondering why we keep talking about the "medical" costs of obesity. What other costs are there? Health economists divide the costs of obesity into two main categories: medical and non-medical.

More than 20%, or one out of every five dollars, spent on health care in the United States is spent on treatment for a medical problem that is caused by obesity. In addition, there are non-medical costs associated with obesity. The non-medical costs are more difficult to calculate than medical costs, but they make obesity an even more expensive disease.

Medical Costs of Obesity

Medical costs, or direct medical costs, are easy to visualize. These costs are what you or your insurance company pay when you or your dependent needs medical treatment because of a health problem caused by obesity. Just to give you an idea, here are a few examples of possible medical costs from obesity:

- Blood sugar testing supplies to monitor type 2 diabetes that was caused by obesity
- Extra visits to a primary care physician to monitor changes in weight and vital signs, such as blood pressure or blood cholesterol levels
- Care from a medical specialist that is required due to any obesity-related health situation. Each of these visits can cost hundreds of dollars even before counting the cost of tests and medical equipment. You might need:
  - Endocrinologists to monitor hormones if you have diabetes
  - Pulmonologists or lung doctors, if you have trouble breathing
  - Sleep doctors if you have sleep apnea

Non-Medical Costs of Obesity

You may not think of the non-medical costs when you think about obesity, but these costs are substantial. They come from work-related problems and from a variety of unexpected sources.

Obesity mainly hurts the economy because of lower overall productivity at work. Absenteeism, or days missed from work, is a huge problem related to obesity. A man who is obese takes 5.9 sick days per year more than a non-obese man, and an average obese woman takes 9.4 extra sick days per year compared to a healthy-weight woman. Absenteeism from obesity really hurts companies and the economy at the local, state, and national levels; on average, it costs $1,000 to $1,200 per obese person per year.

Even while at work, obese individuals may not be as productive. You yourself may be familiar with feeling tired and having more trouble "getting through the day." You are lazy or avoiding effort. More likely, obesity makes you tired by interfering with your sleep and reducing your daytime energy levels. Attending work when you are sick is called "presenteeism." If obesity affects you like an illness and prevents you from doing your best when you are at work, you are experiencing "presenteeism."

Obesity has additional non-medical costs, such as the cost of extra fuel. Gas mileage goes down and costs $4 billion extra per year because of obese drivers and passengers. Airplane passengers pay $5 billion extra per year in additional fuel because of the heavier weights of the average passenger.[7] On the ground, 39 million gallons of additional gasoline are required annually for each extra pound that the average driver weighs.[8] A tragic effect of obesity is that obese individuals are less likely to buckle up, making accidents more devastating. You yourself might regularly skip the seatbelt, because it is too small for you.

Additional prices of obesity come from making society somewhat more accommodating for obese people, although if you are obese, you will probably testify that many more amenities would improve your quality of life! Equipment such as "bariatric chairs" or "bariatric toilets" available in public places can cost more than $1,000 each.

Obesity Is on the Rise

The rate of obesity was relatively constant for many years, but it has sharply increased in recent decades. The rate of obesity worldwide has more than doubled since 1980.9 The same is true in the U.S.; 15% of American adults were obese in 1980, while 34% of adults were obese by 2007–2008.[10]

The number of states with high obesity rates is increasing each year too. The National Center for Health Statistics (NCHS) is part of the Centers for Disease Control and Prevention (CDC). This agency is responsible for keeping records of the nation's health. The NCHS monitors the number of people who are obese each year.

We can summarize this information in *Table 1* so that you can easily see the relationship between obesity rates and medical costs. As Americans become more obese, medical costs also increase.

Year	% of Americans Who Were Obese	Number of States With Obesity Greater Than 30%	Annual Medical Costs Related to Obesity
1998	20%	0	$78.5 billion
2008	33.9%	6	$147 billion
2010	34%	13	$190 billion

Table 1: Relationship between obesity rates and medical costs

Are These Diseases Really Preventable?

The following diseases and conditions are so common and so harmful that it may be hard to believe that they are mostly preventable and that if you are obese, you can greatly reduce your risk of developing these diseases by losing excess body weight. Plus, if you are obese and you already have these conditions, losing weight can help you reverse some of these conditions and reduce your risk of complications from others. BariatricPal.com is a friendly community that is full of real-life examples of people who have gotten healthier by losing weight after getting the gastric bypass. You might want to check out the discussion forums to learn about other people's experiences and ask any questions that you have.

Let's go back to the first part of the definition of an "epidemic": it is a disease. In the U.S., obesity is the second leading cause of death after tobacco. Obesity causes more than 300,000 deaths per year in the U.S. alone.[11] The life expectancy of severely obese individuals is more than 10 years less than that of non-obese individuals.

Health Risks of Obesity

Obesity increases your risk for each of the following conditions that are described. You may already have them, or your doctor may have told you that you are at high risk for them. These diseases and conditions are so numerous that they may seem like a laundry list of diseases and conditions. The problem is that each one of them is real, and one or more of them can impact your life or already is a factor in your life.

Type 2 Diabetes

Diabetes mellitus, or diabetes, is the seventh leading direct cause of death in the U.S. It also causes many deaths due to other diseases, such as kidney disease and heart disease. In 2010 more than 20 million Americans knew that they had diabetes, and another five million were likely living with undiagnosed diabetes, according to the Centers for Disease Control and Prevention.[12] More than 90 percent of people with diabetes have the kind known as type 2 diabetes. The most stunning part is that type 2 diabetes is largely preventable—it is often caused by obesity.[13]

> **Tip**
>
> For more information about types of carbohydrates, their food sources, and their role in nutrition, see Chapter 15, "The RYGB Diet & Nutrition."

What Is Diabetes Mellitus?

Diabetes mellitus is a condition with uncontrolled and higher-than-normal blood sugar levels. When you have diabetes, a high-carbohydrate or high-calorie meal can make your high blood glucose levels go even higher. High blood sugar is called "hyperglycemia" or, literally, "high blood sugar." People with diabetes have hyperglycemia most of the time but can occasionally get "hypoglycemia," or low blood sugar. That happens when your blood glucose levels drop quickly and uncontrollably. You might feel weak or even faint.

Why does this happen? What changes occur when you get diabetes so that your body can no longer control your blood sugar levels? First, let's go over what happens when you are healthy.

Type 1 versus Type 2 Diabetes

Have you ever wondered about the difference between type 1 and type 2 diabetes? They both consist of trouble controlling your blood sugar levels, but they have different causes. Type 1 diabetes is often described as a lack of insulin, while type 2 diabetes is often described as insulin resistance.

Type 1 diabetes has a much stronger genetic component. Your genes are predisposed, or pre-programmed, to be ready to develop type 1 diabetes. You cannot do much to avoid it. Type 1 diabetes develops quickly. It usually occurs in children or adolescents when they get sick with a normal illness, such as a cold. The illness triggers their immune systems to turn against their own pancreas and destroy their insulin-producing beta cells. Without insulin, most of the cells in the body cannot take glucose from the blood, so blood sugar levels stay high. This type of diabetes is sometimes known as "insulin-dependent diabetes," because patients need regular insulin injections for the rest of their lives.

Type 2 diabetes develops slowly. It is often linked to weight gain or obesity. When you consistently eat extra calories—which is true when you are gaining weight—you are consistently breaking down a lot of food into sugar. This sugar goes into your blood. It is a lot to demand of your body to keep your blood sugar levels down when you are constantly placing too much sugar in your body.

At first, your body can keep up with this demand by making and secreting more insulin from your pancreas. For a while, this extra insulin is enough to let the glucose in your blood enter your cells and get your blood sugar back to normal levels. This works okay for a while, but then you start to develop insulin resistance. You may have heard of this; it is just what it sounds like. Your cells are no longer very sensitive to insulin; they are resistant. That means that you need more and more insulin to get the same amount of glucose into your cells and maintain the same blood sugar levels as before.

When you need more and more insulin, you get "hyperinsulinemia," or abnormally high levels of insulin in your blood. Finally, your pancreas can no longer keep up with the high demand for insulin, and your blood sugar levels start to rise. This is a condition called prediabetes, and it can develop into diabetes as your blood sugar levels continue to rise.

When you eat carbohydrates, your digestive system breaks them down into smaller carbohydrate pieces called glucose, which is also a sugar. The glucose gets released into your bloodstream so your blood glucose, or blood sugar, levels increase moderately as a normal part of metabolism.

Most of the cells in your body use glucose for energy. They take the glucose from your blood and bring it inside the cell. This process lets your blood glucose levels go back down to the lower levels they were at before your meal. Most of the cells in your body, including your muscle, liver, and fat cells, depend on insulin to help them carry in glucose from your blood.

In type 2 diabetes, you develop *insulin resistance.* This means that even when insulin is there, your cells do not really recognize it any more. Your cells are not insulin sensitive any more. Insulin no longer is good at helping your cells bring in glucose, so your blood sugar levels stay high.

Complications of High Blood Sugar Levels and Diabetes

Are high blood sugar levels really that important? YES! Glucose in your blood can stick to your blood vessels and other body cells and cause damage. High blood glucose levels can cause a lot of damage. (Diabetes is "uncontrolled" if your blood sugar levels remain high. It is "controlled" if you are on medications or diet therapy to keep your blood sugar levels a little lower.) These are some of the most common complications of uncontrolled diabetes:

- *Heart disease*: Damaged blood vessels are a sign of heart disease. When your blood vessels have glucose stuck to them, they do not function as well. This prevents healthy blood flow to the heart, and you can have a heart attack. Diabetes is also bad for your heart, because it increases your risk for having high cholesterol.

- *Chronic kidney disease*: Your kidneys act as filters for your blood so that waste products can leave your body. The small vessels and nephrons, or little filters, in your kidneys progressively become impaired when you have high blood glucose levels, and you may develop chronic kidney disease. This can lead to needing to go to a hospital to use a dialysis machine to filter your blood multiple times a week.

- *Infections*: When your blood flow is slower or restricted because your blood vessels do not work well, your blood does not clear out toxins as well. Injuries and wounds that would normally be minor can become infected. Diabetes can weaken your immune system, and you can also get more respiratory infections, such as cold and the flu.

- *Peripheral neuropathy*: This condition is also caused by damaged blood vessels from diabetes. You have trouble getting your blood to your legs and feet and may feel numbness or tingling.

- *Amputations*: The result of infections and peripheral neuropathy can be amputations. When you have an infection in your foot and cannot feel it or heal it well, the infection may get so bad that you need to have an amputation. In fact, diabetes is the leading cause of amputations in the U.S.

- *Blindness*: Blood vessels in your eyes can get damaged when glucose attaches to them, so you may eventually become blind. The earlier symptom is blurry vision that progressively gets worse.

Diagnosing Diabetes

- *Fasting Blood Sugar*: Your doctor might use a fasting blood sugar test to diagnose diabetes. This test is standard when you go to the lab in the morning before breakfast. This is how the results are interpreted:

Category	Value
Normal	Less than 100 mg/dL
Impaired fasting glucose (IFT, or prediabetes)	100-125 mg/dl
Diabetes	Greater than 126 mg/dL

Table 2: Interpreting Blood Sugar Tests

- *Oral Glucose Tolerance Test*: Your doctor might also prescribe an oral glucose tolerance test, or OGTT, to diagnose type 2 diabetes. In the test, you drink a solution of 75 grams of glucose dissolved in water.[14] Since glucose is a kind of sugar, this drink is very, very sweet. In fact, it has about twice as much sugar as a 12-ounce can of soda! *Table 3* shows the cut-off values for diagnosing type 2 diabetes from an oral glucose tolerance test.

Time With Respect to Drinking Glucose Water	Normal Value (a Higher Value Is an Indicator of Type 2 Diabetes
Fasting (before drinking)	60 to 95 mg/dl
1 hour after drinking	Less than 200 mg/dl
2 hours after drinking	Less than 140 mg/dl

Table 3: Cut-off values for diagnosing type 2 diabetes from an oral glucose tolerance test

- *A1c, or glycated hemoglobin*: You have probably had this test done if your doctor found that you have diabetes or pre-diabetes, which is a step in the development of full-blown diabetes. The test measures how well you have controlled your blood sugar over the past three months.[15] The value is expressed in terms of percent of red blood cells that have glucose attached to them because of high blood sugar levels. A normal value is less than 6%, and your goal might be less than 7% if you have diabetes. Higher values are more likely to lead to complications of diabetes.

Heart Disease: Heart disease, or cardiovascular disease, is the leading cause of death in the U.S. The heart diseases actually include several different diseases.

- Atherosclerosis is a hardening of the arteries because of the buildup of plaque. It can prevent you from getting enough blood to your arms, legs, heart, or brain.
- Congestive heart failure happens when your heart is too weak to pump enough blood around your body, so you may be tired and out of breath all the time.
- Coronary heart disease happens when your blood vessels narrow so that not enough blood gets to your heart.[16]

Each kind of heart disease can lead to a fatal or disabling heart attack or stroke. A heart attack is when blood flow to your body is blocked because of a blood clot or narrowed arteries. A stroke happens when the blood supply to your brain is cut off so your brain cells start to die from lack of oxygen.

Heart disease is strongly linked to obesity:

- You are much more likely to get heart disease if you are obese.
- You are more likely to get heart disease if you have type 2 diabetes, which is often caused by obesity.
- Your heart works harder to pump blood when you have extra body fat.

Dyslipidemia, or High Cholesterol: Dyslipidemia is a major risk factor for heart disease, and obesity is a major cause. "Dyslipidemia" means abnormal levels of cholesterol and triglycerides in your blood. "Dys" means "abnormal," "lipid" refers to a kind of fat, such as cholesterol and triglycerides, and "emia" refers to your blood.

A lipid panel, or "cholesterol test," is a simple blood test that is used to measure your blood lipid levels. You probably get your lipid panel done regularly when you go to a physical at your doctor's office. These are the components of a lipid test and normal results:[17]

- Total cholesterol should be under 200 mg/dL
- HDL cholesterol should be between 40 and 60 mg/dL, and a higher number is even better. HDL cholesterol is your "good" cholesterol because it helps clear away bad fats from your body.
- LDL cholesterol should be under 130 mg/dL. LDL cholesterol is your "bad" cholesterol, because it can stick in your arteries and cause atherosclerosis from plaque build-up.
- Triglycerides should be under 150 mg/dL. Similar to LDL cholesterol, triglycerides can lead to atherosclerosis.

You have dyslipidemia if any of your values are unhealthy. Dyslipidemia is linked to obesity.

- Obesity increases total cholesterol, LDL cholesterol, and triglycerides
- Obesity lowers HDL cholesterol[18]
- Weight gain leads to dyslipidemia

Hypertension, or High Blood Pressure: Obesity can increase your risk for high blood pressure, or hypertension.[19] More than one-third of U.S. adults have high blood pressure, and many more have prehypertension, or above-normal blood pressure that can soon become hypertension.[20] Your blood pressure is the force of your blood against the walls of your blood vessels, which include your arteries, veins, smaller arterioles and venules, and tiny capillaries.

Most people get their blood pressure measured each time they visit the doctor. Usually a nurse takes your blood pressure when you check in for your appointment. The nurse has you sit down and places a cuff around your forearm. He or she inflates the cuff until you feel it tighten around your arm. Then the nurse slowly releases the cuff and listens carefully for two sounds (or if she is using one of the newer blood pressure machines, she will just wait for the numbers to display on the screen). You get your blood pressure results in two familiar values, which might appear as 150/100.

This fraction is the systolic blood pressure number over your diastolic blood pressure. Here is what each of those really means:

- *Systolic blood pressure*: This is the higher blood pressure value of the two. It is measured when your heart is in systole. That means your heart is contracting to pump blood throughout your body. It occurs once per heartbeat.

- *Diastolic blood pressure*: This is the lower blood pressure value of the two. It is measured when your heart is in diastole, or relaxation. The blood is not being pumped as forcefully through your blood vessels. Each period of diastole occurs when your heart relaxes in between beats. You get one systolic measure (heart contraction) per heartbeat and one diastolic measure (heart relaxation) in between heartbeats. So, if your pulse is 70, you have 70 systolic periods and 70 diastolic periods per minute.

Table 4 shows the different categories for blood pressure as defined by the National Heart, Lung and Blood Institute.[21] Your blood pressure is normal only if *both* your systolic and diastolic blood pressures are normal; that is, if your blood pressure is 120/80 or below. If even one of your values is outside of the normal range, you have prehypertension, stage 1 hypertension, or stage 2 hypertension.

Stage	Systolic		Diastolic
Normal	Less than 120	*And*	Less than 80
Prehypertension	120-139	*Or*	80-89
Stage 1 Hypertension	140-159	*Or*	90-99
Stage 2 Hypertension	160 or higher	*Or*	100 or higher

Table 4: Blood Pressure Range

Obesity can lead to some of the factors that raise blood pressure. For example, obesity can increase your risk for atherosclerosis, or narrow, more rigid blood vessels. Obesity can also increase your pulse rate. Atherosclerosis and a higher pulse rate can both increase blood pressure.

You have probably heard about the link between sodium, or salt, and high blood pressure. Your blood pressure can increase if you eat too much salt. Salt leads to water retention, so the amount of water in your blood increases, and you get more force against your blood vessel walls—or higher blood pressure. Your diet might be high in sodium if you eat a lot of processed and fast foods. A single crispy chicken sandwich from a fast food restaurant can easily have over half the maximum amount of sodium you should have in a day.

High blood pressure has a well-deserved nickname as "the silent killer." You do not feel any early symptoms, so you may not know that you have high blood pressure until conditions such as heart disease, kidney disease, or stroke develop. Heart disease is the leading cause of death in the U.S.; stroke is the fourth leading cause of death; and kidney disease is the ninth top cause of death.[22]

Arthritis: You might think of arthritis as an old person's disease that cannot be prevented. It is true that arthritis is often to blame for the aching joints that many older adults suffer from, but it is also true that arthritis affects many younger people too. In addition, many cases of arthritis have nothing to do with aging; instead, they are caused by obesity. Arthritis can lead to stiffness, swelling, and pain in any of your joints, such as those of your fingers, toes, elbows, knees, and ankles.

Osteoarthritis: Osteoarthritis is the most common kind of arthritis, and 27 million Americans have it, according to the National Institute of Arthritis and Musculoskeletal and Skin Disorders (NIAMS).[23] One way to think about osteoarthritis is wear-and-tear on your joints. These factors can cause arthritis, because they are associated with wear and tear:

- Older age – You have using your joints for a longer time.
- Overuse from exercise – Baseball pitchers might get arthritis in their shoulders, and tennis players develop it in their elbows—you have probably heard of "tennis elbow"!
- Obesity – Your joints are supporting far more weight than they are designed to support.

Gout: Gout is another kind of arthritis that can be caused by obesity, and six million Americans have it. This form of arthritis is caused by uric acid building up in your joints, especially a joint in your toe or another single joint.[24] You are more likely to develop gout if you are obese, do not exercise much, or frequently follow fad diets that are designed for fast weight loss. Gout is also more likely if your diet is poor and if you do not eat enough fruits and vegetables.

You are more likely to get *osteoarthritis* and *gout* if you are obese. If you already have these conditions and are obese, losing weight can help. Why? There are a few reasons:

1. The first reason is pretty simple. Extra body weight places extra stress on your joints. Whenever you walk, stand, or move, your joints have to support your extra body weight. Over time, this can break down the natural supportive cushioning in your joints and cause the pain and swelling of osteoarthritis.

2. The second reason involves chronic inflammation. Arthritis is an inflammatory disease, and obese individuals have more chronic inflammation. Chronic inflammation is different from acute inflammation, which is your body's normal, healthy response to an injury. An example of acute inflammation is when you get a swollen finger as your body tries to heal itself after you jam it into a wall. Chronic inflammation is a risk factor for many chronic diseases, including heart disease and diabetes as well as arthritis. Losing weight can lower your levels of chronic inflammation and help prevent or treat osteoarthritis.

3. The third reason why losing weight can reduce joint pain is that gout is caused by too much uric acid. Your body produces uric acid as a normal part of metabolism, which is when you break down and rebuild your healthy body tissues, which include muscles, bones, and fat. When you are overweight, you have a lot of body tissue, so your metabolism is higher and your body produces more uric acid. This causes uric acid to build up in your joints.

Obstructive Sleep Apnea: When you have obstructive sleep apnea, you stop breathing for seconds or even minutes while you are sleeping. Usually each episode stops when you snort or cough yourself awake. The cycle can repeat itself up to 30 times per hour throughout the night. As you can imagine, you never get a good night's sleep or feel rested when you wake up in the morning. Sleep apnea makes you tired nearly constantly during the day, so you have no energy and cannot focus. Another problem with sleep apnea is that it increases your risk of having a heart attack or stroke. Even scarier, you could die in your sleep when you stop breathing.

More than half of the people with sleep apnea are overweight according to the National Heart, Lung and Blood Institute.[25] Larger throat muscles from being obese block the airways in your throat as you sleep. If you have sleep apnea, your doctor may have told you to use a continuous positive airway pressure, or CPAP, machine overnight to keep your airways open.

Obesity can cause sleep apnea, and sleep apnea can cause more obesity. You are more likely to gain weight when you have sleep apnea, because you are hungrier. So you eat more and are more tired, so you are less active. The more weight you gain, the worse your sleep apnea gets. Losing significant amounts of weight can improve or cure sleep apnea so you do not have to worry about having a heart attack during the night or using your CPAP machine anymore.

Psychological Disorders: *Clinical depression* is more likely in obese individuals. You may feel helpless about your weight and carry that helplessness over to other parts of your life. Other symptoms of depression include:

- Feeling tired
- Not being able to care much about anything
- Not wanting to talk to people
- Feeling unable or unwilling to get up and face the day

Social stigmatization is another of the unfortunate consequences of obesity. You've probably run across more than one person who judges you based on your weight. Many unpleasant people automatically decide that you are stupid or lazy simply because they do not like the way you look. They may do this intentionally or subconsciously, without realizing it, but it hurts you either way.

Poor body image and *low self-esteem* are other common effects of obesity according to the National Institutes of Health.[26] Even though you are a wonderful person with so many unique and valuable qualities, you may not even realize it. All you see are your faults. These feelings of low self-worth can make you binge eat or eat emotionally when you are alone.

Obesity Threatens Quality Of Life

It is no fun being the fat kid, the jolly uncle, or the social outcast. Obesity does not just make your physical health worse. Obesity lowers your quality of life in ways that cannot be diagnosed by your doctor. Obesity can make your life flat-out miserable. Maybe it has made your own life miserable for years.

Obesity affects your daily life. Recent years or your whole life may be a collection of memories of embarrassing moments. Maybe each day is devoted to your attempts to avoid reminders that you are obese. You may spend your time pretending that you do not want to participate in fun things with your friends and family or making up excuses for why you cannot make it to a business meeting. But what are your real reasons for avoiding these occasions? You know that you will not be able to fit into the movie theater seats, that you cannot wear a nice dress to the party, or that your work colleagues will not bother to take you seriously. How do you know? You know from years of experience.

An average day may consist of being the good-natured butt of jokes. These jokes cut you deeply, but you feel obligated to laugh at them because the only thing worse than being the good-natured fat friend is being the fat social recluse. In the best case, the fat jokes come from strangers; in the worst case, they come from your friends, who still have not figured out how much they hurt.

Each day you face people who make you feel bad for being obese. Some people are "kind" enough to "ignore" your looks—they tend to hold eye contact or look anywhere but at you to avoid the appearance of staring at your body. Other people are less considerate and even self-righteous. They make it clear that they think they are better than you and that you are obese because, somehow, you want to be. These are the people who are quite comfortable ordering dessert for themselves and asking you whether "you really feel that you should be eating that bite of pasta, because, well, you don't look like you need it."

You know these and numerous other examples first-hand, so there is no point in repeating them. Let's get to the important parts: what causes obesity, why are you obese, and most important, what are you going to do about it?

Obesity and BMI

Most of us use and hear the term "obesity" all the time, and we have a pretty good idea of what it means. It describes extra body fat that can harm your health and make you uncomfortable in your daily life. But it is important to know that there are different levels of obesity and to know where you fall along the continuum.

Calculating the BMI

Doctors measure obesity by calculating a number called your body mass index, or BMI. Your BMI is a ratio of your weight to the square of your height. This is the formula using pounds and inches:

$$\frac{\text{Weight (pounds) x 703}}{\text{Height (inches)}^2}$$

Do not worry if you are not a numbers person. You do not have to calculate your BMI by hand! You can take a look at the BMI table *(Table 5)* to check your BMI. Find your height in feet and inches along the left-hand side of the table. Trace that row to the right until you get to your weight. Then trace that column upward until you see your BMI in the top row of the table.

Height			Normal Weight: BMI 18.5 to 24.9						Overweight: BMI 26 to 30					
	BMI →	18.5	19	20	21	22	23	24	25	26	27	28	29	30
Feet	Inches													
4	10	89	91	96	100	105	110	115	120	124	129	134	139	144
4	11	92	94	99	104	109	114	119	124	129	134	139	144	149
5	0	95	97	102	108	113	118	123	128	133	138	143	149	154
5	1	98	101	106	111	116	122	127	132	138	143	148	153	159
5	2	101	104	109	115	120	126	131	137	142	148	153	159	164
5	3	104	107	113	119	124	130	135	141	147	152	158	164	169
5	4	108	111	117	122	128	134	140	146	151	157	163	169	175
5	5	111	114	120	126	132	138	144	150	156	162	168	174	180
5	6	115	118	124	130	136	143	149	155	161	167	173	180	186
5	7	118	121	128	134	140	147	153	160	166	172	179	185	192
5	8	122	125	132	138	145	151	158	164	171	178	184	191	197
5	9	125	129	135	142	149	156	163	169	176	183	190	196	203
5	10	129	132	139	146	153	160	167	174	181	188	195	202	209
5	11	133	136	143	151	158	165	172	179	186	194	201	208	215
6	0	136	140	147	155	162	170	177	184	192	199	206	214	221
6	1	140	144	152	159	167	174	182	190	197	205	212	220	227
6	2	144	148	156	164	171	179	187	195	203	210	218	226	234
6	3	148	152	160	168	176	184	192	200	208	216	224	232	240
6	4	152	156	164	173	181	189	197	205	214	222	230	238	246
6	5	156	160	169	177	186	194	202	211	219	228	236	245	253
6	6	160	164	173	182	190	199	208	216	225	234	242	251	260

Obese: BMI 30 to 39.9											
BMI →		31	32	33	34	35	36	37	38	39	40
Height											
Feet	Inches										
4	10	148	153	158	163	167	172	177	182	187	191
4	11	154	158	163	168	173	178	183	188	193	198
5	0	159	164	169	174	179	184	189	195	200	205
5	1	164	169	175	180	185	191	196	201	206	212
5	2	170	175	180	186	191	197	202	208	213	219
5	3	175	181	186	192	198	203	209	215	220	226
5	4	181	186	192	198	204	210	216	221	227	233
5	5	186	192	198	204	210	216	222	228	234	240
5	6	192	198	204	211	217	223	229	235	242	248
5	7	198	204	211	217	223	230	236	243	249	255
5	8	204	210	217	224	230	237	243	250	257	263
5	9	210	217	223	230	237	244	251	257	264	271
5	10	216	223	230	237	244	251	258	265	272	279
5	11	222	229	237	244	251	258	265	272	280	287
6	0	229	236	243	251	258	265	273	280	288	295
6	1	235	243	250	258	265	273	280	288	296	303
6	2	241	249	257	265	273	280	288	296	304	312
6	3	248	256	264	272	280	288	296	304	312	320
6	4	255	263	271	279	288	296	304	312	320	329
6	5	261	270	278	287	295	304	312	320	329	337
6	6	268	277	286	294	303	312	320	329	338	346

Morbid Obese: BMI Over 40											
	BMI →	41	42	43	44	45	46	47	48	49	50
Height											
Feet	Inches										
4	10	196	201	206	211	215	220	225	230	234	239
4	11	203	208	213	218	223	228	233	238	243	248
5	0	210	215	220	225	230	236	241	246	251	256
5	1	217	222	228	233	238	243	249	254	259	265
5	2	224	230	235	241	246	252	257	262	268	273
5	3	231	237	243	248	254	260	265	271	277	282
5	4	239	245	251	256	262	268	274	280	285	291
5	5	246	252	258	264	270	276	282	288	294	300
5	6	254	260	266	273	279	285	291	297	304	310
5	7	262	268	275	281	287	294	300	307	313	319
5	8	270	276	283	289	296	303	309	316	322	329
5	9	278	284	291	298	305	312	318	325	332	339
5	10	286	293	300	307	314	321	328	335	342	349
5	11	294	301	308	316	323	330	337	344	351	359
6	0	302	310	317	324	332	339	347	354	361	369
6	1	311	318	326	334	341	349	356	364	371	379
6	2	319	327	335	343	351	358	366	374	382	389
6	3	328	336	344	352	360	368	376	384	392	400
6	4	337	345	353	362	370	378	386	394	403	411
6	5	346	354	363	371	380	388	396	405	413	422
6	6	355	363	372	381	389	398	407	415	424	433

	BMI →	51	52	52	54	55	56	57	58	59	60
Height											
Feet	**Inches**										
4	10	244	249	254	258	263	268	273	278	282	287
4	11	253	257	262	267	272	277	282	287	292	297
5	0	261	266	271	277	282	287	292	297	302	307
5	1	270	275	281	286	291	296	302	307	312	318
5	2	279	284	290	295	301	306	312	317	323	328
5	3	288	294	299	305	311	316	322	327	333	339
5	4	297	303	309	315	320	326	332	338	344	350
5	5	307	313	319	325	331	337	343	349	355	361
5	6	316	322	328	335	341	347	353	359	366	372
5	7	326	332	338	345	351	358	364	370	377	383
5	8	335	342	349	355	362	368	375	381	388	395
5	9	345	352	359	366	372	379	386	393	400	406
5	10	355	362	369	376	383	390	397	404	411	418
5	11	366	373	380	387	394	402	409	416	423	430
6	0	376	383	391	398	406	413	420	428	435	442
6	1	387	394	402	409	417	425	432	440	447	455
6	2	397	405	413	421	428	436	444	452	460	467
6	3	408	416	424	432	440	448	456	464	472	480
6	4	419	427	435	444	452	460	468	477	485	493
6	5	430	439	447	455	464	472	481	489	498	506
6	6	441	450	459	467	476	485	493	502	511	519

Height		BMI → 61	62	63	64	65	66	67	68	69	70
Feet	Inches										
4	10	292	297	301	306	311	316	321	325	330	335
4	11	302	307	312	317	322	327	332	337	342	347
5	0	312	317	323	328	333	338	343	348	353	358
5	1	323	328	333	339	344	349	355	360	365	371
5	2	334	339	344	350	355	361	366	372	377	383
5	3	344	350	356	361	367	373	378	384	390	395
5	4	355	361	367	373	379	385	390	396	402	408
5	5	367	373	379	385	391	397	403	409	415	421
5	6	378	384	390	397	403	409	415	421	428	434
5	7	390	396	402	409	415	421	428	434	441	447
5	8	401	408	414	421	428	434	441	447	454	460
5	9	413	420	427	433	440	447	454	461	467	474
5	10	425	432	439	446	453	460	467	474	481	488
5	11	437	445	452	459	466	473	480	488	495	502
6	0	450	457	465	472	479	487	494	501	509	516
6	1	462	470	478	485	493	500	508	515	523	531
6	2	475	483	491	499	506	514	522	530	537	545
6	3	488	496	504	512	520	528	536	544	552	560
6	4	501	509	518	526	534	542	550	559	567	575
6	5	514	523	531	540	548	557	565	574	582	590
6	6	528	537	545	554	563	571	580	588	597	606

Table 5: BMI Table

Another way to get your BMI is with an online calculator or mobile smartphone app. The National Heart, Lung and Blood Institute provides a calculator and app for free. Just enter your height and weight, and you will see your BMI: *http://www.nhlbisupport.com/bmi/*

What is your BMI?

Interpreting BMI: Normal Weight, Overweight, and Obesity

So now, what does the number mean? The BMI divisions are as follows:

- ≤ 18.5: Underweight
- 18.5–24.9: Normal Weight
- 25–29.9: Overweight
- 30–39.9: Obesity
- ≥ 40: Morbid Obesity
- ≥ 50: Superobesity

For most people, the healthiest BMI is between 18.5 and 24.9. Looking at the BMI table, this means that a woman who is 5'1" (five feet and one inch) tall is healthiest at a weight between about 100 and 132 pounds, while a 5'9" man is healthiest between 128 and 169 pounds. In our example, the woman would be overweight between 132 and 158 pounds, and the man would be overweight between 169 and 209 pounds. You are at a slight risk for obesity-related health problems when you are overweight. Being in the overweight BMI category also puts you at risk for becoming obese. Being obese puts you at higher risk for health problems.

Continuing with this example, the 5'1" woman is obese between 158 and 211 pounds and morbidly obese above 211 pounds. The 5'9" man is obese above 209 pounds and morbidly obese above 270 pounds. Most people with morbid obesity have significant risk factors for health problems that can lead to diseases and disabilities if they have not already.

Ways to Use BMI

We are spending so much time on BMI, because it will continue to come up throughout the book and your weight loss journey. These are a few of the ways that you will use it:

- BMI helps determine eligibility for gastric bypass or another weight loss surgery. We will go over this in just a moment.

- BMI helps you set healthy long-term weight loss goals. It does not make sense for a short person and tall person to both say they want to end up at the same weight. BMI helps each person set goals that are realistic and can help you live a longer and healthier life.

- BMI helps you measure your weight loss progress. As you lose weight, you will probably want to keep yourself motivated by seeing how your weight loss compares to other bypass patients' progress at the same post-surgery time-points. Again, it does not make sense for you to compare your own weight loss in pounds to someone else's weight loss if they are taller or shorter than you.

- If you are a supporter of a gastric bypass patient, the BMI helps you understand what your loved one is going through. You can use BMI to put yourself in their shoes to realize their starting weight and how well they are doing throughout their journey. Since you may be seeing some pretty dramatic changes in their appearance, the BMI helps you think clearly about the healthy changes they are making.

Superobesity: The Upper Levels of BMI

Extreme obesity or superobesity, can be defined as having a BMI of 50 or greater. This BMI puts you at higher risk for obesity-related diseases than obese individuals with a lower BMI. Bariatric surgery, or weight loss surgery, is becoming more common as a treatment for extreme obesity. When it is done in the right patients, weight loss surgery can lower the risk of death and severe health problems related to obesity.[27]

There are several different types of weight loss, or bariatric, surgery. The gastric bypass is one of the most frequently performed bariatric surgery procedures, with about 200,000 Americans getting it in 2006.[28] The roux-en-Y gastric bypass, which has been around for some time, is the most common type of weight loss surgery. The remaining chapters of this book focus on weight loss surgery and particularly on the gastric bypass.

What Causes Obesity?

Everyone knows that, at some level, obesity is negative. The parts of obesity that hit each individual hardest may vary. For example, the embarrassing, uncomfortable, debilitating, or life-threatening nature of obesity may be worst. We know that we should not become obese. If we are, we know we should lose weight. We even know the rule of successful weight loss—eat less and exercise more.

Unfortunately, losing weight is not so easy. If it were that easy, you would have done it years ago. Better yet, nobody would ever become obese in the first place.

What is going on?

Calorie or Energy Balance

First, let's review the basics of weight control. It is all about calorie balance, or energy balance. This is the balance between the calories you eat and the calories you burn, or expend.

- You gain weight if you eat too many calories and do not burn enough calories.
- You lose weight if you take in (eat or drink) fewer calories and burn (exercise) more.
- You will gain a pound of body weight if you eat an extra 3,500 calories.
- You will lose a pound if you burn off an extra 3,500 calories.

Normal Regulation of Energy Balance

The human brain is naturally programmed to monitor food intake and energy (calorie) balance. When we need energy, we feel hungry and know that it is time to eat. When we have eaten enough, we feel full and know that it is time to stop eating. Then we get hungry again at the next snack or meal time

Energy balance, or calorie balance, makes sense, and human physiology is designed to keep body weight in check. The system has worked for thousands of years to

> **Tip**
>
> In Chapter 16, "Physical Activity to Control Weight Loss," we will go over some reasons why you might think you do not like exercise...and how you can learn to love it. We will also talk about starting an exercise program at any weight and staying safe while exercising.

Calorie Expenditure: How You Burn Calories

Your calorie expenditure is the amount of calories you burn. It comes from:

- Your basal metabolism
- Your physical activity
- The thermic effect of food

Your **basal metabolic rate**, or BMR, is also called your metabolic rate, or metabolism for short. It is the number of calories you burn in a day without doing much of anything. You are always using some energy to stay alive. Your body needs to breathe, pump blood, maintain acid-base balance, and send signals throughout your nervous system.

Your BMR is higher if you are a male, if you are a young adult compared to an older adult, and if you are taller. As you can see, you do not have much control over the factors that affect your BMR. Your BMR can be about 1,000 to 2,500 calories per day, so the range is pretty big. You can use an online calculator to estimate your BMR fairly accurately.

An obese person has a slightly higher BMR than a normal-weight person of the same gender, height, and age but not much higher. That is because fat tissue does not do much compared to muscle. Fat does not have high energy, or calorie, requirements.

Physical activity is another name for exercise. It includes your "purposeful activity," or movements that you make that are extra and beyond your normal movements. A few examples of physical activity are walking, dancing, gardening, playing sports, and swimming. Physical activity can be important to weight loss, because you have a lot of control over the number of calories you burn through exercise. You can burn hundreds of extra calories per day if you are very active, but you will burn almost no calories from physical activity if you are sedentary or sit around a lot. Increasing your physical activity can speed up weight loss. Many obese people say that they do not like to exercise, and this can turn into a vicious cycle. Maybe you do not like to exercise because you are obese and movement feels difficult, awkward, painful, or embarrassing. When you do not exercise, gaining weight is even more of a threat, because you are not burning very many calories each day.

Developing the exercise habit is not easy, but you can do it no matter how out of shape you are. Chapter 16, "Physical Activity to Control Weight Loss," will give you some pointers on getting started with an exercise routine, gaining your confidence, and enjoying the process.

The thermic effect of food, or TEF, is the amount of energy you use to digest your food. It is not much, only about 10 percent of your total calorie intake. This may be about 150 to 250 calories per day. You cannot really change your TEF too much.

See Chapter 15, "The RYGB Diet & Nutrition" for a more complete discussion of calories from carbohydrates, fat, protein, and alcohol.

keep most humans at the right body weight. The problem is that now something is not working. You can tell that it is not working because obesity rates have nearly tripled in the past few decades. More than one-third of American adults were obese in 2010, and 42% are expected to be obese by the year 2030.[29]

Severe obesity, defined as a BMI over 40, was at 0.9% of the adult population in 1990. It jumped to 3.5% by 2008, and is expected to be 9% by 2030.

> **Tip**
>
> See **Chapter 14, "RYGB Diet 101,"** for some examples of the amounts of different kinds of foods you can choose to eat for a certain number of calories. We will also talk about how to choose more filling foods so it is easy to stay within your calorie limit.

Reasons for Gaining Weight

What has gone wrong in the course of only a few short decades? Our genes have not changed much in this short time, since it takes thousands or millions of years for the gene pool to change dramatically. What *has* changed is our lifestyle. This section covers some of the reasons why we overeat and do not exercise enough—leading to obesity.

Food Is Everywhere: Food used to be something you would eat at meals. Meals used to be occasions when you would sit down at the table and eat home-cooked food. Now Americans eat meals and snacks not only at the table but also while driving, working, studying, and socializing. Food is everywhere. Much of it is not healthy or home-cooked. In fact, Americans now spend nearly half of their food dollars outside the home compared to one-third in 1970.[30]

Fast food is available nearly everywhere. If you go to drive-throughs or get delivery, you do not even have to stand up to get it. Convenience stores and gas stations sell high-calorie snacks on nearly every corner. Vending machines with high-sugar and high-fat snacks and high-calorie drinks are in schools, workplaces, and even places that are supposed to be healthy, such as hospitals and fitness centers. Parties, meetings, and family gatherings tend to revolve around food, and saying "no" is considered rude. Avoiding food is nearly impossible no matter how hard you try.

Food Is Cheap: Absolute food prices have dropped in recent decades; you can buy more food with less money.[31] Worse, high-calorie, high-sugar, high-fat food is cheaper than low-calorie, nutritious options, such as fruits, vegetables, and fish. If you are lucky enough to have a steady income, you do not have to think twice before shelling out $5 for a pepperoni pizza (2,500 calories) or $1 for a double cheeseburger (400 or more calories), a 2-liter bottle of cola (800 calories), or a bakery cookie (300 or more calories).

Processed Foods Are Less Filling: Throughout history, humans ate fruits, vegetables, nuts, whole grains, and meats. These are unprocessed foods that tend to make you full before you eat too many calories from them. That is because they are high in fiber and protein. These foods fill you up fast and keep you feeling full for longer after a meal so you do not want to eat again too soon.

Today we eat less fresh food and more processed foods. Food processing is wonderful, because it makes more choices available to us. However, it also encourages us to eat more refined carbohydrates, added sugars, and saturated fats than before. It is very easy to gain weight when you eat refined pasta, prepared foods such as burgers and pizza, sweets such as cake and ice cream, and fried foods such as French fries and doughnuts. They are high-calorie but not very filling, so you can eat tons of calories from these foods before you realize it.

Portions Are Bigger You tend to eat more when you are served a bigger portion. That means you will take in more calories and be more likely to gain weight—without even realizing that you ate more![32] Portion sizes have increased drastically within the past several years, just as obesity rates have increased.

Eating less fresh food and more restaurant food does not just lead to lower nutrient intake. It is also linked to larger portion sizes and overeating. Most restaurants serve about twice what you really should be eating—or often even more than double.[33] Sadly enough, the first reaction, when the food comes, is rarely based on how good or bad it looks. Our first reaction is usually based on the serving size. We are pleased when we get a heaping plate of food and disappointed when the meal is smaller than expected.

We have been trained to think that "bigger" means "better." This dangerous mentality has carried over to irresistibly cheap value meals with high-calorie beverages, appetizers, sides, and desserts that we absolutely do not need. And, of course, there is the famous "all-you-can-eat," which can easily turn into a sort of frantic frenzy to make sure it is worth the money—at the cost of your weight, health, and dignity.

Food Can Be Addictive: Junk food is literally addictive. Eating sugar and other unhealthy foods can cause changes in your hormones and brain chemistry. The result is that you crave even more junk food. Fast food is especially addictive, because it is high in sugar and fat; it tastes good, and it is comforting. [35]

When you get addicted, the part of your brain begging you to eat more is louder than the part of your brain telling you that you have had enough calories. It is a physical addiction that causes withdrawal symptoms. You may get the jitters or feel anxious when you don't get your usual fix.

Another aspect of an addition to fast food is a psychological dependence on it. Food is always on your mind. You may be hungry all of the time or be looking forward to your evening fix of brownies, ice cream, or pizza—whatever high-fat, high-sugar food satisfies that craving. To make things worse, food advertising is everywhere as a constant reminder that you want to eat. Another symptom of psychological dependence on junk food is emotional eating, whether it is to reduce stress, cheer you up, numb your feelings, relieve boredom, or even celebrate a happy event.

Too Much Sitting: Humans are built to move—after all, our ancestors were hunters and gatherers. But we do not move much anymore. Most of us lead a sedentary

> **Tip**
>
> See **Chapter 16, "Physical Activity to Control Weight Loss,"** for ideas on small changes that increase your calorie burn, making time for physical activity, and fun ways to exercise in any climate or neighborhood.

Portion Distortion: Soft Drinks

Soft drinks and pasta both provide great examples of portion distortion.

Sugar-Sweetened (Non-Diet) Soft Drinks

An official serving of a beverage is 8 ounces, or one cup. This has 100 calories and about 7 teaspoons of sugar. A can of cola, which seems miniscule by today's standards, contains 150 calories and 10 teaspoons of sugar.

A "single-serving" bottle of soda, like you might get in a vending machine, officially has 2.5 servings — but let's be serious. Nobody saves a bottle of a soft drink from a vending machine for 2.5 days; you drink it in a few hours and get 250 calories and 16 teaspoons of sugar.

Then we get to the real villains. There is the 32-ounce fountain drink, which theoretically counts as four servings and has 400 calories and 27 teaspoons of sugar. The amount of calories you can get from soft drinks is literally unlimited — because many places allow unlimited refills.

If you drink an extra bottle of soda each day, you will gain one pound every two weeks, or 26 pounds per year.

Pasta

An official serving size of pasta is one ounce of dry pasta, which makes about ½ cup of cooked pasta and has 100 calories. You can have it with ½ cup of tomato sauce, 1 cup of vegetables, and 3 ounces of grilled chicken for 300 calories.

When you order pasta in a restaurant, you are more likely to get 6 ounces of pasta. Along with a generous portion of high-fat meatball sauce and parmesan cheese, the total for this meal is over 1,000 calories. If you add in an appetizer, such as spinach-artichoke dip, sides such as breadsticks, dessert, and a drink, your meal could easily top 2,000 calories.

Source:[34]

lifestyle, with hours of sitting every day and not many calories burned from physical activity. We have cars, remote controls, elevators, and online shopping portals. We go to the grocery store or a restaurant instead of running after our meat, gathering berries, or farming the land.

Not Enough Exercise: Exercise is not built into our daily lives the way it used to be when people hunted or farmed. For most of us, exercise is something that we have to set aside time to do, and it is so difficult to fit in a busy schedule. Sometimes it seems there is no fun exercise to do or something else gets in the way, so exercise gets pushed aside.

Take a moment or two, if you have not already, to think about your own reasons for being obese. Do you live in a neighborhood with more opportunities to buy fast food meals instead of fruits and vegetables? Do you always clean your plate, no matter how much is on it, because your mother told you about starving children in Africa? Do you always order and eat the value menu, because it is cheap and convenient? Do you eat hundreds of extra calories at night because you are bored or lonely or maybe simply because it tastes good? Write down your reasons on the worksheet at the end of this chapter.

Obesity and You: The "I" in Epidemic

Yes, obesity is an epidemic. Yes, a lot of things are stacked up against you, because our environment is obesogenic—it encourages you to become obese by eating too much and not getting enough exercise. But despite this, you have a responsibility for yourself. Your body is your own, and it is time for you to take control.

And you can. No matter how many times you have tried before, you can still try again and make this time a success.

In this section, you will identify some of your own personal reasons for wanting to lose weight so that you can be motivated and ready to put in the dedication that you will need if you are going to succeed with the sleeve.

What Is Your Personal Reason?

So far, most of the information in this chapter is already somewhat familiar to you. You could probably already recite the obesity statistics by heart before even picking up this book; if not, you probably at least knew the patterns. You already knew about calories, healthy eating, exercising, and too much fast food. You could probably already point to a few things in your life that could change and help you lose weight.

But those are not what brought you to this book. You are not here to save a million lives, and you are not here because you are an angry taxpayer protesting the annual cost of obesity in this country. You are not here to learn about why there is a hamburger restaurant on every corner or how the average American lifestyle is different now than hundreds of years ago.

You are here for you, so what is *your own* reason for wanting to lose weight? You are not just concerned about the millions of obese patients, the list of obesity-related diseases, and national health care costs. You are concerned about yourself, as you should be. Think about your own, personal reasons for losing weight. Everyone has a few. Some of the common ones are:

- You want to live long enough to see your son get married or your granddaughter graduate from high school.
- You do not want to live with diabetes, like your mother did, and die as young as she did.
- You want to be able to go clothes shopping with your friends—and buy things in the same stores they do.
- You want to fit into your car without moving the seat back and removing the seat-back cushion while squashing your stomach against the steering wheel.
- You want to be able to order in a restaurant without hearing, even if nobody says it out loud, "Should you really be eating that?"

Take some time to go over your reasons for losing weight. Write them down on the form at the end of this chapter, and keep your list handy. The only way you will ever be successful is if you are motivated so that when the going gets tough, you will be able to remind yourself why you are trying so hard and what the prize will be.

Sometimes you have a bunch of reasons for wanting to lose weight, but one particular incident, what I call the "Ah-Ha! moment," is the final straw. It is what pushes you to go from yo-yo dieting and thinking about a lifestyle change to making the final decision that *I will lose weight.*

These are a few stories of Ah-Ha! moments that I have heard:

- *"I just wanted to look normal so that I could walk down the street and look into store windows without people staring or looking away."*
- *"One day I realized that my obesity was making me take up two seats on the bus so that older people didn't even have a place to sit."*
- *"The day we found out our first child was a boy, I had images of playing catch and hitting fly balls outdoors with my son in a few years. Then I realized my obesity wouldn't let me be active, and I might not even be around to see him play ball."*
- *"I looked in the mirror and saw my mother. At age 45, I looked just like she did at age 45. She was obese like me, and she died of diabetes 5 years later. I didn't want to die, so I knew I had to do something. The gastric sleeve worked for me."*

It Is Time for You to Take Control

Maybe you have put on a brave face every day for years because that is all you know how to do, because you are resigned to being obese, and because diets have not worked for you. Maybe you have never told anyone or even admitted to yourself how miserable you really are because…well, why? Because you are afraid of what will happen? Because you do not know what to do about it? It is time to get going.

Take Control – You Are Worth It!

One of the barriers to losing weight is…you. If you are not careful, you may fall into the trap of being your own worst enemy. You may feel sorry for yourself, or you might feel as though you do not deserve to succeed in weight loss. Or you might just feel like giving up because it seems as though you have tried and failed at every possible weight loss attempt.

No More Excuses

These are just excuses. The truth is that you deserve happiness, health, and a healthy weight. Living a healthy life will take time and effort, and you are worth it. And you can have it. Everyone can find a weight loss method that works for them. Your method may not be the same as your neighbor's, but in the end, you can both achieve the results you want by following the best method for you.

✍ Summary

This chapter provided an introduction to obesity. If you could not before, now you can name specific reasons why obesity is such a problem. It is expensive, it increases the risk of many chronic diseases, and it kills hundreds of thousands of Americans each year.

☛ The personal costs of obesity have probably been plaguing you for years, not only in the form of health problems, but also in your daily life. Your obesity may make you ashamed, interfere with work or other activities that you want to do, or cause people to treat you with disrespect.

☛ This chapter covered a lot of reasons why so many Americans are obese. Many of them, such as too many fast food restaurants and lack of physical activity in daily life, are out of your control. Still, you can take charge of your weight as long as you find and follow a method that is right for you. What method is that? The next chapter will explore different approaches to weight loss and describe the different options for weight loss surgery. Maybe the roux-en-Y gastric bypass is the right choice for you.

Time to Take Action: Set Your Goal and Name Your Reasons

Write your current weight here:

Using the BMI tables in the chapter or a BMI calculator, find out what weight you would need to be at to have a BMI of 25, which is a normal-weight BMI. You will need to know your height for this. Your weight at a BMI of 25 is your goal weight. Write your goal weight here:

Subtract your goal weight from your current weight:

That's the amount of weight you need to lose to get to your goal weight.

Now, write down the reasons you want to hit your goal weight. Examples include having better health, being able to be more energetic around your kids, being more comfortable in your daily life, and fitting into your dream outfit:

Finally, write down a personal, secret reason to lose weight. It is a reason that you have never told anyone and maybe have never let yourself think about too much. It could be something like showing up your mother who put you on a diet when you were 10 years old because she thought you were chubby.

RYGB Patient Story: Jenneliza

Jen from Pennsylvania says getting the Roux-en-Y gastric bypass became a "no-brainer" when her daughter started getting teased for having a fat mom. Jen turned her weight and life around with Roux-en-Y gastric bypass. Her highest weight was 286 pounds. Within a year of surgery, she lost 136 pounds and was enjoying her weight of 150 pounds and a healthy BMI of 24.2! Here is what this mom has to say about her RYGB journey.

On Her Years of Diets, Weight Loss Drugs, and Weight Cycling

I was definitely a yo-yo dieter. In high school, I would fluctuate between 130 and 150 lbs. I would just skip meals and drink Slim-Fast to lose weight. After going to 230 after my first pregnancy, I made it down to 150 in six months by exercising (I was in the Army and had no choice) and with a very low-calorie diet (under 1000 calories per day). Then I went up to 210 pounds after the next pregnancy a year later and went down to 160 for about two years by dieting and using the weight loss drugs phentermine and Xenical. I lost that 50 pounds about a year-and-a-half after the second pregnancy and kept it off for two years. My weight slowly crept up to 210 pounds for a few months after a bad break up and stress at work. Then over the next four years I gained 70 pounds with the stress of being a single mom, nurse, and full time student and having kids in activities. Dieting basically consisted of Slim-Fast or Diet Coke for breakfast, Lean Cuisines for lunch, and Egg Beaters omelets or fish for dinner. Exercising while in the Army was all the typical military exercises: running, sit-ups, pushups, and jumping jacks. I tried Atkins for a little bit twice and just couldn't stick with it longer than two weeks. I'm a milk addict and couldn't get rid of milk, which is a big no-no on Atkins. Atkins was just unreasonable for me. Phentermine worked great and helped me stick with small portions, but the side effects of racing heart and constant dry mouth were terrible. And it's a dangerous medication. The Xenical worked well, too, but the side effects were completely disgusting, and I would never do that again. You can never be more than a few steps from the bathroom when taking it.

On the Decision to Get Weight Loss Surgery and Why RYGB

I saw how successful a few co-workers were with the surgery and was happy for them and jealous at the same time. I was getting closer to 300 pounds, which scared me, and my body fat started to get in my way and slow me down. I couldn't paint my toenails and was afraid of breaking chairs—lots have a 250-lb weight limit. I was afraid to get on amusement park rides and didn't want to go dancing with my girlfriends. I realized over the last year that my weight was keeping me from living life the way I wanted to. To top it off, my kids got picked on for having a fat mom, and one of my psych patients kept calling me "big girl." I just couldn't deny my weight problem anymore.

I chose RYGB because I have seen many people get the lap band and not be successful. Also, the idea of foreign bodies that could erode my tummy or become infected didn't sit well with me.

The vertical sleeve didn't seem extreme enough for me, and duodenal switch was just too extreme. I knew that if I were going to commit to the surgery, then I could not fail. I was worried that the vertical sleeve and band just wouldn't help me lose enough, which to me is failing. I also liked the malabsorption piece of RYGB even though it requires vitamin supplementation.

On Choosing a Surgeon and Paying for Surgery

We only have two bariatric surgeons in my county. The one that I chose has an outstanding reputation, and the other is known for infections and complications. I did not see the need to go out of county for a different one so chose the one with the better reputation, who also operated on my co-workers. I also had the support of a dietitian. For seven months, I attended a monthly two-hour class to prepare for before and after surgery. There were mandatory food logs, individual consultations with the dietitian and bariatric nurse, and mandatory support group meetings.

Insurance paid for everything after my $2000 deductible was met…and that was met within the first month of evaluations and lab work!

On the Surgery Experience

I was surprisingly calm the night before and the morning of surgery. When I woke up, surgery seemed like a dream. The pain and nausea were a 10 on a scale of 10, and I couldn't believe what I had just done. The first day was the worst pain I've ever had – worse than my two C-sections and the three other abdominal surgeries I had. I had such a hard time getting the gas out, and then when it started, I had terrible diarrhea from the liquid diet, but I was too scared of throwing up or bruising my staples to want to advance to food.

On Support, Triumphs, and Challenges

My friends and family have been very supportive and encouraging. They weren't very helpful after that first week, but that's okay because I don't like to ask for help. I didn't have any problems at home or work, but my 11- and 9-year-olds had to make their own soup and sandwiches for the first week because I just wasn't up to cooking. My best moments have been every little moment when I feel able to move easier and just feel smaller – it's priceless! My worst moments?

- *Eating chicken too fast and having terrible pain in my chest (pouch) and vomiting for hours*

- *Dumping for the first time and having to take a nap on a beautiful Sunday afternoon instead of going to the pool…I learned that it not worth that half of an English muffin!*

On the RYGB Diet

I'm still adjusting to the post-surgery diet. I am afraid to try meats, but I'm so sick of eggs. Most days I just have herbal tea and stevia for breakfast. I'll usually have string cheese or cottage cheese for lunch. Dinner is on the go four nights a week due to my children's sports practices, so I will usually do string cheese for dinner. Other nights I will just have some kind of soup or tuna salad or poached eggs for dinner. Sugar-free ice pops are a good evening treat. Crockpot black bean chili is very pouch–friendly, and soy meats seem to work well. I use three cans black beans, a pack of chili starter mix, a can of diced fire-roasted tomatoes, dried onion flakes, a pack of ranch mix, and a bag of soy meat (like boca crumbles). I like to top it with cheddar, guacamole, and plain Greek yogurt. It's definitely pouch-friendly comfort food! I also make a breadless crab cake.

Some of Jen's Recipes

Breadless Crab Cake

(makes 8 servings)

- *1 egg*
- *16 oz can crab meat*
- *3 tbsp light mayo*
- *2 tbsp either Old Bay (by far the best!) or Phillips seasoning*
- *1–2 tbsp parsley depending on your preference*
- *2 twists each of salt and pepper or to taste*
- *1–2 tbsp lemon juice*
- *1 tsp dry mustard (optional)*

Combine all ingredients. If you're in the pureed foods phase, you can mix this in the food processor, which means you can save money by buying the backfin or claw meat. Use an ice cream scoop to make ¼-cup servings. I like to sprinkle Old Bay on top. Broil about 8 minutes or until done. I make them in foil muffin cups so they can be individually frozen and pulled out for quick work lunches. They're great with a little yellow mustard on the side!

High Protein Ranch Dip

1 packet ranch dip mix
Plain nonfat Greek yogurt (usually 16 oz.)
Mix according to directions using Greek yogurt instead of sour cream

High Protein Onion Dip

1 packet onion soup mix
Plain nonfat Greek yogurt (usually 16 oz)
Mix according to directions using Greek yogurt instead of sour cream

Tips from a Successful RYGB Patient

- *Get as much information as you can from reliable sources.*

- *Don't believe everything you read online or hear from others. Sometimes the wrong information can be dangerous. When you think something is wrong, get it checked out.*

- *Follow your instructions from your surgeon. If you don't, your surgeon will hold you accountable if things don't go as planned.*

- *Don't stress out about this too much. Celebrate your bravery and commitment to a healthier you!*

1   Epidemic. Merriam-Webster. Web site. http://www.merriam-webster.com/dictionary/epidemic. Accessed November 9, 2012.

2   Centers for Disease Control and Prevention: Overweight and Obesity http://www.cdc.gov/obesity/index.html. Updated 2012, November 6. Accessed November 9, 2012.

3   Obesity and Overweight. Fact Sheet No. 311. World Health Organization. Web site. http://www.who.int/mediacentre/factsheets/fs311/en/index.html. 2012, May. Accessed November 9, 2012.

4   Global Health Risks. World Health Organization. http://www.who.int/healthinfo/global_burden_disease/global_health_risks/en/index.html. 2009, December. Accessed November 9, 2012.

5   Finkelstein E, Trogdon JG, Cohen JW, Dietz W. Annual medical spending attributable to obesity: payer-and service-specific estimates. Health Affairs. 2009;28(5):w822-w831.

6   Reuters. Study: obesity adds $190 billion in health costs. MSNBC. Web site. http://today.msnbc.msn.com/id/47211549/ns/today-today_health/t/study-obesity-adds-billion-health-costs. 2012. Accessed June 15, 2012.

7   Reuters. Study: obesity adds $190 billion in health costs. MSNBC. Web site. http://today.msnbc.msn.com/id/47211549/ns/today-today_health/t/study-obesity-adds-billion-health-costs. 2012. Accessed June 15, 2012.

8   Barth L. U.S. obesity problem impacts automobile safety and fuel economy. Consumer Reports. Web site. http://news.consumerreports.org/cars/2010/08/-us-obesity-problem-impacts-automobile-safety-and-fuel-economy-.html. 2010, August 12. Accessed November 9, 2012.

9   Obesity and Overweight. Fact Sheet No. 311. World Health Organization. Web site. http://www.who.int/mediacentre/factsheets/fs311/en/index.html. 2012, May. Accessed November 9, 2012.

10 Ogden CL, Carroll MD. Prevalence of overweight, obesity and extreme obesity among adults: United States, trends 1960-1962 through 2007-2008. NCHS E-Stat, Centers for Disease Control and Prevention. Web site. http://www.cdc.gov/nchs/data/hestat/obesity_adult_07_08/obesity_adult_07_08.htm. Updated 2011, June 6. Accessed November 9, 2012.

11 Allison DB, Fontaine KR, Manson JE, Stevens J, Vanitallie TB. Annual deaths attributable to obesity in the United States. JAMA. 1999;282(16)1530-8.

12 Diabetes data and trends. Centers for Disease Control and Prevention. http://apps.nccd.cdc.gov/DDTSTRS/default.aspx. 2010. Accessed November 9, 2012.

13 Diabetes overview. National Diabetes Information Clearinghouse. Web site. http://diabetes.niddk.nih.gov/dm/pubs/overview/. 2012, April 4. Accessed November 9, 2012.

14 Dugdale DC, Zieve D. Glucose tolerance test. Medline Plus, National Library of Medicine. Web site. http://www.nlm.nih.gov/medlineplus/ency/article/003466.htm. Updated 2012, June 2. Accessed November 11, 2012.

15 Topiwala S, Dugdale DC, Zieve D. HbA1c. Medline Plus, National Library of Medicine. Web site. http://www.nlm.nih.gov/medlineplus/ency/article/003640.htm. Updated 2012, April 29. Accessed November 11, 2012.

16 Conditions. American Heart Association. Web site. http://www.heart.org/HEARTORG/Conditions/Conditions_UCM_001087_SubHomePage.jsp. Accessed November 2012.

17 Dugdale DC, Zieve D. Coronary risk profile. Medline Plus. http://www.nlm.nih.gov/medlineplus/ency/article/003491.htm. Updated 2012, June 3. Accessed November 11, 2012.

18 Adult Treatment Panel III. (2001). Executive summary of the third report of the National Cholesterol Education Program (NCEP) expert panel on detection, evaluation, and treatment of high blood cholesterol in adults (Adult Treatment Panel III). National Institutes of Health. Retrieved from http://www.mayoclinic.com/health/hdl-cholesterol/CL00030/NSECTIONGROUP=2

19 High blood pressure and kidney disease. National Heart, Lung and Blood Institute. Web site. http://kidney.niddk.nih.gov/kudiseases/pubs/highblood/. Updated 2010, September 2. Accessed November 11, 2012.

20 High blood pressure. Centers for Disease Control and Prevention. Web site. http://www.cdc.gov/bloodpressure/. Updated 2012, September 6. Accessed November 11, 2012.

21 What is high blood pressure? National Heart, Lung and Blood Institute. Web site http://www.nhlbi.nih.gov/health/health-topics/topics/hbp/. 2012, July 12. Accessed November 11, 2012.

22 Leading causes of death, 2009. FastStats, Centers for Disease Control and Prevention. Web site. http://www.cdc.gov/nchs/fastats/lcod.htm. Updated 2012, October 19. Accessed November 11, 2012.

23 Handout on health: osteoarthritis. National Institute of Arthritis and Musculoskeletal and Skin Diseases, National Institutes of Health. Web site. http://www.niams.nih.gov/Health_Info/Osteoarthritis/default.asp. 2010. Accessed November 11, 2012.

24 Questions and answers about gout. National Institute of Arthritis and Musculoskeletal and Skin Diseases, National Institutes of Health. Web site. http://www.niams.nih.gov/Health_Info/Gout/default.asp. 2010 Accessed November 11, 2012.

25 What Is Sleep Apnea? National Heart, Lung and Blood Institute. Web site. http://www.nhlbi.nih.gov/health/health-topics/topics/sleepapnea/. 2012, July 10. Accessed November 11, 2012.

26 Obesity Education Initiative. Clinical guidelines on the identification, evaluation and treatment of overweight and obesity in adults: the evidence report. National Heart, Lung and Blood Institute, National Institutes of Health. NIH No. 98-4083.1998.

27 Christou NV, Sampalis JS, Liberman M, Look D, Auger S, McLean APH, MacLean LD. Surgery decreases long-term mortality, morbidity and health care use in morbidly obese patients. Ann Surg. 2004;240(3):416-424.

28 Blackburn GL, Hutter MM, Harvey AM, Apovian CM, Boulton HRW, Cummings S...Annas CL. Expert panel on weight loss surgery: executive report update. Obesity, 2009;17(5):842-862.

29 Finkelstein EA, Khavjou OA, Thompson H, Trogdon JG, Pan L, Sherry B, Dietz W. Obesity and severe obesity forecasts through 2030. Am J Prev Med, 2012;Jun;42(6):563-70.

30 Young LR, Nestle M. The contribution of expanding portion sizes to US obesity epidemic. Am J Public Health. 2002;92(2):246-249.

31 Finkelstein EA, Khavjou OA, Thompson H, Trogdon JG, Pan L, Sherry B, Dietz W. Obesity and severe obesity forecasts through 2030. Am J Prev Med, 2012;Jun;42(6):563-70.

32 Diliberti N, Bordi PL, Conklin MT, Roe LS, Rolls BJ. Increased portion size leads to increased energy intake in a restaurant meal. Obes Res. 2004;12(3):562-8.

33 Condrasky M, Ledikwe JH, Flood JE, Rolls BJ. Chefs' opinions of portion sizes. Obesity (Silver Spring). 2007;15(8):2086-2094.

34 Garber, A.K., & Lustig, R.H. Is fast food addictive? Current Drug Abuse Reviews. 2011; 4(3):146-62.

35 Condrasky M, Ledikwe JH, Flood JE, Rolls BJ. Chefs' opinions of portion sizes. Obesity (Silver Spring). 2007;15(8):2086-2094.

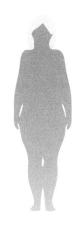

2

Options for Losing Weight: Diets, Exercise, Weight Loss Drugs, and Surgery

The science behind losing weight is simple. You lose weight when you consume fewer calories than you use. That is called a calorie deficit. Weight loss really is that straightforward, but it is definitely not easy! If you are considering or you have had weight loss surgery, you already know from experience that losing weight is difficult. This chapter will cover each of the possible options for weight loss and how well they work.

Losing Weight Is Tough

These are the approaches you can take to losing weight:

- *Diet:* You can change your diet so that you are eating fewer calories.
- *Exercise:* You can be more active so that you are burning more calories.
- *Weight loss drugs:* These may decrease your appetite so that you eat fewer calories; they can speed up your metabolism so that you burn more calories; and/or they can cause malabsorption or interfere with digestion so that you do not absorb all of the calories from your food.
- *Weight loss surgery:* This is a weight loss tool that has helped hundreds of thousands of very obese people lose weight, and it may be able to help you. There are many different types of weight loss surgery. This chapter will explain the most common ones, and then the rest of the book will focus on the roux-en-Y gastric bypass.

You are probably already familiar with these weight loss options and have already tried one or more of them. By the end of the chapter, you will have a better idea of why you have not been able to find a long-term weight control solution. You will be ready to consider carefully whether you might be a good candidate for weight loss surgery and the gastric bypass.

Why Dieting Alone Can't Help

Since you are considering weight loss surgery, you have undoubtedly tried countless diets that have not worked for you. You are not alone. More than 95 percent of diets fail eventually.[1] They may help you lose a little bit of weight or even get you to your goal weight, but they do not help you keep the weight off.

Common Types of Diets

There are many approaches to dieting, but what they all have in common is that each weight loss diet restricts calories in some way. That is true for any weight loss diet that helps you lose body fat. We are not talking about crash diets that help you lose 10 pounds in a couple of days. When you lose weight that fast, you are just losing water weight and maybe some lean muscle but not much body fat.

This chart shows just a few of the common approaches to dieting, how they help you cut calories, and their pros and cons.

Table 6: Common approaches to dieting, how they help you lose weight, and some of their strengths and limitations

Approach	How Calories Are Reduced	Benefits	Disadvantages
Calorie Counting Diets	You count your calories and stay within your daily limit. A "regular" low-calorie diet has at least 1,200 calories per day, and some medically supervised very low-calorie diets have even fewer.	• It is straightforward, and it makes sense: Keep your calorie intake lower your calorie output (expenditure) and you will lose weight. • You do not have to cut out specific foods or food groups as long as you stay within your calorie limits. • You can have the occasional treat as long as you stay within your calorie limits.	• It is a hassle. You have to add up each calorie that you eat and try to figure out the calories you burn each day. • You do not always know the number of calories in a food.
Prepackaged Meals (e.g., Nutrisystem and Jenny Craig)[2]	Portion control: You only eat the meals and snacks that are delivered in your weekly shipment, plus a few approved snacks throughout the day.	• You do not have to cook fancy meals. • You do not have to measure portions from multi-serving packages or from large recipes. • You get to "eat the whole bag" because each bag (or carton) has only one serving. • Menus are often designed to provide balanced nutrition so you do not have to worry about your nutrient intake.	• It is expensive. You have to pay for the food, for delivery, and often for each pound that you lose. • You do not necessarily learn the skills you need to select your own healthy foods and proper portions. • The menu options can become boring.
Low-Carbohydrate Diets and Sugar-Free Diets	You cut out nearly all carbohydrates, which are sources of calories. If you normally eat foods like potatoes, pasta, bread, desserts, fruit, beans, and cereal, a low-carb diet is almost certain to reduce your total calorie intake, even though you are eating meat, cheese, and nuts. A variation of a low-carbohydrate diet is a diet without added sugars or refined grains, so you avoid pasta, desserts, and white bread.	• They can keep you from being tempted by trouble foods if you are one of those people who cannot stop at one serving of starchy or sugary foods such as potatoes, pasta, or brownies. • They can be easier to follow because the emphasis on food types rather than precise portions. • They discourage some unhealthy refined foods, such as sweets.	• They can cause nutrient deficiencies from a limited diet. • They can be high in saturated fat from meat and cheese. • They discourage some healthy carbohydrates, such as whole grains, beans, and fruit. • They can get boring and cause you to quit. • You are likely to regain the weight when you go off the diet.

Low-Fat Diets	This is a traditional diet approach. Fat has more calories per gram than protein and carbohydrates, so cutting out fat helps you cut out a lot of calories.	• It encourages fruits, vegetables, whole grains, beans, fat-free dairy products, and lean proteins. • It leaves you with a wide variety of options. • It discourages fatty junk food, such as fried foods, pizza, doughnuts, and hamburgers.	• Low-fat, high-carbohydrate diets can be bad for your blood sugar and cholesterol. • It can be boring and unsatisfying. • It does not distinguish between healthy and unhealthy carbohydrates; sugar is an unhealthy carbohydrate and a fat-free food. • It does not distinguish between healthy and unhealthy fats.
Single Food-Focused Diets	These unhealthy diets help you lose weight because you cut out most types of foods. Examples include cookie diets, which might include a few cookies plus a single daily meal; the grapefruit diet, which consists of large quantities of grapefruit to fill you up; and the cabbage diet, which has you eating low-calorie cabbage and vegetable soup with some beef or chicken.	• They are simple. • You do not have to count. • The diet prevents you from eating many "problem" foods, so you are less likely to get started and be unable to stop eating.	• It is not nutritious. • It can be dangerous. • You will not lose weight in the long term.
Meal Replacement Diets	These diets are similar to food-focused diets. You might have a diet bar or shake to replace two or even three of your regular meals.	• It is convenient and easy. You do not have to cook. • They can satisfy your sweet tooth if you like standard chocolate-flavored bars and shakes.	• They are boring. • They are made up of highly processed foods. • You will probably regain the weight when you go off of the diet because the diet does not teach you portion control or healthy eating habits. • You may be hungry from eating bars instead of meals.

Table 6: Common approaches to dieting

Why Do Diets Not Work?

Some people are able to lose weight and keep it off with diet, but most people are not. If you are reading this book, you are probably among the majority who are not. Why has dieting not worked for you? These are a few common reasons why diets fail, and you may recognize them as part of your own story.

1: They Are Temporary

You follow the diet to the letter, achieve your goal weight, and then "go off your diet." Guess what? As soon as you start to go back to your "regular" eating habits, you go back to your "regular" weight. A successful eating plan for maintaining a healthy weight needs to be a lifestyle change, not a short-term program. The gastric bypass is designed to be a permanent procedure, and your weight control success with the bypass depends on eating well for life.

2: You Feel Deprived and Quit

A lot of diets forbid your favorite foods, but you still want them. You might break your low-carbohydrate diet because you love pasta, go off a low-sugar diet because you love apple pie, go off a prepared meals diet because you have friends over for dinner, or break a low-fat diet because you want a piece of pizza. Or you may want to go out to eat with friends at a restaurant, but you cannot find anything that is allowed on your diet. Once you sneak in the first forbidden food, you might fall into the all-or-nothing trap.

3: The All or Nothing Trap

Some people have an all-or-nothing approach. They feel that giving in to a single French fry makes the day and diet a failure, and therefore it is pointless to continue. These people might reason that as long as they had a forbidden fry, they might as well have the whole order…and a cheeseburger and milkshake too. By the time they are done, they think of themselves as failures and continue to eat badly instead of getting back on track at the next meal.

4: You Are Still Hungry

You might not be doing well at diets, because they do not fill you up. You might eat the right amount of calories to lose weight or maintain your weight, but you are still hungry, so you eat some more. This is actually more likely to happen in obese people than in normal-weight people. The brains of skinny people might get the "stop eating" signals from their stomachs quickly. You might not be so lucky, so your brain does not know to "stop eating" until you have eaten more calories than you really need. The gastric bypass can decrease hunger and make you feel full more quickly.

> **Tip**
>
> See **Chapter 14, "RYGB Diet 101,"** for meal planning help and information on characteristics of healthy diets to control your calories and meet your nutritional needs.

Diets are great in theory, but they do not seem to work in practice. There is still hope, though, and failing at a diet—or many diets—does *not* make you a failure or condemn you to lifelong obesity.

Why Exercise Won't Help You Lose Weight

What about exercise? Like dieting, exercising is another approach to weight loss that seems foolproof—and is in theory but not in practice.

How It Works: Theory behind Exercising to Lose Weight

Exercise more, maintain or lower your calorie consumption, and lose weight. It is a simple concept.

Why Exercise on Its Own Is Not Effective

You can look at tables or use calculators to estimate the calories you can burn per hour of physical activity. Someone that weighs 240 pounds can burn 305 calories per hour walking at a speed of 2 miles per hour, and you can increase that to nearly 470 calories in an hour by walking at 3.5 miles an hour. All you would have to do to lose one to two pounds per week is walk an hour in the morning and an hour in the evening.

Some of these numbers seem pretty impressive, right? They are, until reality hits. It is almost impossible to lose weight just by exercising. These are some of the reasons why.

1: It is Difficult to Burn a Lot of Calories with Exercise

The calories you burn from exercise might be a lot lower than you would expect. You may find that you are not physically able to walk as fast as you are hoping for or for as long. Even if you can, you may not enjoy it or might not have time for it, which means you probably will not be doing it every day. You might start off expecting to burn 1,000 calories a day, for a weight loss of 2 pounds per week, by walking briskly for two hours per day. You might find out that you are only able to manage one hour of slow walking on five days each week—or about the amount of exercise needed to lose ½ pound per week. Eventually, you might get discouraged and give up.

2: Bad Food Choices Usually Outweigh Exercise

It is tough to burn enough calories to balance out bad food choices. The calories that you can burn during physical activity are not that high compared to calories you can eat within minutes. This table can give you an idea of how much you would have to exercise to burn off the calories from certain food choices—and that is just to *balance* them out, not to *lose weight*!

Table 7: Is It Worth It? Take a look at these foods, their calorie counts, and the amount you would have to exercise to burn off these foods. The bottom line is that you need to exercise a lot to burn off the calories from these foods.

To Balance	You'd have to burn	A 200-pound person can burn the calories by:
Small beef burrito	420 calories	Playing tennis for an hour
Slice of large pepperoni pizza	300 calories	Biking moderately for an hour
1 buffalo wing with 1 ounce dipping sauce	270 calories	Moderate walking for an hour
1 large chocolate chip cookie	210 calories	Playing tennis for 30 minutes
1 large slice triple chocolate cheesecake	830 calories	Moderate walking for three hours

Table 7: Sample of foods and calorie counts

3: Sticking to an Exercise Program Is Challenging

You have probably tried an exercise program once or a thousand times before. You start out enthusiastically but within days, weeks, or even months, you start to fade. It may be because you are unmotivated or because you are not seeing results. It can also be because you are bored. Obesity may make your boredom worse by limiting the variety of activities you *can* do or *want* to do. Some activities may be painful, too hard, or simply embarrassing because you feel conspicuous or awkward in your body. So exercise is not a reliable obesity cure.

Do not get the wrong impression here. Exercise is wonderful and necessary for health. It makes your heart healthier, improves your insulin sensitivity, helps you think better, and reduces stress. But exercise on its own is not a complete, successful weight loss program.

> **Tip**
>
> Chapter 1, "Obesity – A Widespread Disease," talks about insulin sensitivity, blood sugar control and type 2 diabetes Chapter 16, "Physical Activity to Control Weight Loss," has a discussion of the benefits of exercise, how many calories different activities can burn, and how to design an exercise program.

What You Need To Know About Weight Loss Drugs

Everyone wants a cure-all medication because it seems so easy…just pop a pill and watch your problems disappear. Wouldn't it be nice if a pill could "cure" obesity in the same way painkillers make your headaches and muscle cramps go away? Unfortunately, it is not that easy. Scientists have been searching for obesity drugs for years, and they have not yet found the perfect formula.

How Weight Loss Drugs Work

As mentioned at the beginning of this chapter, there are a few different ways that weight loss drugs can work. Some products have one or more of these effects:

- *Appetite suppressants*: These drugs suppress your appetite so that you do not eat as much. They work by increasing the amount of serotonin and catecholamines in your brain. These chemicals are neurotransmitters that help you feel full and satisfied.

- *Metabolism boosters*: They can increase your metabolism so that you burn more calories. Similar to caffeine, they may work by increasing your heart rate and breathing rate.
- *Nutrient absorption blockers*: They can reduce the amount of nutrients from food so that you do not absorb all of the calories that you are eating. Fat blockers grab onto the fat in your food so that you cannot absorb as much of it from your stomach or small intestine. Carb blockers, or starch blockers, interfere with salivary amylase, an enzyme in saliva that starts breaking down carbohydrates from food. The effects of carb blockers are minimal,

since most digestion of carbohydrates takes place after you swallow.

> **Tip**
>
> Chapter 1, "Obesity – A Widespread Disease," reviews the metabolic rate, or your metabolism
> Chapter 8, "Roux-En-Y Gastric Bypass Costs, Insurance, and More," has guidance for navigating your insurance policy and financing weight loss surgery.

What Weight Loss Drugs Are Available?

Table 8 lists some of the weight loss drugs available that the FDA has approved to be marketed as weight loss drugs.[3]

Drug	How it Works	FDA Approval	Side Effects
Orlistat	Decrease nutrient absorption (blocks fat)	Approved for use for up to one year in adults and children over age 12 years; Xenical is prescription; Alli is over-the-counter (OTC)	Need to restrict dietary fat intake to avoid severe diarrhea; may lead to vitamin and mineral deficiencies or cramping
Phentermine ("fen-fen")	Appetite suppressant	Approved for use for up to 12 weeks in adults; OTC	Raises blood pressure and heart rate; nervousness; insomnia
Diethylpropion (Tenuate)	Appetite suppressant	Approved for use for up to 12 weeks in adults; OTC	Raises blood pressure and heart rate
Lorcaserin (Lorqess)	Appetite suppressant	Approved for use for up to one year; prescription	May cause birth defects
Qsymia (formerly known as Qnexa) (phentermine and topiramate)	Appetite suppressant	Approved as a prescription drug by the FDA in July of 2012[4]	Increased pulse and blood pressure; dizziness; constipation; birth defects; dry mouth
Phendimetrazine	Appetite suppressant	Approved for use for up to 12 weeks in adults; OTC	Nervousness and insomnia
Belviq (lorcaserin hydrochloride)	Appetite suppressant	Approved in June 2012 as prescription drug[5]	Headaches; nausea; dizziness; heart complications

Table 8: Weight loss drugs (FDA approved)

There are a few other drugs available that may help you lose weight, but the FDA has not yet approved them to be labeled as weight loss drugs. They are approved for other conditions, and using them for weight loss is an example of "off-label drug use." The FDA does not believe that they are safe and effective enough to be approved for weight loss. *Table 9* provides some examples of medications that are used off-label for weight control.

Drug (Generic Name)	Main (FDA-approved) Purpose	Side Effects
Topiramate	Prevent seizures	Numbness; changes in taste
Metformin	Diabetes: control blood sugar	Dry mouth; metallic taste; nausea; weakness
Zonisamide	Prevent seizures	Fatigue; nausea; headache; dry mouth; dizziness
Bupropion	Depression treatment	Dry mouth; sleeplessness

Table 9: Examples of medications that may help you lose weight (not FDA approved)

Weight Loss Drugs: Not the Solution

Weight loss drugs are not likely to provide a long-term solution to your obesity. This is how the weight loss drug market currently stands:

- There are not many options.
- They can cause side effects and complications.
- Their results are not that impressive if you have a lot of weight to lose. You can expect to lose about 10 to 15 pounds in 12 weeks, or about three months, if you take weight loss drugs and follow the recommended diet.
- Weight loss might not last. The limit for using many of these drugs is 12 weeks to a year, and you probably will not hit your goal weight during that time. After that, your hunger will increase and your metabolism will decrease back to their pre-drug levels.

Get the Lowdown on Weight Loss Surgery

Diets nearly always fail, physical activity alone is not enough to get you to your goal weight, and a safe and effective weight loss medication does not yet exist. What is left? Weight loss surgery is a last resort for many obese individuals. Thousands of patients have had the gastric bypass and are quickly losing weight and, more important, are keeping it off.

Myths and Realities of Weight Loss Surgery

Most people do not know much about weight loss surgery. Maybe you do not know much about it either, or you did not until you started considering it. *Table 10* identifies some common myths surrounding weight loss surgery and explains the truth about each.

Myth	Reality
All weight loss surgery is the same.	There are many different kinds of weight loss surgery, as you will see in the next section. There is roux-en-Y gastric bypass, duodenal switch, adjustable laparoscopic gastric banding, and vertical sleeve gastroplasty, just to name a few.
Bariatric surgery is a complicated and unusual medical procedure.	Hundreds of thousands of bariatric surgeries are performed each year. Surgery usually takes one to two hours. Many weight loss surgery patients leave the hospital within days, and patients return to work within weeks. Many surgeries now are laparoscopic, or minimally invasive, with only a few small incisions.
The only medical professional that you will be interacting with is your surgeon.	Your entire medical team is important. In addition to your surgeon, your weight loss surgery team includes a dietitian, nurses, and mental health professionals. You will work closely with your team before and after your surgery.
Bariatric surgery is the easy way out for lazy people.	Losing weight is hard work, whether or not you have weight loss surgery. Most surgeons only accept patients who have tried many diets and have been unable to keep the weight off. The surgery is a tool to help you eat less, but it only does part of the work. You do the rest.
You will never eat normal food again.	Within days after surgery, you transition to solid foods. Eventually, most patients can eat any kind of food. You may need to limit high-fat and high-sugar foods to avoid dumping syndrome. Another key is to limit your portion sizes.
Weight loss surgery causes long-term health complications.	Serious complications from bariatric surgery performed in a reputable clinic are very rare, although they can happen. Some kinds of bariatric surgery can lead to risk for nutrient deficiencies. You need to take dietary supplements for life to prevent deficiencies.
Weight loss surgery is a quick option for losing weight.	Successful weight loss with bariatric surgery is a lifetime commitment. You will need to follow the healthy diet that your dietitian recommends. It may take years to achieve your goal weight, and you should follow your new diet for life.
No insurance plans cover weight loss surgery.	Some insurance plans cover all or part of weight loss surgery if you meet certain criteria and approach your surgery and financial payments as required by your plan.

Table 10: Weight loss surgery-Myths Vs. Reality

How Does Weight Loss Surgery Work?

There are two main ways that a weight loss surgery can help you lose weight: restriction and malabsorption.[6] In addition, some bariatric surgeries, including the gastric bypass, can reduce your hunger by changing your hormone levels.

Restrictive Weight Loss Surgery

All bariatric surgeries include restrictive components to limit your food intake. The way they work is by making your stomach smaller. Your stomach is like a food storage container. When it fills up at the end of the meal, it sends signals to your brain that you are full. When your stomach is smaller as a result of a restrictive weight loss procedure, it fills up faster and sends the signal to your brain. You feel full sooner, before you have eaten as much food as you would have eaten before surgery.

Examples of restrictive weight loss surgeries include the following:

- Vertical banded gastroplasty (VBG)
- Vertical sleeve gastrectomy (VSG), laparoscopic sleeve gastrectomy (LSG), or gastric sleeve
- Sleeve plication, or laparoscopic greater curvature plication
- Gastric bypass (GB), roux-en-Y gastric bypass (RYGB), or laparoscopic roux-en-Y gastric bypass (LRYGB). This book focuses on the roux-en-Y gastric bypass.
- Adjustable gastric banding (AGB) and laparoscopic adjustable gastric banding (LAGB)

Malabsorptive Weight Loss Surgery

Some surgeries are both restrictive and malabsorptive. Malabsorptive procedures reduce the absorption of calories and nutrients from food to help you lose weight. The surgeon alters your gastrointestinal tract to exclude part of the small intestine. The small intestine is where a lot of absorption occurs, so skipping over it lets your body absorb fewer nutrients and calories into your body.

Examples of malabsorptive weight loss surgeries include:

- Roux-en-Y gastric bypass (RYGB)
- Biliopancreatic bypass diversion (with or without duodenal switch) (BPD-DS). This surgery is a two-step process. The first step is the vertical sleeve gastrectomy, and the second step involves rearranging the digestive system to reduce nutrient absorption.

Suppressing Your Hunger

Some kinds of weight loss surgery may reduce your hunger and increase your feelings of fullness. The procedures affect different hormones in your body that are involved in hunger.[7] After the surgery, some patients report less hunger and fewer cravings for high-sugar foods. The RYGB is a surgery that reduces levels of at least one of your hunger hormones. Upcoming chapters will discuss that in more detail.

Learning the Facts before Deciding on Weight Loss Surgery

The number of annual surgeries in the U.S. has skyrocketed since 1990, when 16,000 patients underwent some type of weight loss surgery. By 2003, 103,000 patients had bariatric surgery; and in 2008, there were 220,000 weight loss surgeries.[8] As weight loss surgery becomes more common, more information is known about the safety and effectiveness of weight loss surgery.

Only some obese individuals are good candidates for weight loss surgery. You need to meet certain criteria before a surgeon will recommend and agree to perform bariatric surgery on you. In most cases, you have to have a BMI of 40 or have a BMI over 35 and a health condition due to your obesity. You also need to have documentation that you have tried diets before, and they have not worked for you. Most of all, you need to be ready to make the lifestyle changes that are required for success with weight loss surgery.

> **Tip**
>
> Chapter 1, "Obesity – A Widespread Disease," introduces BMI. We will go over specific criteria for qualifying for the Roux-En-Y in Chapter 3, "All About the Roux-En-Y Gastric Bypass (RYGB),"

You may also need to postpone your weight loss surgery or consider other options if any of these descriptions are true for you.

- You are pregnant or are planning to become pregnant within the next year.
- You have a severe medical condition that can be made worse with surgery.
- You abuse alcohol or drugs.
- You are unwilling to commit to a lifetime of careful food choices.

Open versus Laparoscopic Surgery

The two main surgery categories are laparoscopic and open. Today, most weight loss surgeries are laparoscopic instead of open. You and your surgeon will decide which is best for you, so you might want to learn a little bit about each one. This section describes each of them briefly, and the rest of the book will continue to mention laparoscopic and open surgeries.

Open Surgery

Open surgery is what probably comes into your mind when you think about surgery. The surgeon makes an incision, or cut, into your abdomen to get access to your stomach and the rest of your gastrointestinal tract. After finishing the bariatric procedure, the surgeon sews up the incision.

Laparoscopic Surgery

Laparoscopic surgery is a technique that lets the surgeon make smaller incisions than in open surgery. It is classified as a minimally invasive surgical procedure. Your surgeon makes a few small incisions in your abdomen and inserts a camera (the laparoscope) and the surgery instruments. Then the surgeon uses a camera to see your insides and the surgical tools on a screen. The surgeon controls the thin surgical tools instruments by remote control. For most people, laparoscopic surgery is safer and has a lower risk of complications than open surgery. Many bariatric surgeries today are laparoscopic.

Risks of Weight Loss Surgery

Bariatric surgery patients face risks and complications from the surgical procedure and from the after-effects.

Risks of Surgery

Weight loss surgery has the same risks as any other kind of surgery. However, the risks are usually lower with weight loss surgery because it is a minor procedure compared to some other kinds of surgical procedures. These are some of the risks:

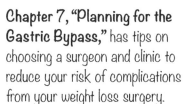

Tip

Chapter 7, "Planning for the Gastric Bypass," has tips on choosing a surgeon and clinic to reduce your risk of complications from your weight loss surgery.

- *Embolism or blood clot*: Within the days following surgery, your risk of blood clots increases, and you could have a stroke or heart attack.

- *Infection*: Surgery requires one or more incisions, and you can be infected any time you have an open wound. Furthermore, obesity increases your risk of infections. You can reduce your risk by choosing a doctor at a clinic that you trust and following your surgeon's instructions for keeping your incision(s) protected and clean.

- *Death*: Death is always a risk when going into surgery, but weight loss surgery is relatively safe compared to other kinds of surgery. Fewer than one in 200 patients die from weight loss surgery.[9]

Later Risks

Unfortunately, the rapid weight loss that is normal after successful weight loss surgery increases your risk for some medical conditions, such as gallstones. To prevent this, your surgeon may remove your gallbladder during your surgery. Your gallbladder helps digest fat, but it is not a necessary organ. You can digest fat without it too.

Another possible risk for weight loss surgery patients is depression. This can happen even when you are losing the amount of weight that you had hoped for. Depression can occur because underlying issues that were not caused by your weight start to surface. Another possibility is that depression is your reaction to how differently people treat you when you lose weight. The risk of depression makes it even more important for you to see a psychologist before getting approved for the surgery. Your after-care team should also be very careful to monitor you for signs of depression and get you help if you need it.

How Your Body Gets Nutrients from Food

Weight loss surgery alters your digestive tract. To understand these changes and how they can help you lose weight, it is helpful to understand normal metabolism, or how your body gets nutrients from food when you eat.

Digestion and Absorption

Digestion and absorption are necessary parts of metabolism because you cannot just put entire foods directly into your body's cells. First, you have to *digest* food. This includes breaking it down into smaller components, such as fractions of larger fats and carbohydrates and proteins, and releasing other nutrients, such as vitamins and minerals. Next, your body needs to *absorb* the nutrients, or get them out of the GI tract and into your body. A basic idea of how food is digested helps explain how each type of weight loss surgery works. This discussion will not get too technical, so do not worry if you are not an expert in physiology and anatomy.

The Gastrointestinal Tract

The gastrointestinal tract, or GI tract, is the series of tubes and compartments that food travels through as it goes from your mouth to your colon (*See Figure 1*).[10] Your body absorbs nutrients from food as it passes through your GI tract. The remainder of the food becomes waste and is excreted as feces and urine. Following is a list of the parts of the digestive tract and a description of what happens as food passes through each one.[11]

- *Mouth*: Chewing grinds food into smaller pieces and mixes it with saliva so you do not choke when you swallow. Saliva also has a minor role in starting to break down some of the starches, or carbohydrates, in your food. The mouth is where carb blockers or starch blockers, discussed earlier in the chapter, have their effects.

- *Esophagus:* Food enters the esophagus, or throat, when you swallow. Not much digestion happens in the esophagus; it is mainly just a tube that pushes food from your mouth to your stomach.

- *Stomach:* The stomach is an expandable pouch that stores food from your meal. Hydrochloric acid in the stomach breaks food down into smaller particles. The stomach mixes your food with digestive juices to continue the digestive process. Carbohydrates and proteins are largely broken down in the stomach. The stomach slowly empties the partially digested food into your small intestine. Your stomach is very important in sending hunger and fullness signals to your brain. A full stomach tells your brain that it is time to stop eating, and an empty stomach tells your brain that you are hungry. Bariatric surgeries, such as the vertical sleeve gastrectomy, that make the stomach smaller can reduce hunger and make you feel full sooner.

- *Small intestine:* The small intestine is so important to nutrition because this is where most of your nutrients are absorbed. That means that they go from your GI tract, across the wall of the small intestine, and into your bloodstream. Proteins, carbohydrates, fats, vitamins, and minerals all get absorbed from the small intestine. Food enters the small intestine at the portion called the duodenum, which is the portion closest to the stomach. The next portion of the small intestine is called the jejunum, and the last part, just before the large intestine, is the ileum. By preventing some of the fat from being broken down, fat blockers reduce the amount of fat that you absorb in the small intestine.

- *Large intestine:* Most of the "food," or material, that gets to the colon consists of waste products that will be excreted. Some of the dietary fiber that you have eaten is fermented by healthy bacteria in your large intestine. Not much nutrient absorption occurs from your large intestine.

- *Rectum and anus*: Waste products leave your body as feces.

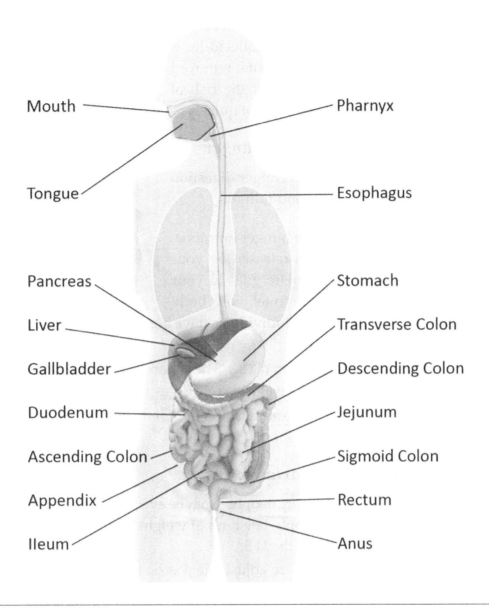

Figure 1: The Digestive System

Food enters your GI tract by entering your mouth when you eat or drink. Food begins in your mouth; it moves through your gastrointestinal tract as it is broken down and you absorb the nutrients. Any food that is not absorbed is excreted through the anus as waste.

Digestive Juices

Various organs produce digestive juices that mix with your foods and help break them down into nutrients that your body can use.

- *Stomach*: Your stomach produces stomach acid, or hydrochloric acid, which breaks down food. It also produces enzymes to help digest carbohydrates and proteins.
- *Pancreas:* Enzymes from your pancreas break down carbohydrates, proteins, and fats.
- *Liver*: Your liver secretes bile, which helps digest fat.

- *Gallbladder*: The gallbladder stores bile until you eat a meal with fat or cholesterol. Your gallbladder is not an essential organ, and sometimes it is removed during weight loss surgery to avoid the risk of getting gallstones when you lose weight quickly.

Hormones Related to Digestion and Hunger

Your body produces hormones that trigger digestion and also affect your levels of hunger and fullness.

> **Tip**
>
> See **Chapter 1, "Obesity – A Widespread Disease,"** for a discussion of the role of insulin in carbohydrate metabolism and its relationship to diabetes. **Chapter 4, "RYGB & It's Potential Benefits,"** discusses how the gastric bypass affects some of these hormones to help you lose weight.

- *Ghrelin:* Ghrelin is known as the hunger hormone. This hormone is produced and released by your stomach when it is empty. Ghrelin goes to your brain and stimulates your brain to tell your body that you are hungry. Some obese individuals have higher levels of ghrelin than normal-weight people.

- *Gastrin, secretin, and Cholecystokinin (CCK):* These hormones sense the presence of food and signal your organs to produce and secrete digestive juices when you eat.

- *Peptide YY (PYY):* This hormone comes from your GI tract and tells your brain that you are full after eating.

Types of Weight Loss Surgery (Bariatric Surgery)

As the list of myths pointed out, many people — maybe even you before starting to consider bariatric surgery — think that there is only one kind of weight loss surgery. However, at least five types of surgery are performed in the U.S.

The four most common in the U.S. are adjustable gastric band, roux-en-Y gastric bypass, vertical sleeve gastrectomy, and biliopancreatic diversion with duodenal switch.[12] You might also hear about the vertical banded gastroplasty, which is becoming less common, and sleeve plication, which is relatively new. This part of the chapter summarizes these procedures so you can understand their differences.

The book focuses on the roux-en-Y gastric bypass. We will talk about it in detail in the next chapter and throughout the rest of the book. In this chapter, we will just introduce it briefly along with the other kinds of weight loss surgery.

Where Can I Get More Information?

Everyone can use some good advice when making a decision as important as weight loss surgery. Understanding each of the different kinds of bariatric surgery and their pros and cons can be confusing. If you are considering surgery, BariatricPal.com is an excellent resource. You can communicate with a friendly and welcoming community of bypass patients, experts, and surgeons.

Vertical Banded Gastroplasty: Restrictive

Vertical banded gastroplasty, or VBG, is also known as stomach stapling. It is a restrictive type of bariatric surgery. The patient feels full sooner and is unable to eat as much food. Immediately after surgery, the stomach pouch holds only one tablespoon, or one-half ounce, of food.

This bariatric procedure, developed by Dr. Edward Mason from the University of Iowa, dates back to 1982. Laparoscopic vertical banded gastroplasty has been introduced since then, but 90 percent of vertical banded gastroplasty surgeries in the U.S. are still open surgeries, which have a higher risk of complications than laparoscopic procedures.

The open or laparoscopic surgery takes one to four hours and requires general anesthesia.[13] You may need to stay in the hospital for up to five days after surgery. Using open or laparoscopic methods, the surgeon makes a cut in the stomach wall coming down from a starting point a few inches below the esophagus. The surgeon staples the stomach so that the small usable pouch is only about 10 to 15 percent of its original size. The surgeon inserts a band, which seals off the large part of your stomach from the small pouch. The large pouch is no longer usable.

Common short-term risks that occur can within the days and weeks after vertical gastroplasty include nausea and vomiting, injury to the spleen, and an incisional hernia. You may also get dehiscence, which is when your staples are displaced or loosened so that the cut in your stomach lining is opened. Over the long term, you may experience continued nausea, heartburn, and depression. Vertical banded gastroplasty is less effective than other forms of weight loss surgery, with less than a 50 percent rate of maintaining weight loss after 10 years. Because of its dangers and poor weight loss results compared to other bariatric procedures, the VBG is no longer common.

Vertical Sleeve Gastrectomy: Restrictive

Vertical sleeve gastrectomy is also known as a sleeve gastrectomy, the gastric sleeve, and greater curvature gastrectomy.[14] Your stomach pouch size is reduced to 15 percent of the original size so that it fills up faster and you feel full faster. The VSG was originally done as the first step of a two-surgery procedure known as the biliopancreatic diversion with duodenal switch bypass (BPD-DS). When surgeons saw how effective the VSG could be, they started to do the gastric sleeve as its own weight loss surgery. It is often done laparoscopically in the U.S.

The vertical sleeve gastrectomy usually takes one to two hours. The hospital stay is about two to seven days. A vertical sleeve gastrectomy is similar to a vertical band gastrectomy, but instead of folding over the stomach, as in the VBG, the surgeon *removes* 80 to 85 percent of your stomach in the VSG. The surgeon uses the remaining portion of your stomach to make a tube-shaped sleeve that goes from the esophagus to your small intestine. Finally, the surgeon stitches closed the sleeve in your stomach and uses a sealant to prevent leaks. Because your stomach is removed rather than folded or stapled, the VSG is irreversible.

After the procedure, the size of your sleeve is only 15 to 20 percent of the original size of your stomach. The sleeve gastrectomy is a restrictive procedure because the small sleeve fills up quickly when you eat so that your brain realizes that you are full. This bariatric surgery does not interfere much with nutrient absorption, so it is not considered a malabsorptive procedure. However, the vertical sleeve gastrectomy can reduce your appetite because of its effects on some of your hormones. For example, your stomach produces a hormone called ghrelin, which sends signals to your brain to make you feel hungry. When the majority of your stomach is removed, the amount of ghrelin in your body is decreased so you do not have as many hunger signals.

Along with the normal risks of surgery, specific risks of vertical sleeve gastrectomy include internal injury to your organs during surgery and leaking between the stitches that are supposed to seal up your sleeve. If you get scarring inside your abdomen as you heal, the scar tissue can eventually block your bowel, or colon or large intestine, and cause constipation in the future. You may develop gastritis, or inflammation and pain in your stomach, ulcers, and heartburn. If you eat too much food at once, you will probably end up vomiting.

Vertical sleeve gastrectomy is a relatively safe surgery, especially for very obese patients that need a two-step process instead of undergoing gastric bypass all at once. You can lose most of your excess weight within two or three years with a vertical sleeve gastrectomy, but the procedure itself may not be enough for all patients. Some individuals with a vertical sleeve gastrectomy eventually choose to have their surgeries converted into a biliopancreatic diversion with duodenal switch (BPD-DS).

Sleeve Plication: Restrictive

Sleeve plication is also known as laparoscopic greater curvature plication or gastric imbrication. This relatively new technique is similar to vertical sleeve gastrectomy, but no part of your stomach is actually removed.[15] Instead, the part that will not be used is sutured shut. The sleeve plication is usually performed on patients with a BMI of less than 50. Your surgeon might recommend a vertical sleeve gastrectomy if your BMI is over 50.

For a laparoscopic greater curvature plication, the surgeon makes small incisions into your abdomen to be able to place the instruments. The surgeon uses a line from below your esophagus to above your small intestine. The large pouch of your stomach is sutured, or folded in, along that line, so it can't be used anymore. The usable pouch of your stomach will be about 15 percent of its original size, and the rest of your stomach is folder over and held shut. The procedure takes two to four hours.

Some of the benefits compared to the vertical sleeve gastrectomy are a shorter hospital stay and less of a risk of nutritional deficiencies. Plus, there is no insertion of an object into your body—you do not have a ring or tube or staples in your body. This means that there is no risk of things getting loose or having a defective part inside of you. Some of the possible complications of sleeve plication are an inability to digest food properly and swelling of the stomach from the procedure. It may also cause gastroesophageal reflux disease, or GERD, which you may feel as heartburn. GERD increases your risk of developing esophageal cancer. Also, it is not widely used in patients with a BMI over 50.

Laparoscopic Adjustable Gastric Banding: Restrictive

Laparoscopic adjustable gastric banding is the least invasive type of weight loss surgery because it does not alter your body physiology. This is the only bariatric procedure that is both adjustable and reversible. The LAP-BAND® system, made by Allergan,[16] and REALIZE™ adjustable gastric band, made by Ethicon Endo-Surgery,[17] are FDA-approved medical devices for the treatment of obesity. The lap-band can be used in lower-BMI patients and has been approved for patients with a BMI as low as 35.

A typical laparoscopic adjustable gastric banding procedure takes 30 to 60 minutes, and you may go home on the same day. Some patients spend a night or more in the hospital. [18] The surgeon makes three to five cuts in your abdomen to insert the laparoscope and other instruments. The gastric band is a silicon tube that goes around the upper part of your stomach and divides it into a small upper pouch and a large lower pouch. The upper pouch is about 15 percent of the size of the original stomach, and the lower pouch is 85 percent. When you eat, food goes into the upper pouch, called the stoma. The gastric band is tight enough around the stomach to keep the food from passing quickly into the lower stomach. The stoma fills up quickly so you feel full soon.

The lap-band has a lower rate of complications than some other weight loss surgeries. For example, compared to roux-en-Y gastric bypass and biliopancreatic diversion with a duodenal switch (discussed below), the lap-band had less than half the rate of mild complications, such as nausea, and less than one-tenth the rate of serious complications, such as organ injuries.[19] Most lap-band patients do have some form of mild complications, such as vomiting, diarrhea, or gastroesophageal reflux.

The surgeon can adjust the band by filling it with saline solution, or salt water, to make it tighter. That makes it more restrictive. You may need it deflated to increase the size of your stomach during times when you need more nutrients, such as during pregnancy. The lap-band does not cause dumping syndrome or lead to nutrient deficiencies.

It may take three or four adjustments for the surgeon to be able to inflate the band to the exact right pressure to restrict food intake enough to help you lose weight but not so tight that you vomit a lot. Another drawback is that the lap-band can be displaced and require another surgery to reposition or replace the band. The lap-band helps you lose weight more slowly than the other kinds of weight loss surgery. It may take you three or more years to get to your goal weight while following a strict diet. Of course, all of the weight loss surgeries require you to pay attention to your diet.

Roux-en-Y Gastric Bypass: Restrictive and Malabsorptive

Roux-en-Y gastric bypass (RYGB) is the most common type of gastric bypass weight loss surgery.[20] It is restrictive because it shrinks the size of your stomach pouch. It is malabsorptive because it changes your digestive tract so that you absorb fewer nutrients from food. After the surgery, your stomach pouch is the size of a walnut and the bottom of your stomach is attached to the jejunum, or middle portion, of your small intestine instead of the ileum, or upper, portion.

The roux-en-Y surgical procedure takes two to four hours. It can be open or laparoscopic. Similar to the restrictive procedures discussed above, the surgeon closes off most of the stomach with staples or a band, leaving just a small functional pouch. Then the surgeon attaches the bottom of the small pouch to the jejunum, or middle of the small intestine, rather than to the ileum. It takes three to five weeks to fully recover from RYGB and get back to your usual activities.

Right after surgery, your stomach pouch will be able to hold one to two ounces of food, or about 15 to 20 percent of your former stomach capacity. That is the restrictive part of roux-en-Y. The "gastric bypass" results from the small stomach emptying into the jejunum, therefore "bypassing" the majority of your original stomach ("gastric" is a term referring to your stomach).

The malabsorptive part of the surgery comes from the "roux-en-Y" part. The term describes the final anatomical appearance of your surgery. Your gastric pouch is called the roux limb, and the "Y" shape is formed by the three arms coming together at a junction. The three arms are:

- Your small stomach pouch that holds food
- Your large stomach pouch that secretes digestive juices
- The jejunum of your small intestine that receives food from the small pouch

Roux-en-Y gastric bypass can help you lose more than half to three-quarters of your excess body weight within one to two years. The surgery also helps to resolve diabetes or reduce its severity. Roux-en-Y patients have increased levels of CCK, which is one of the hormones that helps you digest food and tells your brain that you are full. Gastric bypass tends to increase the hormone peptide YY, which is another hormone that tells your brain that you are full.

RYGB reduces nutrient absorption by making food avoid your duodenum, which is where a lot of nutrient absorption usually takes place. That helps you lose weight, but it can also cause nutritional deficiencies if you do not take supplements. You will need to be monitored by a dietitian or doctor for the rest of your life to make sure you do not get anemia, osteoporosis, or vitamin deficiencies. Roux-en-Y gastric bypass can be a good choice for individuals that tend to overeat sweets because you cannot eat them after the surgery. Eating sweets after gastric bypass can lead to dumping syndrome, with symptoms of cramping, nausea, and diarrhea. This can happen if you eat sweets because the sugars do not get digested properly when your food leaves your stomach faster.

The remainder of this book focuses on the roux-en-Y gastric bypass. We will cover each portion of it in more detail later.

Biliopancreatic Diversion with Duodenal Switch: Restrictive and Malabsorptive

Biliopancreatic diversion with duodenal switch, or BPD-DS is technically a form of gastric bypass surgery, but it is less common than roux-en-Y. With BPD-DS, your stomach pouch becomes smaller and nutrient absorption decreases because food bypasses part of the small intestine and your digestive juices are rerouted.

This surgery is more extensive than laparoscopic roux-en-Y gastric bypass or simple restrictive weight loss surgeries. It is a two-step process. The first step is similar to a vertical sleeve gastrectomy, but less of your stomach is removed. The remaining stomach portion stays at about half of your original stomach size, compared to only 15 percent of the original size in the other procedures. The BPD-DS can be done in super-obese patients.

The second part of the surgery is the diversion and switch. Your small intestine is divided into two parts. One part, the alimentary limb, gets connected to the bottom of your stomach. The rest of your small intestine, now called the biliopancreatic limb, is attached to the bile duct. Food travels down the alimentary limb into your colon without being absorbed in the biliopancreatic limb. Digestive juices are free to flow from your biliopancreatic limb to your alimentary limb. This means food is digested (broken down) but not absorbed (taken into your body). This is how the BPD-DS causes nutrient malabsorption.

The biliopancreatic diversion with duodenal switch is one of the bariatric surgeries with the most rapid weight loss in the first year or two. It is also likely to have good results for long-term weight loss and prevention of weight regain. And this procedure is good for patients with an initial BMI of more than 55 because it works so well. The biliopancreatic diversion with duodenal switch helps to prevent dumping syndrome, or diarrhea, because of the digestive juices that come through the biliopancreatic limb and digest your food.

The biliopancreatic diversion with duodenal switch has some drawbacks though. It may lead to chronic diarrhea. There is also a high risk of chronic malnutrition because of the reduced absorption of nutrients. An iron deficiency causes anemia, and calcium deficiency causes osteoporosis, or the increased risk of fractures, especially in your hips, back, and wrists. Dumping syndrome can occur in BPD-DS, especially if you eat high-sugar foods.

Summary of Types of Weight Loss Surgery

Table 11 summarizes the different kinds of weight loss surgeries described above. It may be a handy resource to review as you read this book. It will help you compare the bypass to the other surgeries at a glance.

Name (and alternate names)	Description	Notes
Vertical Banded Gastroplasty (Stomach Stapling)	The surgeon divides the stomach into two parts by using staples so that you cannot eat as much. Your pouch is 10 to 15% of its original size.	This surgery can be done open or laparoscopically. It is less effective than other types of bariatric surgery. Risks include nausea, vomiting, and dehiscence, or displacement of staples.
Vertical Sleeve Gastrectomy (Gastric Reduction, Gastric Sleeve, The Sleeve)	The surgeon reduces your stomach to 15% of its original size by surgically removing the rest of your stomach.	This surgery helps reduce food intake by restricting your stomach size and reducing levels of a hunger-increasing hormone called ghrelin. The Sleeve was originally part of a two-step procedure for biliopancreatic diversion with duodenal switch gastric bypass but has been effective on its own. It can cause bleeding and gastritis.

Name (and alternate names)	Description	Notes
Sleeve Plication	Sleeve plication is similar to a vertical sleeve gastrectomy because it reduces your stomach size to about 15% of its original size. However, your stomach is sewn shut, not removed.	This relatively new type of weight loss surgery has results comparable to gastric bypass, but it is safer and has fewer side effects. Since your stomach is sutured and not removed, there is less chance of nutrient malabsorption and internal bleeding than with the gastric sleeve, but it is less well-studied.
(Laparoscopic) Adjustable Gastric Banding	The adjustable gastric band goes around the tube from your throat to your stomach. The surgeon inflates the tube with saline solution to narrow it and reduce your food intake.	Adjustable gastric banding is a restrictive procedure that does not cause nutrient deficiencies. This approach is the only weight loss surgery approach that is both adjustable and reversible. It is FDA-approved as an obesity treatment. It may be the best choice for some lower-BMI patients.
Roux-en-Y Gastric Bypass (gastric bypass, RYGB)	This surgery reduces your stomach size to about one ounce. The surgeon then connects your stomach to the jejunum of your small intestine. Roux-en-Y gastric bypass can be a laparoscopic or open procedure.	Roux-en-Y is restrictive and malabsorptive. Patients lose about 70% of excess body weight within the first year. This surgery is known for its resolution of diabetes, and it alters your hormone levels for a result of reduced hunger. It raises the risk for nutrient deficiencies.
Biliopancreatic Diversion with Duodenal Switch Gastric Bypass	This surgery is a two-step process. The first step is the vertical sleeve gastrectomy, which reduces stomach size. The second step reroutes your digestive tract so food goes from your small stomach to your lower small intestine. The rerouting procedure also alters the effects of digestive juices, such as bile.	The approach works in three ways. It reduces stomach size (restrictive); it reduces nutrient absorption by avoiding the small intestine; and it interferes with absorption by altering bile and other digestive juices. It can lead to anemia and osteoporosis because of reduced absorption of iron and calcium.

Table 11: Summary of types of weight loss surgery

✍ Summary

This chapter introduced some of the different approaches to weight loss. We talked about why weight loss surgery may be the only realistic option for effective, long-term weight loss for you.

☛ For many people, dieting does not work, because it is temporary and can lead to yo-yo diets.

☛ Exercise is healthy and a great way to support additional methods for losing weight, but you probably cannot burn enough calories to lose weight very fast from exercise without other weight loss methods.

☛ Weight loss drugs seem appealing, but you may not lose weight very fast with them. Plus, many weight loss medications are only approved for short-term use — between 12 weeks and one year — and they have side effects that can be serious.

☛ Weight loss, or bariatric, surgery can be a good tool to help you lose weight. Procedures can be restrictive, to shrink the size of your stomach, and malabsorptive, to reduce the absorption of nutrients from food. Weight loss surgeries have the same risks as any surgical procedures. Additional complications depend on which surgery you choose and may include nausea, internal bleeding, leaks, obstructions, and nutritional deficiencies.

Time to Take Action: Your Past Weight Loss Attempts and the Future

List the diets and weight loss pills that you have tried over the years.

....

....

....

Describe your weight loss results. Include how much you typically lost, how long the diet lasted, and when you started to regain the weight.

....

....

....

Why have the diets not worked for you? Your answer might be because you were too hungry, too bored, unmotivated to continue, or unable to afford them or take the time to prepare the right foods.

....

....

....

After reading this chapter, do you think weight loss surgery is the right choice for you? YES/NO

If you think weight loss surgery is right for you, do you understand that weight loss surgery is only a tool? YES/NO

Do you understand that your own diet decisions will determine your weight loss success after bariatric surgery? YES/NO

Finally, are you ready at this point in your life to commit to lasting weight loss and a lifestyle change that will require a lot of effort? YES/NO

If not, what is holding you back?

....

....

....

1   Phelan S, Hill JO, Lang W, Dibello J, Wing RR. Recovery from relapse among successful weight maintainers. American Journal of Clinical Nutrition. 2003;78(6):1079-1084.

2   This book is not affiliated with Nutrisystem or Jenny Craig, which are branded companies.

3   Weight-Control Information Network. Prescription medications for the treatment of obesity. National Institute of Diabetes and Digestive Kidney Diseases. Web site. http://win.niddk.nih.gov/publications/prescription.htm. Updated 2010, December. Retrieved December 7, 2012.

4   FDA approves weight management drug Qsymia. Food and Drug Administration. Web site. http://www.fda.gov/NewsEvents/Newsroom/PressAnnouncements/ucm312468.htm. 2012, July 17. Accessed November 14, 2012.

5   Food and Drug Administration. FDA approves Belviq to treat some overweight or obese adults. Web site. http://www.fda.gov/NewsEvents/Newsroom/PressAnnouncements/ucm309993.htm. 2012, June 27. Accessed December 7, 2012.

6   Bennet JMH, Mehta S, Rhodes M. Surgery for morbid obesity. Postgraduate Medical Journal. 2007;83(975):8-15.

7   Rao RS. Bariatric surgery and the central nervous system. Obes surg. 2012;22(6):967-78.

8   Weight-Control Information Network. Longitudinal assessment of bariatric surgery. National Institute of Diabetes and Digestive Kidney Diseases. NIH No. 04-5573. 2010. http://win.niddk.nih.gov/publications/labs.htm.

9   Kissler HJ, Settmacher U. Bariatric surgery to treat obesity. Semin Nephrol, 2013;33(1):75-89.

10 National Digestive Diseases Clearinghouse. Your digestive system and how it works. NIH 08-2681. http://digestive.niddk.nih.gov/ddiseases/pubs/yrdd/. 2012.

11 Truesdell D. Digestion and absorption. The Gale Group, MacMillan Reference. Healthline. Web site. http://www.healthline.com/galecontent/digestion-and-absorption. Published 2004. Accessed November 15, 2012.

12 Weight-Control Information Network. Bariatric surgery for morbid obesity. National Institute of Diabetes and Digestive Kidney Diseases. NIH Publication No. 08-4006. http://win.niddk.nih.gov/publications/gastric.htm. 2011. June. Accessed December 7, 2012.

13 Frey, R. Vertical banded gastroplasty. Healthline. Web site. http://www.healthline.com/galecontent/vertical-banded-gastroplasty. 2004. Accessed December 7, 2012.

14 Nall R. Vertical sleeve gastrectomy. Healthline. Web site. http://www.healthline.com/adamcontent/vertical-sleeve-gastrectomy#1. 2012, July 25. Accessed November 16, 2012.

15 Gebelli JP, de Gordejuela AGR, Badia AC, Medayo LS, Morton AV, Noguera CM. Laparoscopic gastric plication: a new surgery for the treatment of morbid obesity. Cirugia Espana. 2011;89(6):356-61.

16 FDA expands use of banding system for weight loss. Food and Drug Administration. Web site. http://www.fda.gov/NewsEvents/Newsroom/PressAnnouncements/ucm245617.htm. 2011, February 16. Accessed November 16, 2012.

17 Realize Band-P070009. Food and Drug Administration. Web site. http://www.fda.gov/NewsEvents/Newsroom/PressAnnouncements/ucm245617.htm. 2007, September 28. Accessed November 16, 2012.

18 Nall R. Laparoscopic adjustable banding. Healthline. Web site. Retrieved from http://www.healthline.com/adamcontent/laparoscopic-gastric-banding. 2012, July 25. Accessed November 16, 2012.

19 Parikh MS, Laker S, Weiner M, Hajiseyedjavadi O, Ren CJ. Objective comparison of complications resulting from laparoscopic adjustable banding. Journal of the American College of Surgeons. 2006;202(2):252-61.

20 Laberge M. Gastric bypass. Healthline. Web site. http://www.healthline.com/galecontent/gastric-bypass. 2004. Accessed November 16, 2012.

3

All About The Roux-En-Y Gastric Bypass (RYGB)

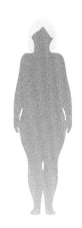

Chapter 2 discussed why losing weight is so difficult. It talked about some of the diets, exercise programs, and weight loss drugs that you may have already tried in the past to lose weight. They may have been successful for a while until you went off them and gained the weight back, or they might not have worked at all for you.

If traditional diets, exercise, and weight loss drugs are not the solution for your weight, weight loss surgery — or bariatric surgery — might be. As introduced in the previous chapter, bariatric surgery may help you to:

- Lose weight.
- Keep it off.
- Improve your health profile.
- Be more successful long-term than with just diets, exercise, and/or weight loss drugs.

The gastric bypass is one of the most common weight loss surgeries in the U.S. and around the world.[1] Nearly half of bariatric surgeries in the U.S. are RYGB.[2] The surgery is:

- Designed to be a permanent change to your body
- A restrictive procedure that helps you eat less
- A malabsorptive procedure that reduces your calorie and nutrient absorption
- Similar to other weight loss surgeries in its effectiveness
- Likely to improve certain health conditions

This chapter will go into more detail on the RYGB so that you can make an informed decision about whether you want this surgery. The chapter answers these questions:

- What is the Roux-en-Y gastric bypass?
- How can the surgery help you lose weight?
- What is the RYGB procedure?

By the end of the chapter, you will have a clear picture of the Roux-en-Y gastric bypass procedure. You will be closer deciding whether or not you are still interested in the gastric bypass.

> **Tip**
>
> **Take your time!** This chapter contains many details. We include them so that you can find answers to your questions, but you do not have to read every detail if you are not interested. We suggest that you just skim the parts of the chapter that are too technical for now. You can always come back later when you have specific questions.

Restrictive, Malabsorption, and Hunger Hormones: How Roux-en-Y Gastric Bypass Can Help You Lose Weight

The Roux-en-Y gastric bypass is a restrictive and a malabsorptive procedure. It is restrictive because, after surgery, your stomach pouch is very small. It fills up faster, and you are not able to eat as much. It is malabsorptive because food does not enter the upper portion of the small intestine, where a significant amount of nutrient absorption normally occurs. In addition, the RYGB may affect some of your gut hormones and reduce your hunger.

Restriction to Help in Weight Loss after RYGB

The large size of the normal stomach can contribute to weight gain. The normal adult stomach has a volume of one to two liters—that is four to eight cups, or up to half a gallon or 64 ounces! That means that you can eat up to a half gallon of food—*per meal*—before your stomach fills up. That is a lot of food! As an example, a cup of fried rice, mashed potatoes, or macaroni and cheese each have 200 to 300 calories.[3] Add to those three cups a cup of ice cream at 300 calories, and this meal can contain 1,300 calories! Think about eating three of these meals per day, along with a few snacks, and you can understand why gaining weight is so easy! You could be at 3,000 or more calories per day, when you really only need about 2,000 (or more or less, depending on your body size and activity levels). You could potentially be eating thousands of extra calories if you eat until your stomach is full three times a day. Each time you eat 3,500 calories more than you need, you gain a pound of body fat.

Does your stomach size really matter for weight control? Yes! In fact, on average, normal-weight individuals report feeling full when their stomachs contain only 1.1 liters, while obese participants in the same study on average are not full until their stomachs contained 1.9 liters.[4] If you never feel full and you think your hunger and a large stomach pouch are causing your weight problems, the Roux-en-Y gastric bypass may be a worthwhile option because it makes your stomach pouch smaller.

In the gastric bypass procedure, the surgeon closes off the majority of your stomach pouch, leaving the functional portion of your stomach with a volume of only one to two ounces right after surgery. That is only a fraction the size of your original stomach size. The intention is to reduce the amount of food that you want to eat or are physically able to eat. This idea is known as restriction. Meals and snacks must be small to avoid feeling sick or having side effects. The result of eating less is weight loss.

If you are considering gastric bypass after many failed diet attempts, you have probably already tried eating smaller meals as a weight loss strategy. If you have lost and regained the same weight multiple times, you may be wondering how the bypass can turn out any differently than your previous weight loss efforts. The answer is that the gastric bypass actually changes your stomach size. As long as you do not stretch your pouch after surgery, it will continue to restrict your food intake.

What Is Roux-En-Y Gastric Bypass, How It Works, and the Surgical Procedure

Before surgery, food that you swallow travels down your throat, into your stomach, and into the duodenum (the upper part of the small intestine) and then the jejunum (middle portion of the small intestine) en route to the ileum (lower portion of the small intestine just above the colon, or large intestine). A significant amount of nutrients is absorbed from food in the duodenum and jejunum. After gastric bypass, food goes directly from the stomach to the lower part of the small intestine, therefore skipping the duodenum and part or all of the jejunum.

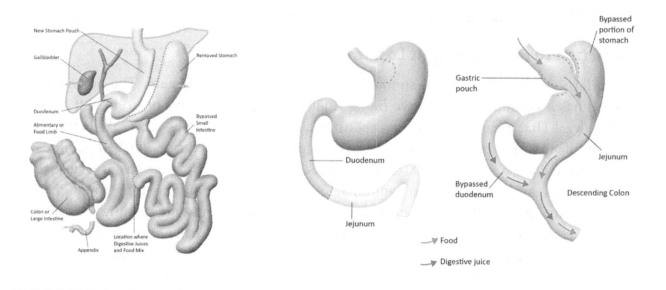

Figure 2: Nutrient Malabsorption to Help in Weight Loss after RYGB

This is an illustration of the regular stomach (left) versus the bypass. The J-shaped regular stomach, before surgery, has a large pouch shown here toward the right side of the stomach. That large pouch is where food normally sits after you eat a meal. You do not feel full until the stomach pouch is full. After RYGB, your stomach pouch is much smaller, so there is no big pouch for a lot of food to sit in. Instead, the theory is that you will feel full when your small stomach pouch is full—and the small pouch is only a few tablespoons in size! Gastric bypass also has another important difference from your original stomach. Before surgery, food that you eat passes from your stomach to the top of your small intestine. After surgery, food passes from your stomach into the middle of your small intestine so fewer nutrients are absorbed.

Gastric bypass can reduce the absorption of protein by about one-quarter and fat by two-thirds.[5] Protein has 4 calories per gram, and fat has 9 calories per gram. Preventing such large proportions of protein and fat from being absorbed reduces the amount of calories your body receives and helps you lose weight.

Although it can accelerate weight loss, nutrient malabsorption has some potential disadvantages. The first is that in addition to decreasing your calorie absorption, it also decreases absorption of essential nutrients. You are at higher risk for deficiencies of nutrients such as protein, calcium, and vitamin B12 as well as vitamins A, D, E, and K, which require adequate fat for proper absorption.[6]

The second negative effect of nutrient malabsorption is that it can cause dumping syndrome, with symptoms of nausea, diarrhea, shakiness, and confusion. Dumping syndrome is the result of food reaching the lower part of the small intestine when it is still relatively undigested because it has bypassed the upper part of the small intestine. High-sugar, high-fat foods are more likely to cause dumping syndrome. Some RYGB patients consider it a benefit of surgery because it gives you extra motivation to avoid these high-calorie, unhealthy foods. Later chapters will discuss dumping syndrome and how to avoid it.

Changes in Hunger Hormones to Help in Weight Loss after RYGB

Along with making your stomach smaller and interfering with nutrient absorption, roux-en-Y gastric bypass may help you lose weight in a third way. It changes the levels of some of your body's hormones that affect how hungry or full you feel. After RYGB, you are likely to feel more satisfied or full after a meal because of increases in certain hormones, such as peptide YY (PYY) and glucagon-like peptide-1 (GLP-1).[7] Ghrelin is known as the hunger hormone because high levels of ghrelin in your bloodstream make you feel hungry.[8] Levels of ghrelin may decrease after RYGB,[9] leading to less hunger, although the effects may be insignificant[10] and only last for a few months after surgery.[11]

Your Responsibilities and the RYGB: Success Is up to You

Here is another reminder that the gastric bypass is only a tool for weight loss; it is up to you to decide whether to use the tool by following the prescribed weight loss surgery diet. If you cheat on the diet, your weight loss results will not be as good, and you will have a higher risk for complications. Something else to consider is that your stomach pouch can stretch. It starts out at a very small fraction of your original stomach size, but it can stretch over time if you continuously eat too much. Follow these guidelines to improve weight loss and lower your risk of complications:

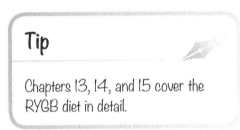

Tip

Chapters 13, 14, and 15 cover the RYGB diet in detail.

- Do not eat *too much* (a high volume of) food
- Choose low-calorie foods
- Do not eat too frequently
- Avoid beverages with or immediately before or after meals
- Drink low-calorie or calorie-free beverages
- Eat only when you are hungry
- Stop eating when you are full

Overview of the Roux-en-Y Gastric Bypass (RYGB)

Chapter 2, *"Options for Losing Weight: Diets, Exercise, Weight Loss Drugs, and Surgery,"* introduced the RYGB. To summarize, the surgeon divides your stomach into a small upper portion and a larger lower portion, which gets stapled shut so that food cannot enter it and it is unusable. The small portion of the stomach is then attached to the middle or lower part of your small intestine. When you eat after RYGB, food goes into the small stomach pouch and directly to the middle or lower portion of your small intestine, thus bypassing the upper part of the small intestine.

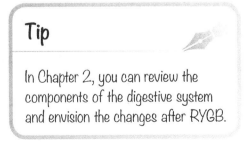

Tip

In Chapter 2, you can review the components of the digestive system and envision the changes after RYGB.

Now that you know how the Roux-en-Y gastric bypass can help you lose weight, this section will describe the actual procedure and what happens in the operating room when you go in for surgery. We will start with the surgeon and other healthcare workers in the operating room so you know who is who.

Key Players in the Operating Room

The surgeon and a few other important figures are responsible for performing your surgery safely and well. You will have at least one appointment with your surgeon and probably meet the other surgical team members before surgery.

- The *surgeon* has the lead role. The surgeon directs the other members of the team, makes the incisions into your abdomen, controls the laparoscopic medical tools, and makes important decisions, such as any changes to plans in the surgical cuts. Compared to the other members of the surgical team, you will probably work more closely with your surgeon both before and after surgery.

- The *anesthesiologist* is responsible for administering the general anesthesia to put you to sleep so that you remain unconscious during the procedure. Anesthesiologists are fully licensed physicians with special training. A good anesthesiologist:

  - Provides the right type and amount of anesthesia so that it is enough to help you fall asleep quickly but not so much that you are groggy for too long after the procedure.[12]

  - Monitors your heart rate and other vital signs during surgery.

  - Monitors and helps to reduce your pain levels after surgery.

- Two *surgeon assistants* are present in the operating room to assist the surgeon.[13] Typically, one stands on each side of you as you are on your back on the operating table. The surgeon assistants help out by handing the surgeon tools as necessary, helping to inflate the abdominal cavity with gas so the surgeon has room to work, watching the screen with the images from the laparoscopic camera, and alerting the surgeon if anything does not look right.

Laparoscopic versus Open Surgery: What is the Difference?

When you think of a traditional surgery, you probably envision open surgery. In open surgery, the surgeon cuts into the abdomen through the skin and tissues to gain direct access to your inner stomach cavity. The surgeon performs the surgery directly and operates the tools with his or her own hands. An open surgery in the abdominal cavity, such as the RYGB, is also known as a laparotomy.

Most bariatric surgeries today are laparoscopic. Laparoscopic surgery is minimally invasive because the surgeon only makes a few small cuts into your abdomen. Through these incisions, the surgeon inserts a laparoscope, or tiny camera, and some tiny tools. The surgeon can "view" the surgery site on a screen that displays images from the laparoscope and can operate the tools using remote controls instead of directly placing his or her hands within the patient's stomach cavity.

These are some of the advantages of laparoscopic procedures compared to open procedures:

- *Faster recovery time*: Only a few small incisions have to heal; you do not have slow-healing injuries to your muscles as in open surgery.
- *Less pain*: Deeper incisions into your muscles during open surgery are more painful than surface incisions as they heal.
- *Less risk of infection*: Open surgery requires deeper cuts and a wide open stomach cavity. It is easier to get infections during or after surgery than laparoscopic surgery, where your inner body is not exposed to the air.
- *Faster surgical procedure*
- *Less time in the hospital*
- *Smaller scars*: Smaller, shallower cuts in laparoscopic surgery lead to smaller, less visible scars than deeper cuts in open surgery.

Laparoscopic surgery is usually preferred, but as this chapter will soon discuss, open RYGB is a safer option.

The Roux-en-Y Gastric Bypass Operation

You already know the basics of RYGB. Briefly, your stomach pouch becomes smaller, and food bypasses the upper part of the small intestine. This section provides more details about the procedure. If you are the type of person that does not like to think about surgery, you can skip this section.

Laparoscopic RYGB Procedure[14]

You, the patient, will be lying on your back, unconscious from anesthesia. The surgeon will make a few incisions in your abdomen and place five ports, or small devices that go under the skin. During surgery, these medical ports hold the skin and other tissues in place so the surgeon can easily see and access the surgery site. The surgeon carefully inserts the laparoscope—that is the tiny camera that will let the surgeon visualize what is happening—through the slits in your abdomen.

The surgeon or a surgeon's assistant creates a pneumoperitoneum by pumping carbon dioxide gas to inflate the peritoneum, or lining around your stomach. The pneumoperitoneum gives the surgeon space to work.[15]

What Is a Pneumoperitoneum and Why Do You Get One?

"Pneumo" means "air," and "peritoneum" refers to the lining around your abdominal cavity. "Pneumoperitoneum" happens during laparoscopic surgery when you have carbon dioxide gas pumped into your abdominal cavity. This helps inflate it so the surgeon has room to work—remember, the beauty of the laparoscopic technique is that you only have tiny incisions in your abdomen.

The pneumoperitoneum allows the laparoscopic procedure to occur so that you do not have to have a longer and riskier open surgery. However, there are a few side effects or complications that can happen as a result of having the pneumoperitoneum:

- Nausea, vomiting, and pain after the surgery, especially in your shoulders and neck

- Thromboembolism, or a blood clot that can block blood flow to a leg, arm, your heart, or brain

- Severe headaches until all of the extra gas has left your body

Source:[16]

The surgeon creates a small stomach pouch of about one ounce or less by stapling closed the majority of your stomach. The surgeon then finds the ligament of Treitz, which connects the jejunum to the diaphragm and is a marker for where the duodenum ends and the jejunum begins. The surgeon attaches the small stomach pouch to a place on the jejunum about 30 centimeters (1 inch) beyond (below) where the ligament of Treitz attaches to the small intestine. This is the Roux-en-Y limb. The upper portion of the small intestine gets attached to form the biliopancreatic limb.

Stitches are used to close the seams. To finish up, the surgeon tests to make sure that the seams are tight.

A short-limb Roux-en-Y gastric bypass has a Roux-en-Y limb that is about 30 centimeters below the ligament of Treitz. In a longer-limb RYGB, the Roux-en-Y limb begins as much as 150 centimeters below the ligament of Treitz.[17] The longer-limb procedure leads to greater nutrient malabsorption because more of the small intestine is bypassed. It is used in patients with more weight to lose.

Laparoscopic Roux-en-Y Gastric Bypass (LRYGB) versus Open RYGB

Nowadays laparoscopic RYGB is more common.[18] The procedure can take about two to four hours, and the average hospital stay is about two to seven days. The exact time for surgery and how long you will spend in the hospital vary by surgeon and patient. Compared to open surgery, the laparoscopic procedure is easier on your body in multiple ways. The incisions are smaller, and the procedure is quicker. Recovery is quicker, and you have a lower risk of infections during surgery.

However, some patients are unable to have the laparoscopic procedure and instead need an open RYGB.[19] Your surgeon may know this before starting your surgery, or the surgeon may make the decision to convert your laparoscopic procedure into an open procedure during the middle of surgery.

When might you need an open procedure?

- If you have a weak heart or trouble with your lungs: They may not be able to tolerate the pneumoperitoneum, or carbon dioxide gas in your abdominal cavity, that is necessary for the laparoscopic procedure.[20]

- If you are at a higher BMI than some of the other patients your surgeon sees: Your surgeon may have difficulty making the necessary incision(s) into your abdomen to properly position the laparoscope, surgical instruments, and medical ports.

- If your surgeon has trouble placing or manipulating the laparoscope or other laparoscopic instruments in your abdomen: You might be converted to an open procedure during surgery.

Why Is the Pneumoperitoneum a Challenge for Your Circulatory System?

During a laparoscopic procedure, surgeons pump carbon dioxide gas into your abdominal cavity to create a pneumoperitoneum and have more space to work. However, the need for this extra gas is tough on your circulatory (or cardiovascular) system, and so some RYGB patients are not candidates for the laparoscopic procedure. Instead, they would need the open procedure. Extra carbon dioxide is a challenge because:

- Your heart needs to beat faster to pump more blood.

- Your lungs need to breathe faster to exchange more air between your body and the outside environment.

- Your blood vessels have added stress because of difficulties with venous return, or getting blood back to your heart from your legs and other body parts.

Cholecystectomy and Gastric Bypass

A cholecystectomy is the removal of your gallbladder. The procedure is relatively common to get during your weight loss procedure. Nothing is wrong with your gallbladder. Instead, removal of the gallbladder is performed to reduce your risk of developing gallstones later. Rapid weight loss, which occurs after successful gastric bypass surgery, can increase your risk for gallstones if your gallbladder has not been removed.

Gallstones occur when bile accumulates in your gallbladder and forms hard balls like pebbles.[21] These gallstones can obstruct your bile duct, which is part of the system that allows digestive juices to get from your liver and pancreas to your stomach and small intestines. Gallstones can cause abdominal pain, diarrhea, and vomiting after you eat fatty foods.

Rapid weight loss is a major risk factor for gallstones. A successful weight loss surgery helps you lose weight much more quickly than you would with diet alone, so you are at higher risk for gallstones after RYGB. Your surgeon may discuss the risk of gallstones with you before your surgery and recommend removing your gallbladder while performing the gastric bypass procedure.

Gallbladder removal is not a very high-risk operation. Your gallbladder can be removed during a laparoscopic or an open procedure, so it will not complicate your procedure and recovery. Also, even though your gallbladder is normally involved with digestion, you can still digest your food properly without it. Not all RYGB patients get their gallbladders removed; your surgeon should discuss this with you.

More Roux-en-Y Gastric Bypass Facts

Now you know how the RYGB is performed and how it can help you lose weight. This surgery is such an important decision in your life, though, that we are adding a few more tidbits to keep in mind as you continue to consider the procedure.

Gastric Bypass Is Intended to Be Permanent

The Roux-en-Y gastric bypass is intended to be permanent. In theory, it is reversible. None of your stomach or the rest of your gastrointestinal tract is actually removed from your body during the RYGB procedure, so if necessary, the surgery can be reversed. However, this is only a realistic option if the original surgery goes wrong. When you plan for RYGB, plan for it to be permanent.

What RYGB Does and Does Not Do

Gastric bypass is not magic, but it is a potentially powerful tool against obesity. It is designed to help you lose a lot of weight if you avoid complications and follow your healthcare team's instructions for success. This is what the gastric bypass can do:

- Provide a constant reminder to limit your food intake because you may experience dumping syndrome if you overeat and overfill your small stomach pouch.
- Increase your satiety, or feelings of fullness, by increasing your levels of hormones called PYY and GLP-1.
- Dramatically changes your regular digestive process so fewer nutrients from your food are digested and absorbed.
- Increase your risk for dumping syndrome, malnutrition, and other complications for the rest of your life.

These are some things that RYGB does not do. It does not:

- Lose weight for you. The work is up to you; you still need to follow a strict diet plan if you want to hit your weight loss goals.
- Prevent you from making poor choices, because it is up to you to choose healthy foods.

☞ **Summary**

- ☞ After reading this chapter, RYGB should be something that you can clearly picture in your head. That will help you think carefully about whether gastric bypass still sounds like the answer to your obesity. You are not quite ready to make an informed decision about the surgery yet, though.

- ☞ The next chapters will get more personal in the sense that they will help you decide whether RYGB is right for you.

- ☞ Chapter 4 discusses the amount of weight loss that you can expect after RYGB as well as other potential benefits of the surgery.

- ☞ Chapter 5 presents some of the drawbacks, such as side effects and complications, that RYGB can cause.

- ☞ In Chapter 6, you will learn about eligibility criteria for this surgery and additional factors that are important when you are considering Roux-en-Y gastric bypass.

- ☞ After reading the next three chapters, you will be in a better position to make a decision on whether it is for you.

Time to Take Action: Gastric Bypass and You

Now that you understand how the gastric bypass procedure can help you lose weight and how the surgical procedure works, are you still considering this surgical procedure for weight loss? YES /NO

What did you learn in this chapter that has encouraged you to continue considering the gastric bypass as a tool for weight loss?

....

....

....

What else do you need to know before you are ready to decide whether or not to get RYGB?

....

....

....

What are you worried about that is holding you back from committing to Roux-en-Y gastric bypass?

....

....

....

Are you ready to make the commitment to get weight loss surgery? YES / NO

Describe what makes you feel that you are mentally prepared to make the necessary lifestyle changes to succeed with bariatric surgery.

....

....

....

1   Buchwald H. ASBS 2004 consensus conference statement: bariatric surgery for morbid obesity: health implications for patients, health professionals and third-party payers. Surgery for obesity and related diseases, 2005;371-381

2   Hutter MM, Schimer BD, Jones DB, Ko CY, Cohen ME, Merkow RP, Nguyen NT. First report from the American College of Surgeons – Bariatric Surgery Center Network laparoscopic sleeve gastrectomy has morbidity and effectiveness positioned between the band and the bypass. Ann Surg. 2012;254(3):410-422.

3   National nutrient database for standard reference. National Agricultural Library, Agricultural Research Service, USDA. 2012, January 30. Accessed August 30, 2012 from http://ndb.nal.usda.gov/

4   Geliebter A. Gastric distension and gastric capacity in relation to food intake in humans. Physiol Behav. 1988;44(4-5):665-8.

5   Aills L, Blankenship J, Buffington C, Furtado M, Parrott, J. ASMBS Integrated health nutritional guidelines for the surgical weight loss patient. Surgery for Obesity and Related Diseases, 2008; S73-S108.

6   Mechanick MD, Kushner RF…Dixon J. American Association of Clinical Endocrinologists, The Obesity Society, and American Society for Metabolic & Bariatric Surgery medical guidelines for clinical practice for the perioperative nutritional, metabolic, and nonsurgical support of the bariatric surgery patient. Obesity, 2009;17(S1):S3-72.

7   Morinigo R, Moize V, Musri M, Lacy AM, Navarro S, Marin JL…Vidal J. Glucagon-like peptide-1, peptide YY, hunger and satiety after gastric bypass surgery for morbid obese subjects. JCEM, 2006;91(5):1735.

8   Inui A, Asakawa A, Bowers CY, Mantovani G, Laviano A, Meguid MM, Fujumiya M. Ghrelin, appetite and gastric motility: the emerging role of the stomach as an endocrine organ. 2004;18(3):439-456.

9   Chronaiou A, Tsoli M, Kehagias I, Leotsinidis M, Kalfarentzos F, Alexandrides TK. Lower ghrelin levels and exaggerated postprandial peptide—YY, glucagon-like peptide-1 and insulin responses after gastric fundus resection in patients undergoing Roux-en-Y gastric bypass: a randomized clinical trial. Obes Surg. 2012 Nov;22(11):1761-70. doi: 10.1007/s11695-012-0738-5.

10 Barazzoni R, Zanetti M, Nagliati C, Caittin MR, Ferreira C, Giuricin M…de Manzini N. Gastric bypass does not normalize obesity-related changes in ghrelin profile and leads to higher acylated ghrelin fraction. Obes (Silver Spring), 2012.

11 Peterli R, Steinert RE, Woelnerhanssen B, Peters T, Christoffel-Courtin C, Gass M…Beglinger C. Metabolic and hormonal changes after laparoscopic roux-en-Y gastric bypass and sleeve gastrectomy: a randomized, prospective trial. Obes Surg, 2012;22(5):740-8.

12 Physicians and surgeons. The Bureau of Labor Statistics. Web site. http://www.bls.gov/ooh/healthcare/physicians-and-surgeons.htm. 2012, March 29. Accessed September 1, 2012.

13 Moy J, Pomp A. Laparoscopic sleeve gastrectomy for morbid obesity. American Journal of Surgery. 2008;196(5).

14 Figueredo EJ, Yigit T, Oelschlager BK, Pellegrini CA. Laparoscopic roux-en-Y gastric bypass for morbid obesity. MedGenMed, 2006;8(1):63.

15 Neudecker J, Sauerland S, Neuebauer E, Expert Panel. The European Association for Endoscopic Surgery clinical practice guideline on the pneumoperitoneum for laparoscopic surgery. Surg Endosc. 2002;16(7):1121-43.

16 Neudecker J, Sauerland S, Neuebauer E, Expert Panel. The European Association for Endoscopic Surgery clinical practice guideline on the pneumoperitoneum for laparoscopic surgery. Surg Endosc. 2002;16(7):1121-43.

17 Buchwald H. ASBS 2004 consensus conference statement: bariatric surgery for morbid obesity: health implications for patients, health professionals and third-party payers. Surgery for obesity and related diseases, 2005;371-381

18 Buchwald H. ASBS 2004 consensus conference statement: bariatric surgery for morbid obesity: health implications for patients, health professionals and third-party payers. Surgery for obesity and related diseases, 2005;371-381

19 Holzheimer RG, Mannick JA, eds. Complications of laparoscopic surgery. Surgical Treatment, Evidence-Based and Problem-Oriented. Munich:Zuckschwerdt; 2001.

20 Neudecker J, Sauerland S, Neuebauer E, Expert Panel. The European Association for Endoscopic Surgery clinical practice guideline on the pneumoperitoneum for laparoscopic surgery. Surg Endosc. 2002;16(7):1121-43.

21 Cholecystectomy – Open and Laparoscopic. Medline Plus. Web site. http://www.nlm.nih.gov/medlineplus/tutorials/cholecystectomyopenandlaparoscopic/htm/_no_50_no_0.htm Accessed September 2, 2012.

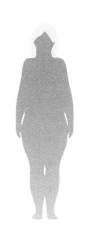

4

RYGB & It's Potential Benefits

Chapter 3 explained how gastric bypass can help you lose weight and what happens during surgery. At this point, you may be leaning toward getting Roux-en-Y gastric bypass or even fairly sure that you will get it. You are hoping that it is your answer to years of struggling with obesity, just like it has been the answer for thousands of patients. But you still need more information before making your final decision about RYGB. This chapter and Chapter 5 will help you understand the benefits and risks of surgery so that you can make an informed decision.

This chapter discusses the possible benefits of RYGB, including weight loss, improved health, and better quality of life.

- Weight loss after gastric bypass: how much, how quickly, and how likely
- Physical health benefits: better health and fewer medications
- Going beyond the numbers: quality of life is just as important

This chapter will help you form realistic expectations for the gastric bypass and possible weight loss.

Weight Loss

How much weight will I lose? The best way to answer this question is with averages because nobody knows how much weight *you*, a unique individual, will lose after surgery. Just a few factors that affect your own weight loss are your starting weight and BMI, how closely you follow your RYGB diet instructions, your exercise program, and your follow-up care. This section presents some of the average weight loss numbers from various research studies. Your own results with RYGB depend on your own choices. The more consistent you are with your diet, the more likely you are to hit your weight loss goals.

Ways to Measure Weight Loss

As you read this book and continue to gather information on the gastric bypass online and from other sources, you might run across more ways of measuring weight loss than just number of pounds lost. Each individual has a different amount of weight to lose, and using specific terminology can help make comparisons between people easier. The following measures of weight loss are some of the more common ones. You can refer back to this list as you read through this chapter and do your own research on the bypass.

Pounds Lost

This simple measure is probably how you measure your own weight loss. The problem is that people that have more weight to lose are likely to lose more weight. An average loss of, for example, 100 pounds after five years is very different if the average starting weight was 250 pounds than if the average starting weight was 400 pounds.

Ideal Body Weight Is Only an Estimate

Your ideal body weight falls within a range. You can be just as healthy with a BMI of 20 or 21 as you can with a BMI of 23 or 24, so you do not *have to worry about setting your goal weight at that exact BMI of 22. It is okay if you end up a few pounds below or above the "ideal" of 22 as long as you are eating healthy foods and feeling great.*

Excess Weight Loss (EWL)

Excess weight is the number of pounds that you weigh above a number called your ideal body weight. By definition, the ideal body weight is the weight of someone at your height with a BMI of 22, which is right in the middle of the normal, healthy range of 18.5 to 24.9. So, let's say, for example, that your height is 5 feet, 4 inches. Your ideal body weight, or your weight with a BMI of 22, is 128 pounds (you can check that on the table in chapter one or use an online calculator). If you weigh 228 pounds, you are 100 pounds above your ideal body weight. This means that your excess weight is 100 pounds.

- *Your excess weight loss or EWL*: is the amount of this "excess weight" (the 100 pounds in the above example) that you lose after weight loss surgery. It is expressed in percent. Going back to the above example, let's say that you start off with a pre-surgery weight of 228 pounds, or an excess weight of 100 pounds. If you lose 60 pounds within the first year after your gastric bypass surgery, you will have an excess weight loss (EWL) of 60 percent. Your excess weight loss will be 100 percent when you hit your goal weight of 128 pounds. Excess weight loss is usually expressed in terms of percent so that you can know how much weight loss to expect and compare your weight loss progress to the progress of people with different starting weights and different amounts of excess weight.

- *Excess BMI Loss (EBMIL)*: Remember how the BMI is a way to compare your own weight to someone else's, even if you both have different heights? (If not, take a look at Chapter 1 for an explanation of BMI.) Well, the EBMIL has a similar idea. Your excess BMI is defined as the BMI you have over an "ideal BMI" of 22. So, if your pre-surgery BMI is 62, your excess BMI is 40. The excess BMI loss is the percent of excess BMI you lose. Let's say you get down to a BMI of 32 after surgery. That means that you have lost 30 BMI points, or 30 out of your initial 40 excess BMI points. That is an EBMIL of 30 divided by 40, or 75 percent.

- *Sufficient weight loss*: There is no single definition for this. Researcher may define it by the following:
  - number of pounds lost, such as 75 within a year
  - EWL, such as 40 percent in a year
  - BMI, such as BMI under 35[1]
  - certain EBMIL, such as 50 percent

- *Other common measurements include the following*:
  - Waist circumference, often measured in inches
  - Percent body fat, or the weight of your fat divided by your total body weight. A normal body fat percent range is 14 to 24 percent for men and 21 to 31 percent for women.

How Much Weight Do People Lose After Gastric Bypass?

While nobody can tel you exactly how much weight *you* will lose, you can get an idea by looking through results of research studies that track patients who get RYGB. These are some of the weight loss numbers that have been reported.[2]

Excess Weight Loss (EWL)

- After one to two years, the average excess weight loss (EWL) in various studies ranged from 48 percent to 85 percent excess weight loss after one year.
- After three to five years, the EWL range was 53 to 77 percent.
- After 7 to 10 years, various studies found EWL to be 25 to 68 percent. To put that in perspective, an EWL of 68 percent is a loss of 68 pounds for a 5'4" woman whose starting weight was 228 pounds.

Long-limbed RYGB has greater weight loss on average.[3] As Chapter 3 explains, long-limbed RYGB causes more:

- After one to two years, the average EWL was 53 to 74 percent.
- After three to five years, various studies reported average EWL of 55 to 74 percent.

Additional Weight Loss Numbers

The following statistics are reported in a variety of research studies:

- Excess BMI loss of 63 percent, or a decrease from an average starting BMI of 44 to a BMI of 32[4]
- After two years, a decrease in BMI from a starting average of 48 to an average of 43[5]
- Many RYGB patients lose 100 pounds in the first year.

As you look through these numbers, remember that they vary greatly because of differences in surgeons, techniques, follow-up care, and patient characteristics, such as starting weight, age, gender, overall health, and adherence to the prescribed diet.

More to Think About

These are a few additional considerations:

- Your weight loss will be delayed if you have complications during or after surgery.
- Weight loss often slows or stops after one to two years.

- About one-quarter of weight loss surgery patients regain significant weight after a couple of years.[6]
- Weight loss depends on your diet.
- Revisional RYGB, or RYGB as a second weight loss surgery attempt, leads to less weight loss than in patients that are getting RYGB as a first weight loss surgery.[7]
- The amount of weight you can expect to lose after RYGB is comparable to weight loss after the vertical sleeve gastrectomy (gastric sleeve) and adjustable gastric band (lap-band).[8] Initial weight loss is likely faster with RYGB.

Weight Loss Depends On You!

Not all weight loss surgery patients hit their weight loss goals. And some of the patients that do hit their initial weight loss goals find themselves regaining the weight. What happens in that case? Your choices depend on the reason why you are not controlling your weight as well as you had hoped. These are some of the possible reasons and the actions to implement to take charge.

Unrealistic Expectations

Prevent disappointment and possible failure by keeping your weight loss goals realistic. Roux-en-Y gastric bypass is not a quick fix for obesity. You might not hit your goal weight within a year or even two or more years. Weight loss will not be easy or automatic. Staying on track requires you to change your diet and stay focused.

Poor Diet

You can regain weight if you are not honest with yourself about your diet. Do not sneak in foods or beverages that are not allowed or eat oversized portions. Monitor yourself carefully to prevent mistakes that can slow weight loss or lead to weight gain. Accidental diet blunders are likely once you become accustomed to the RYGB diet and are less careful about each bite. You may *think* you have memorized the entire diet or that you can estimate ("eyeball") portions without measuring them, but bad habits can creep in. Be sure to follow the instructions from your surgeon and/or dietitian. Another great tip, if your weight loss is not on track, is to check in with BariatricPal.com for advice from other weight loss surgery patients who thought they were following their diets but realized that they were making mistakes that were hurting their weight loss.

Lack of Restriction – Stretching of the Pouch

Your small stomach pouch, formed from the upper portion of your original stomach, consists of a stretchable material. Right after surgery, the small pouch has a capacity of about an ounce, so it can only hold tiny amounts of food. Over time, though, if your meals are too big or you drink fluids with meals and snacks, the pouch can stretch so that you no longer feel full on a small amount of food.

Poor Support

Inadequate post-surgery support can make you lose motivation and leave you without the information you need to meet your weight loss goals. Choose a surgeon with a comprehensive aftercare program. If you already had gastric bypass surgery and you need more support, do not be afraid to look to another surgeon, clinic, or peer support group for help. BariatricPal.com is another source of support, where you can get information and advice from thousands of other RYGB patients.

RYGB Simply May Not Work for You

For a variety of other reasons, some patients do not lose their desired amount of weight with RYGB. Revisional surgery is one option for patients that tried following the RYGB diet and still were unable to lose weight. You might get revisional surgery to get your gastric bypass redone as a long-limbed gastric bypass. Another type of conversion is a band-over-bypass, or adjustable gastric band inserted around your stomach pouch.

Reminder: Weight Loss Depends on You!

As you have seen, your possible weight loss falls within a wide range; that is, you might lose only a few pounds, or you might hit your goal weight within the first year of getting the RYGB. The amount of weight that you lose is largely up to you. These steps can increase your chances of losing your goal amount of weight:

- Following the diet that your surgeon, dietitian, or clinic recommends
- Exercising regularly
- Choosing an experienced surgeon for your procedure
- Taking your post-surgery aftercare program seriously[9]

Other Factors Affecting Your Weight Loss after RYGB

You play the largest role in your own success with RYGB, but other factors also affect your weight loss.[10] Chapter 5 will explore more deeply how you can use this information to your advantage before and after surgery. Factors affecting your weight loss include the following:

- Surgeon differences: technique and experience
- Degree of comprehensiveness of your post-surgery follow-up care plan
- Biological factors – You are more likely to hit your weight loss goals, for example, if your pre-surgery BMI is lower, if you do not have type 2 diabetes before surgery, and if you are normally physically active. You can be aware of these factors and adjust your weight loss expectations in order to avoid disappointment.

Benefits of RYGB: Potential Changes in Hormone Levels

Chapter 3 introduced the changes in hormone levels that can happen after RYGB and that can help you lose weight. This section outlines some of the current information on various hunger hormones and how their levels can change after RYGB. In general, Roux-en-Y gastric bypass appears to reduce hunger and increase satiety in many patients.

Changes in Hormone Levels after RYGB

A hormone is a chemical that is produced in one part of your body and affects other parts of your body. Hormones come from a variety of organs, such as the liver, thyroid, pancreas, hypothalamus, adrenal gland, and stomach, and they affect almost everything in your body, including growth and development, metabolism of energy and nutrients, hunger, mood, sleep, and immune function.

Roux-en-Y gastric bypass may be able to help you lose weight and improve your health because of its effects on some of your hormones related to metabolism and hunger.

Peptide-YY (PYY): PYY increases your feelings of fullness after a meal. Levels are higher in obese individuals than normal-weight people, leading to less satisfaction. Levels of PYY tend to increase after getting the gastric bypass, and this can contribute to your weight loss. [11,12] However, not all RYGB patients have higher PYY after RYGB. [13]

Glucagon-Like Peptide-1 (GLP-1): Glucagon-like peptide-1, or GLP-1, is a gut hormone that helps you feel full. Levels of GLP-1 are lower between meals and higher after meals. A high amount of GLP-1 tends to make you eat less. Obese individuals have lower levels of GLP-1—and greater hunger—than normal-weight individuals. The Roux-en-Y gastric bypass may raise your GLP-1 levels,[14] which might increase your post-meal satiety[15] and help you lose weight. Together, GLP-1 and PYY are part of the "ileal brake." It is called that because these hormones work to make you feel full when food gets toward the farther end of your small intestine—the ileum.

Leptin: Leptin is a hormone that comes from your fat cells and is involved in appetite control. Leptin may reduce appetite. However, obese individuals tend to have higher leptin levels than normal-weight individuals, and leptin may have altered effects in the body. The RYGB may improve the effects of leptin on your appetite and lower your leptin levels, making them more similar to those of normal-weight people. [16]

Ghrelin: Ghrelin is also known as the hunger hormone. It is produced and secreted by cells in your stomach, and it makes you feel hungry. You have higher levels of ghrelin circulating in your bloodstream before meals to make you feel hungry. Levels decrease after meals so you feel full. However, obese individuals tend to have higher levels of ghrelin—more potential for hunger—than normal weight individuals. Levels can decrease after RYGB,[17] but they can return to pre-surgery levels within a year.[18] Some studies find that RYGB does not affect ghrelin levels. Vertical sleeve gastrectomy, or VSG, is a weight loss surgery option that decreases ghrelin more than the roux-en-Y gastric bypass does.[19]

Insulin: As discussed in the section on diabetes in Chapter 1, insulin is mainly responsible for regulating your blood sugar levels. Later in this chapter, we will describe how RYGB's effects on insulin can improve your blood sugar control. Insulin is relevant here, too, because it increases your hunger. Insulin levels may decrease after getting weight loss surgery,[20] helping you to feel less hungry.

Bottom Line: RYGB, Hormones, and Hunger

Hormones can get complicated, but you do not have to know everything from the above descriptions. These are the main points:

- RYGB can reduce your hunger by changing the levels of some of your hormones.
- These changes are not the same for every patient.
- Many additional factors affect your hunger.
- The amount of hunger you will have after RYGB is unpredictable.

Beyond Weight Loss: More Potential Benefits of RYGB

Weight loss is not the only measure of success after RYGB, although it is your main reason for getting the surgery. Compared to patients that get gastric bypass surgery, obese individuals that are eligible for RYGB but do not opt for weight loss surgery have a higher risk of death from any cause.[21] RYGB can lead to a variety of additional benefits, such as better physical and psychological health as well as a better social life.

Possible Health Benefits of the Gastric Bypass

Do you remember some of the obesity-related chronic conditions introduced in Chapter 1? They include type 2 diabetes and high blood sugar; heart disease, high blood pressure, and cholesterol; asthma; and osteoarthritis. Losing weight, which is what you will be doing after RYGB, can prevent, delay, or reverse these and other conditions.

Type 2 Diabetes and Blood Sugar Levels

Nearly all cases of type 2 diabetes are related to obesity, and most RYGB patients with high blood sugar levels before surgery see improvements in their blood sugar levels, insulin levels, and glycated hemoglobin (HbA1C, or A1C) after surgery.[22] These benefits are partly because of weight loss, but the RYGB procedure itself can lead to improved blood sugar control within days of surgery before any weight loss occurs.[23] The effects appear to last for years after surgery,[24] and most patients experience these benefits.[25]

What kind of improvements might you see?

- Reduced need for medications or the ability to get off your medications entirely (but always remember, only change your medication dosage with your doctor's recommendation)
- Lower blood glucose and A1C values, meaning that you are at lower risk for diabetes complications such blindness, heart disease, kidney disease, and infections
- Lower insulin levels, which is a sign of better glucose control[26]
- Decreased levels of glucagon-like peptide-1 (GLP-1) and peptide-YY (PYY), leading to a healthier (smaller) insulin response[27]

With or without the gastric bypass, losing weight can contribute to these benefits. However, the improvements in your blood sugar control after RYGB are greater than in patients who do not get weight loss surgery. In addition, the improvements can happen more quickly, within days of surgery and before you have had a chance to lose much weight. RYGB is more effective at improving blood sugar control than the laparoscopic adjustable gastric band (Lap-Band or Realize Band) and the vertical sleeve gastrectomy (VSG or gastric sleeve).

Roux-en-Y Gastric Bypass and Heart Disease

Weight loss and the Roux-en-Y gastric bypass surgery can be powerful weapons in fighting heart disease, the top killer of Americans. Major risk factors for heart disease that are related to obesity include high blood pressure and dyslipidemia, or high total cholesterol, high LDL cholesterol, high triglycerides, or low HDL cholesterol. If you are in the high-risk zone for heart disease or stroke, your numbers will likely improve as you lose weight.

- Obese individuals are about twice as likely to have coronary heart disease as normal-weight individuals, so losing weight reduces your risk. [28]
- High blood pressure, or hypertension, is likely to decrease after RYGB.[29,30]
- Blood cholesterol and triglycerides: Total cholesterol, "bad" LDL cholesterol, and triglycerides are likely to decrease, and HDL can increase after getting RYGB. [31,32] These improvements an last for years. [33]

A Word about the RYGB and Medications

Among the biggest benefits of losing weight is that you may be able to lower your dose of medications, go off of some medications entirely, or prevent health conditions that caused you to need medications in the first place. Examples include medications to lower cholesterol, blood sugar, and blood pressure, and prescription steroids or non-steroidal anti-inflammatory drugs (NSAIDs) to reduce joint pain from osteoarthritis and asthma medications. There are many benefits of avoiding or reducing your prescriptions:

- You do not have to remember to order and refill prescriptions.
- You do not have to remember to take your medications at the proper time.
- You do not have to pay for medications. A single medication for controlling blood sugar can be $1 to $5 or more per day—or $2,000 per year!

Another benefit of avoiding medications is that you will not need to worry about their side effects.

- Blood pressure medications (anti-hypertensives) can lead to muscle and joint pain, nausea, constipation and diarrhea, fatigue, and dizziness.
- Cholesterol-lowering medications, such as statins, can cause muscle and joint pain and weakness, nausea, diarrhea, liver disease, and memory loss.

- Glucose or type 2 diabetes medications: These can lead to hypoglycemia (low blood sugar), diarrhea, gas, and weight gain.
- Steroids, such as those for fighting osteoarthritis and asthma, can lead to bone mineral density loss and osteoporosis, which is a high risk for bone fractures.
- Some asthma medications lead to dry mouth and throat.
- Many NSAIDs are rough on your stomach and can lead to ulcers or stomach discomfort.
- The continuous positive airway pressure, or CPAP, is not a pill, but it is a treatment for an obesity-related disorder: sleep apnea. Getting rid of your CPAP machine will make sleep more comfortable.

You should not ever alter your dose or stop taking a prescription drug or other treatment without your doctor's recommendation. That can lead to even more serious side effects.

Sources:[34,35,36]

Other Improvements in Your Physical Health after the RYGB

Even more improvements in your physical health can result from losing weight. They are the opposite of the problems caused by obesity that we described in Chapter 1.

- **Sleep apnea:**[37,38] You will be able to breathe better at night as you lose weight and do not have as much fat blocking your throat and airways. If your sleep apnea is resolved, you would be able to sleep through the night without waking up and gasping for air. You might be able to stop using an annoying continuous positive airway pressure, or CPAP, machine without worrying that you will stop breathing in the middle of the night.
- **Gastroesophageal reflux disease (GERD):**[39] GERD is a chronic condition with frequent heartburn. It occurs when the highly acidic contents of your stomach backtrack up into your lower esophagus and you feeling a burning sensation in your chest. If you have GERD before surgery, gastric bypass might reduce or get rid of your symptoms for these reasons:
  - *You lose weight:* When you lose weight, you do not have as much fat pushing against your stomach (or stomach pouch) as you did before surgery. This means that you are not as likely to have the contents of your full stomach forced back up into your esophagus after a meal.
  - *No more wolfing down food:* Eating too quickly can lead to reflux. After RYGB, you eat more slowly.
  - *Meals are smaller:* Your stomach pouch is only a fraction of the size of your original

stomach, so your meals are smaller. Smaller meals can help you prevent heartburn and GERD.

- *Different food choices:* Fatty and fried foods, alcohol, and caffeinated beverages are all common triggers for heartburn and GERD, and these foods are not allowed or are strictly limited on the weight loss surgery diet.[40]

- **Asthma:** Losing weight can help you overcome asthma and other respiratory problems that you had before surgery. That is because extra fat in your abdomen and in the area near your airways can make breathing difficult.

- **Osteoarthritis:** Carrying around so much extra body weight can cause joint pain, and losing weight can reduce your pain and increase your mobility. Your energy levels can increase, too, because you are not hauling around so many extra pounds.

Additional Benefits from RYGB: Better Quality of Life

Some potential benefits of RYGB are less definable but just as important. Your Quality of Life score reflects the fact that life is more than numbers on a scale and medical lab test results. Your quality of life, also known as QoL, is an overall indicator of how good your life is. It considers your physical health in addition to your social life, your psychological health, and how well you can move around to do the things you want to do.

Measuring QoL

Researchers measure QoL with a variety of tests. They have slight variations but address the same general questions. One study that found dramatic improvements in quality of life after the gastric bypass asked these questions as part of its QoL assessment. These questions are known as the Moorehead-Adult Quality of Life Assessment.

Question	Answer Scale (on a Continuum)
Usually I feel	Very bad → very good about myself
I enjoy physical activities	Not at all → very much
I have satisfactory social contacts	None → very much
I am able to work	Not at all → very much
The pleasure I get out of sex	Not at all → very much
The way I approach food	I live to eat → I eat to live

Source: [41]

Why does the QoL tend to improve after you get the RYGB? [42]

Besides the weight loss and physical benefits, it affects nearly every aspect of your life.

- *You feel better about yourself.* You are proud of how you look. Confidence in your ability to control your eating can translate into confidence that you can succeed in other aspects of your life.

- *Your social life may improve.* Many other people will notice that you are a happier and more capable person, and they will enjoy being around you more than before. You will also be better able to keep up with the group during fun activities than when you were morbidly obese.

- *Life is easier.* To put it more formally, you are more functional. You can move around without struggling instead of having your obesity hold you back. Chances are, you will have better attendance at work, and each day will seem easier and more enjoyable.

Many factors contribute to an improved QoL when the RYGB becomes a successful tool for weight loss. However, it is important to remember that not all RYGB patients have better quality of life or are glad they got the procedure done. The most prudent advice is to make sure that you are getting the RYGB for the right reasons and that you are a good candidate for the surgery. It is a weight loss tool, not a magical cure for obesity. You need to make lifestyle changes — long-term — to achieve weight control.

Why Do the Numbers Not Add Up?

As you continue to research RYGB, you will probably start to notice something a little strange. The numbers change. One website, for example, might tell you that there is a 90% risk of having your diabetes in remission post-surgery, while another site might say 80%. The more research you do, the more you will notice that the numbers vary between sources. You may have already noticed the apparent discrepancies in this book! Why does this happen? It is not a mistake, and we are not lying to you. It is because there are different sources of data and different ways of calculating the numbers.

Clinical Trials versus Estimated Figures

Sometimes the information comes from clinical trials. These are carefully-planned research studies to investigate patients who get weight loss surgery. Before surgery, surgeons ask their patients if they are willing to participate in the study. During the entire time of the study, which might be for six months or a year or more after surgery, surgeons and other researchers ask patients about all of their complications. At the end of the study, they try to answer these or similar questions:

- Which side effects or complications occurred? In how many patients?
- Is there a difference between patients who got certain complications and those who did not?
- How much weight did the average patient lose over the course of the study?
- Is there a difference between patients who lost their target amount of weight and those who did not?
- Were there any other benefits to the surgery, e.g., health or mood improvements?

Clinical trials are great because they provide trustworthy information, but they have a big problem. They are too small. Clinical trials focusing on RYGB might include only 10 or 20 or 50 patients, which just is not that much compared to the thousands of obese patients that got RYGB. Some of the figures describing complication rates or weight loss success come from estimates based on reports from thousands of patients that have told their surgeons that they are having trouble. That is great because there is a lot of data but not so good because it is not too well controlled. One patient might call to report diarrhea while another patient with the same symptoms might not. This is different from a clinical trial when all patients promise to report all symptoms. So the numbers coming from clinical trials and patient reports can be different.

More Reasons Why Different Research Studies Can Have Different Results

There are other reasons for different numbers from different studies:

- Small number of people in the study. Let's say a study includes 10 participants, and one develops a serious infection after surgery. That is a 10% infection rate. Another study might include 1,000 participants and have 10 people develop a serious infection. That is a 1% infection rate. The more people in the study, the more accurate the results in general.
- Differences between patients. A study whose patients have lower pre-surgery BMIs, for example, usually finds lower complication rates and better weight loss than studies with higher-BMI patients.
- Average age of participants. Older adults tend to have more complications than younger adults.
- Slight differences in surgical procedures. More experienced surgeons and laparoscopic surgery usually lead to fewer complications.
- How good the aftercare program is. A better post-surgery care program leads to more weight loss, patients that are more likely to stick to their diets, and fewer complications.

What This Means for You

You are not an obesity researcher; you are not looking to make comparisons between studies. All you want is to make the best decision for you. It is not always easy or even possible to interpret the numbers. Hopefully you have already guessed the next piece of advice, because it is the first thing that should come to mind by now when you have questions. The advice? Talk to your doctor, a surgeon, and anyone else with the background to give you good individual advice. Your surgery decision needs to be based on your own circumstances. You can also gather information from online communities, such as BariatricPal.com, to get a feel for what their RYGB experiences are.

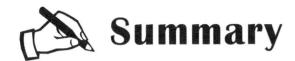 # Summary

- This chapter provided an overview of some of the likely benefits of the gastric bypass from weight loss to improved health, more self-confidence, and a better social life.

- The next chapter examines the negative aspects of the gastric bypass and the potential complications and side effects. The information is critical for you to be able to make the right personal decision about the RYGB.

- It is important as you read to remember that each person is an individual. Your own weight loss results, health consequences, and the remainder of your gastric bypass experiences can be better, worse, or simply *different* than someone else's. Predicting your own outcomes is impossible, but you can get a much better handle on the likely results when you do more research. So keep on reading — the next chapter is waiting!

Time to Take Action: How Do You Feel about RYGB Now?

This chapter covered some of the potential benefits of gastric bypass that you might experience if the surgery goes smoothly and you follow your surgeon's instructions. Let's take a look now at how you are feeling about the RYGB.

Do you recognize the amount of weight that you can reasonably expect to lose if you follow the RYGB diet? YES / NO

Is this an amount of weight that you would be happy with? YES / NO

Do you understand the additional health benefits that can happen after getting the gastric bypass? YES / NO

Are these health conditions of concern to you? YES / NO

The Roux-en-Y gastric bypass is just a tool for losing weight. You are responsible for making the RYGB diet work for you. For each of the following responsibilities, describe what you, the individual patient, must do if you want to write your own RYGB success story.

Diet

Exercise

Self-care

Patience/persistence

RYGB Patient Story: Panda

Panda is a 44-year-old single mom with two daughters. She struggled for years with weight loss, depression, and other health issues and says her Roux-en-Y gastric bypass surgery has enabled her to overcome these challenges. She lost over 100 pounds with the surgery and is now far below her high weight of 285 pounds. Now, at 5'6" tall and 159 pounds, her BMI is a normal 25. Some of her greatest support has come from the BariatricPal.com discussion forums, which she visits daily to give and receive advice and encouragement. Panda is happy to talk about her faith and her success in hopes of helping others who are struggling with obesity or the RYGB.

On Health Problems and the Decision to Get Surgery

I had been treated by a psychologist as well as a psychiatrist for many years for major depression and high anxiety. The acid reflux that I was having and the sleep apnea were making my life miserable. I was tired all of the time. I had uncontrolled asthma, plus I was in pain management for herniated discs in my back. Despite those ailments, I didn't have high blood pressure or diabetes.

What made me decide to have the surgery was because I prayed to God to help me lose weight, and bariatric surgery was the direction He sent me. Since the seventh grade, I had tried every weight loss fad, method, and craze out there. You name it, and I guarantee you I've tried it. I say that God led me to the bariatric surgery because I had never even consciously thought about it, although I have a couple of acquaintances that have had it. My story isn't as dramatic as others, and I came to be here through a road less travelled, but I truly believe that it was God who led me to this journey. I once saw a talk show about a woman who prayed herself thin, and it made sense to me. All things are possible through Christ, so why not weight loss?

One day out of the blue, I sat at my computer and looked up a number locally to a bariatric surgeon, and the next thing you know, I was attending the mandatory seminar. I learned that you had to have co-morbidities to be a candidate for my insurance, although I did weigh a whopping 285 lbs at 5'6" and wore a size 20 tightly. Within two months I had a surgery date. One month later I had surgery. It all happened so fast that it was almost surreal. Of course, they say that when I arrived at the seminar, my having all of the required paperwork completed as well as my medical records for the past ten years helped speed things along as well. I had already done all of their leg work for them all the way down to a current mammogram.

On Her Improved Physical and Mental Health Since Surgery

Surgery changed my life drastically in ways that all of the above mentioned ailments are gone or alleviated to the point of no longer being a nuisance. For example, I still have asthma, but it is not an issue at the moment. I used to always say there must be a lot of fat around my heart because I felt like I was suffocating. Now, I exercise daily. This has helped with the depression so much that I no longer am on medications for it. I have no more severe back or joint pain; I can even bend over and touch my toes now. I no longer snore or have sleep apnea. I have no acid reflux, which means I don't have to take pills for that. Most importantly, I don't mind looking at myself in the mirror anymore.

On Overcoming Self-Doubt

My biggest challenge, as with most RGYB patients, has been self-doubt. I have wondered whether I could succeed this time after so many failed attempts at weight loss. Did I have enough self-discipline to go through with this journey? Could I commit to a rigorous exercise plan five days a week? Was I ready to let go of my love affair with food? All of these questions plagued my mind daily and often still do.

One thing I would say to anyone struggling with their weight loss would be to believe in yourself because you are God's greatest gift, and through Him, all things are possible. Even for those who may not believe in Him, believing in something is better than not believing at all…so why not believe in yourself? Your mind is a magnet for wonderful things. Good thoughts bring good things.

1   Catheline JM, Fysekidis M, Dbouk R, Boschetto A, Bihan H, Reach G, Cohen R. Weight loss after sleeve gastrectomy in super superobesity. J Obes. 2012.

2   Mechanick MD, Kushner RF…Dixon J. American Association of Clinical Endocrinologists, The Obesity Society, and American Society for Metabolic & Bariatric Surgery medical guidelines for clinical practice for the perioperative nutritional, metabolic, and nonsurgical support of the bariatric surgery patient. Obesity, 2009;17(S1):S3-72.

3   Mechanick MD, Kushner RF…Dixon J. American Association of Clinical Endocrinologists, The Obesity Society, and American Society for Metabolic & Bariatric Surgery medical guidelines for clinical practice for the perioperative nutritional, metabolic, and nonsurgical support of the bariatric surgery patient. Obesity, 2009;17(S1):S3-72.

4   Edholm D, Svensson F, Naslund I, Karlsson FA, Rask E, Sundborn M. Long-term results 11 years after the primary gastric bypass in 384 patients. Surg Obes Related Dis. 2012.

5   Adams TD, Pendleton RC, Strong MB, Kolotkin RL, Walker JM, Litwin ES…Hunt SC. Health outcomes of gastric bypass patients compared to nonsurgical, nonintervened severely obese. Obesity, 2010;18(1):121-130.

6   Leitman IM, Virk CS, Avgerinos DV, Patel R, Lavarias V, Surick B, Holup JL, Goodman ER, Karpeh MS Jr. Early results of trans-oral endoscopic plication and revision of the gastric pouch and stoma following Roux-en-Y Gastric Bypass Surgery. JSLS. 2010 Apr-Jun; 14(2): 217–220.

7   Mor A, Keenan E, Portenier D, Torquati A. Case-matched analysis comparing outcomes of revisional versus primary laparoscopic Roux-en-Y gastric bypass. Surg Endoscop, 2012.

8   Hutter MM, Schimer BD, Jones DB, Ko CY, Cohen ME, Merkow RP, Nguyen NT. First report from the American College of Surgeons – Bariatric Surgery Center Network laparoscopic sleeve gastrectomy has morbidity and effectiveness positioned between the band and the bypass. Ann Surg. 2012;254(3):410-422.

9   Buchwald H. ASBS 2004 consensus conference statement: bariatric surgery for morbid obesity: health implications for patients, health professionals and third-party payers. Surgery for obesity and related diseases, 2005;371-381

10 Kaplan LM, Seeley RJ, Harris JL. Myths associated with obesity and bariatric surgery – myth 5: patient behavior is the primary determinant of outcomes after bariatric surgery. 2012;9(8):8-10.

11 Morinigo R, Moize V, Musri M, Lacy AM, Navarro S, Marin JL…Vidal J. Glucagon-like peptide-1, peptide YY, hunger and satiety after gastric bypass surgery for morbid obese subjects. JCEM, 2006;91(5):1735.

12 Peterli R, Steiner RE, Woelnerhanssan B, Peters T, Christoffel-Courtin C, Gass M, Kern B, von Flueee M, Beglinger C. Metabolic and hormonal changes after laparoscopic roux-en-Y gastric bypass and sleeve gastrectomy: a randomized, prospective trial. Obes Surg. 2012;22(5):740-748.

13 Ramon JM, Salvans S, Crous X, Uig S, Goday A, Benaies D, Trillo L…Grande L. Effects of roux-en-y gastric bypass vs sleeve gastrectomy on glucose and gut hormones: a prospective randomized trial. J Gastroinstest Surg, 2012;16(6)116-22.

14 Morinigo R, Moize V, Musri M, Lacy AM, Navarro S, Marin JL…Vidal J. Glucagon-like peptide-1, peptide YY, hunger and satiety after gastric bypass surgery for morbid obese subjects. JCEM, 2006;91(5):1735.

15 Peterli R, Steinert RE, Woelnerhanssen B, Peters T, Christoffel-Courtin C, Gass M…Beglinger C. Metabolic and hormonal changes after laparoscopic roux-en-Y gastric bypass and sleeve gastrectomy: a randomized, prospective trial. Obes Surg, 2012;22(5):740-8.

16 Ramon JM, Salvans S, Crous X, Uig S, Goday A, Benaies D, Trillo L…Grande L. Effects of roux-en-y gastric bypass vs sleeve gastrectomy on glucose and gut hormones: a prospective randomized trial. J Gastroinstest Surg, 2012;16(6)116-22.

17 Chronaiou A, Tsoli M, Kehagias I, Leotsinidis M, Kalfarentzos F, Alexandrides TK. Lower ghrelin levels and exaggerated postprandial peptide—YY, glucagon-like peptide-1 and insulin responses after gastric fundus resection in patients undergoing Roux-en-Y gastric bypass: a randomized clinical trial. Obes Surg. 2012 Nov;22(11):1761-70. doi: 10.1007/s11695-012-0738-5.

18 Peterli R, Steinert RE, Woelnerhanssen B, Peters T, Christoffel-Courtin C, Gass M…Beglinger C. Metabolic and hormonal changes after laparoscopic roux-en-Y gastric bypass and sleeve gastrectomy: a randomized, prospective trial. Obes Surg, 2012;22(5):740-8.

19 Peterli R, Steiner RE, Woelnerhanssan B, Peters T, Christoffel-Courtin C, Gass M, Kern B, von Flueee M, Beglinger C. Metabolic and hormonal changes after laparoscopic roux-en-Y gastric bypass and sleeve gastrectomy: a randomized, prospective trial. Obes Surg. 2012;22(5):740-748.

20 Peterli R, Steiner RE, Woelnerhanssan B, Peters T, Christoffel-Courtin C, Gass M, Kern B, von Flueee M, Beglinger C. Metabolic and hormonal changes after laparoscopic roux-en-Y gastric bypass and sleeve gastrectomy: a randomized, prospective trial. Obes Surg. 2012;22(5):740-748.

21 Adams TD, Pendleton RC, Strong MB, Kolotkin RL, Walker JM, Litwin ES…Hunt SC. Health outcomes of gastric bypass patients compared to nonsurgical, nonintervened severely obese. Obesity, 2010;18(1):121-130.

22 Adams TD, Pendleton RC, Strong MB, Kolotkin RL, Walker JM, Litwin ES…Hunt SC. Health outcomes of gastric bypass patients compared to nonsurgical, nonintervened severely obese. Obesity, 2010;18(1):121-130.

23 Proczko-Markuszewska M, Stefaniak T, Kaska L, Kobiela J, Sledziński Z. Impact of Roux-en-Y gastric bypass on regulation of diabetes type 2 in morbidly obese patients. Surg Endosc. 2012 Aug;26(8):2202-7. doi: 10.1007/s00464-012-2160-4.

24 Edholm D, Svensson F, Naslund I, Karlsson FA, Rask E, Sundborn M. Long-term results 11 years after the primary gastric bypass in 384 patients. Surg Obes Related Dis. 2012.

25 Mechanick MD, Kushner RF…Dixon J. American Association of Clinical Endocrinologists, The Obesity Society, and American Society for Metabolic & Bariatric Surgery medical guidelines for clinical practice for the perioperative nutritional, metabolic, and nonsurgical support of the bariatric surgery patient. Obesity, 2009;17(S1):S3-72.

26 Peterli R, Steiner RE, Woelnerhanssan B, Peters T, Christoffel-Courtin C, Gass M, Kern B, von Flueee M, Beglinger C. Metabolic and hormonal changes after laparoscopic roux-en-Y gastric bypass and sleeve gastrectomy: a randomized, prospective trial. Obes Surg. 2012;22(5):740-748.

27 van Rutte PWJ, Luyer MDP, de Hingh IHJT, Nienhuijs, SW. To sleeve or not to sleeve in bariatric surgery? ISRN Surgery. 2012.

28 Gagnon L, Sheff Karwacki EJ. Outcomes and complications after bariatric surgery. AJN. 2012;112(9):26-36.

29 Yaghoubian A, Tolan A, Stabile BE, Kaji AH, Belzberg G, Mun E, Zane E. Laparoscopic Roux-en-Y gastric bypass and sleeve gastrectomy   achieve comparable weight loss at 1 year. Am Surg, 2012;78(12):1325-8.

30 Adams TD, Pendleton RC, Strong MB, Kolotkin RL, Walker JM, Litwin ES…Hunt SC. Health outcomes of gastric bypass patients compared to nonsurgical, nonintervened severely obese. Obesity, 2010;18(1):121-130.

31 Adams TD, Pendleton RC, Strong MB, Kolotkin RL, Walker JM, Litwin ES…Hunt SC. Health outcomes of gastric bypass patients compared to nonsurgical, nonintervened severely obese. Obesity, 2010;18(1):121-130.

32 Mechanick MD, Kushner RF…Dixon J. American Association of Clinical Endocrinologists, The Obesity Society, and American Society for Metabolic & Bariatric Surgery medical guidelines for clinical practice for the perioperative nutritional, metabolic, and nonsurgical support of the bariatric surgery patient. Obesity, 2009;17(S1):S3-72.

33 Edholm D, Svensson F, Naslund I, Karlsson FA, Rask E, Sundborn M. Long-term results 11 years after the primary gastric bypass in 384 patients. Surg Obes Related Dis. 2012.

34 Dugdale DC, Zieve D. High blood pressure medications. Web site. http://www.nlm.nih.gov/medlineplus/ency/article/007484.htm. Updated 2011, June 10. Accessed September 10, 2012.

35 Humphries A, Workman T, Balasubramanyam A, Fordis M. Medicines for type 2 diabetes: a review of the research for adults. Web site. http://effectivehealthcare.ahrq.gov/index.cfm/search-for-guides-reviews-and-reports/?pageaction=displayproduct&product ID=721. 2011, June 30. Accessed September 10, 2012.

36 Mayo Clinic staff. Statins: are these cholesterol-lowering medications right for you? http://www.mayoclinic.com/health/statins/ CL00010. 2012, March 13. Accessed September 10, 2012.

37 Adams TD, Pendleton RC, Strong MB, Kolotkin RL, Walker JM, Litwin ES…Hunt SC. Health outcomes of gastric bypass patients compared to nonsurgical, nonintervened severely obese. Obesity, 2010;18(1):121-130.

38 Edholm D, Svensson F, Naslund I, Karlsson FA, Rask E, Sundborn M. Long-term results 11 years after the primary gastric bypass in 384 patients. Surg Obes Related Dis. 2012.

39 Yaghoubian A, Tolan A, Stabile BE, Kaji AH, Belzberg G, Mun E, Zane E. Laparoscopic Roux-en-Y gastric bypass and sleeve gastrectomy achieve comparable weight loss at 1 year. Am Surg, 2012;78(12):1325-8.

40 Snyder-Markow G, Taylor D, Lenhard MJ. Nutrition care for patients undergoing laparoscopic sleeve gastrectomy for weight loss. J Am Diet Ass. 2010;110(4):600-7.

41 Keren D, Matter I, Rainis T & Lavy A. Getting the most from the sleeve: the importance of post-operative follow-up. Obesity Surgery. 2011;21(12):1887-1893.

42 Adams TD, Pendleton RC, Strong MB, Kolotkin RL, Walker JM, Litwin ES…Hunt SC. Health outcomes of gastric bypass patients compared to nonsurgical, nonintervened severely obese. Obesity, 2010;18(1):121-130.

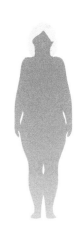

5

Roux-en-Y Gastric Bypass: Risks and Considerations

Chapter 4 focused on Roux-en-Y gastric bypass surgery's potential benefits, including the possibility of dramatic weight loss, improved health, and a better quality of life. These tantalizing benefits can be yours with RYGB, but the surgery also has risks. This chapter goes over some of the possible problems of RYGB:

- Complications from the open or laparoscopic RYGB surgical procedure
- Complications from Roux-en-Y gastric bypass

This is another chapter that will be pivotal in your decision on whether to get RYGB. By the end of it, you will be better able to balance its benefits against its risks so that you can make your decision confidently.

Risks of the Roux-en-Y Gastric Bypass

This section examines some of the risks from the surgery and complications that can develop later. This information will help you know what to expect and what can happen if you get the gastric bypass. An important question when deciding about RYGB—and all other medical procedures—is whether the positives outweigh the negatives.

All Surgical Procedures Have Risks

All surgeries, including laparoscopic and open gastric bypass, have risks. These are some of the risks:[1]

- Allergic reaction to anesthesia.[2]
- Excessive bleeding or hemorrhage during or after the procedure if you are prone to bleeding or if your body does not respond well. [3]
- Infections that occur during surgery because of a non-sterile surgical environment. Organs, such as the bladder, kidneys or lungs, and surgical cuts can get infected.
- Blood clots, heart attack, or stroke during or for days after surgery, which are more likely if you stopped taking blood thinners before surgery to prevent excessive bleeding.

Surgery Can Cause Death

Nobody wants to think about it, but surgery can be fatal. The rate of death in bariatric surgery is 0.15 to 0.64 percent. Among RYGB patients, the rate of death during or shortly after surgery is about 0.15 to 0.44 percent, or about 1 in every 300 to 700 patients.[4] As many as one to two percent of all bariatric surgery patients die within a year of surgery.[5,6] The leading causes are pulmonary embolisms (blood clot in your lungs), heart attacks, other heart complications, and severe infections, or sepsis. Leakage, excessive bleeding (hemorrhage), and bowel obstruction can also cause death.

Risks of Laparoscopic versus Open Surgery

Laparoscopic surgeries, or minimally invasive procedures, have lower risks than open procedures. You are less like to have excessive blood loss or get infections. The laparoscopic procedure does, however, cause more pain due to the need for pneumoperiosteum, or carbon dioxide gas pumped into your abdominal cavity. Also, patients with heart or lung conditions may not be able to tolerate the procedure and may need an open surgery instead. Chapter 3 talked about pneumoperiosteum in detail.

Risks from RYGB

The gastric bypass can lead to a variety of complications, ranging from simply unpleasant to very serious. This section describes some of them. Keep in mind that most of the following complications are the ones that patients actually tell their surgeons about. As you read through them, remember that some other patients may have experienced less serious complications without reporting them. These may include milder cases of nausea, vomiting, diarrhea, and stomach pain. Most bariatric surgery patients experience at least some of these symptoms.

Staple Line or Anastomotic Leak

After the gastric bypass procedure, the small stomach pouch that was created from the upper portion of your stomach is attached to your small intestine. The route that food travels from your stomach to your small intestine should be sealed. Leaks occur when the seal is not tight, and food and other contents of your gastrointestinal tract can escape into the rest of your body. As many as 17 percent of RYGB patients, or one in six patients, develop leaks.[7] Between 0.4 and 5% of patients get anastomatic leaks, which are more serious.[8]

A poorly performed surgery can cause leaks, and your surgeon should test for leaks during surgery. One way is to place a brightly colored dye in the stomach pouch. If you have a leak, the dye will leave your gastrointestinal tract, and the surgeon will be able to see it and fix it. Your chances of leaks from surgery are lower with laparoscopic than open procedures.[9]

After surgery, you can get tested for a leak using a fluorescent dye that can be seen using x-ray equipment.[10] Dehiscence, or splitting of the staple lines, is a common cause of post-surgery leaks. You can reduce your risk by choosing a skilled surgeon and by taking your recovery seriously. Later chapters discuss the post-operative diet and how to recover from surgery.

Leaks are serious complications, and you should tell your surgeon if you think you may have one. You might have stomach pain, bloating, low blood pressure, or frequent urination.[11] A leak can lead to infections and peritonitis, or inflammation of the lining around your abdominal cavity. This occurs when the bacteria from your digestive tract leak into the abdominal cavity. Symptoms of peritonitis include nausea, vomiting, thirst, and fever.[12] You can get gangrene or go into shock if you do not get your leak treated. Another risk is an intraperitoneal adhesion, or the formation of thick scar tissue,[13] which can eventually cause your large intestine to be blocked or obstructed.

A stent may be enough to treat an acute leak or one that does not have symptoms.[14] A stent is a small tube that can be used in small spaces in your body.[15] It can be placed using an endoscope so you do not need another surgery. For a leak, the doctor might coat the stent with a medication and hope that your leak gets stopped up within 30 days.[16] If not, you will probably need another surgery. The exact procedure that your surgeon will recommend depends on whether your leak is toward the top of the stomach pouch (known as a "proximal leak") or nearer the bottom of your small intestine (a "distal leak").

Possible Complications

Strictures and Related Complications: A stricture is a narrowing, or con"strict"ion, of some part of your gastrointestinal tract, such as your stomach, small intestine, or large intestine (bowel). Strictures prevent food from passing through easily. Excessive vomiting is a main symptom. You will probably have trouble keeping your food down because it will get stuck at the location of your stricture. Strictures can appear shortly after surgery but are more likely to develop weeks or months after surgery. They can usually be treated with endoscopy but sometimes require surgery.

Small Bowel Obstruction and Hernia: Small bowel obstructions are strictures that are usually caused by internal hernias. A hernia occurs when an organ pokes through into a space where it does not belong. The part of the RYGB procedure where the surgeon creates the roux limb can trigger hernias that obstruct the bowel. Between one and 10% of RYGB patients develop hernias or bowel obstruction.[17,18,19] Laparoscopic RYGB and more rapid weight loss increase your risk for hernias. Symptoms can include nausea, vomiting, lower abdominal pain, and bloating. Small bowel obstruction is difficult to diagnose, and you may need laparoscopic surgery to diagnose and treat one.

Gastrojejunostomy Anastomotic Strictures: A stricture can be toward the lower end of the stomach pouch, near where it attaches to the jejunum of the small intestine. This is called a gastrojejunostomy anastomotic stricture, and it occurs in 2.9 to 23% of RYGB patients.[20] Like the other complications of RYGB, your personal risk varies depending on factors such as your surgeon's experience and your own individual characteristics, including starting weight, age, and compliance with the RYGB diet. You need to get strictures treated if you are vomiting to avoid dehydration and malnutrition.

Roux-en-O Loop: In Roux-en-Y gastric bypass, the Y symbolizes the shape formed by your surgeon. One of the upper two limbs is the roux limb, or connection from the small stomach pouch to the mid or lower part of the small intestine; the other upper limb of the Y is the dead-end portion of your stomach that is no longer used. The bottom part of the Y is your lower small bowel. A roux-en-O loop is a rare complication, but it can be devastating. It occurs if the roux limb accidentally cuts off the other upper limb of the Y.

Dumping Syndrome: Dumping syndrome is a mixed blessing for RYGB patients. It feels like a curse when you get it because you feel so sick. However, it can help you lose weight because it forces you to limit your food intake. About three-quarters of RYGB patients develop dumping syndrome at least once,[21] and 12% of RYGB patients get severe dumping syndrome.[22] Most patients learn how to avoid dumping syndrome over time, and often it gets less severe on its own. That does not mean you should eat the foods that cause it, though! If you do, you will end up eating more sugar, fat, and calories than you need, and your weight loss will slow down.

Reason for Dumping Syndrome after Gastric Bypass

You can get symptoms of dumping syndrome when food from your stomach empties too quickly into your small intestine, which is common after RYGB. Compared to before gastric bypass, food not only passes more quickly from the stomach into the small intestine, but food also bypasses the majority of the small intestine, which is where a lot of digestion and absorption previously occurred. So food can be largely undigested when it gets to your small intestine.

- Undigested food leads to a higher-than-normal amount of sugar in the small intestine. To compensate, water is pulled in, and you get diarrhea and other symptoms.
- Undigested food leads to changes in your levels of gastrointestinal hormones and insulin.

Symptoms of Dumping Syndrome[23]

Early symptoms of dumping syndrome occur during or just after a meal. These include:

- Nausea
- Vomiting
- Diarrhea
- Cramps
- Feeling unexpectedly full
- Rapid heart rate
- Faintness, shakiness, or lightheadedness

Late symptoms occur one to three hours after you eat. It can include:

- Sweating
- Faintness, shakiness, or lightheadedness
- Hunger
- Confusion

Lower Your Risk of Dumping Syndrome

Following your RYGB diet carefully reduces your risk of experiencing dumping syndrome. Keep your portion and meal sizes in check; do not drink fluids when you eat solid foods or just before or after meal times, and use the following guidelines when choosing your foods:

- Limit high-fat, high-sugar foods such as the following:
  - Sweetened foods, such as pastries, desserts, candies, sweetened cereals, ice cream, dried fruit, and sweetened canned fruit
  - Sugary beverages, such as sugar-sweetened teas, coffees, sports and energy drinks, fruit drinks and juices, chocolate milk, and lemonade

- Avoid very hot and very cold foods
- Limit sugars, such as white sugar, brown sugar, molasses, honey, and corn syrup
- Read food package labels
  - Choose low-fat and fat-free foods when possible.
  - Choose foods with no more than five grams of sugars per serving.

Sugar substitutes are usually okay. They include:

- Sucralose (yellow packet; Splenda)
- Stevia (green packet; Truvia)
- Saccharine (pink packet; Sweet n Low, Sugar Twin)
- Aspartame (blue packet; Equal and Nutra-Sweet)
- Sugar alcohols, such as maltitol, xylitol, and sorbitol (although excess consumption can have a laxative effect unrelated to dumping syndrome)

Nutritional Deficiencies

Nutritional deficiencies and the supplements you will need after RYGB will be discussed in detail in later chapters. You should at least be aware of them now, though, as you continue to weigh the benefits and risks of RYGB. An adequate diet is not just about protein, as you will learn. The vast majority of RYGB patients experience deficiencies of at least one vitamin or mineral.[24]

Gastric bypass is more likely to cause nutritional deficiencies than lap-band or gastric sleeve surgery because it interferes more with your nutrient absorption.[25] You are also at risk for deficiencies because of low food intake on your rapid weight loss diet. To prevent deficiencies, you will need to focus on getting key nutrients, and your dietitian or surgeon may recommend supplements.

These are some of the vitamins and minerals that can be of concern after weight loss surgery.[26] Later we will go over the food sources and consequences of deficiency for each of these nutrients in more detail.

- *Vitamin B12*: Deficiency can lead to anemia and permanent neurological damage.
- *Calcium:* Deficiency can lead to osteoporosis, or low bone mineral density, and a high risk fractures.
- *Vitamin D:* Deficiency can lead to osteoporosis.
- *Beta-carotene (plant-based sources of vitamin A):* This is not likely to have deficiency symptoms but indicates a poor intake of fruits and vegetables.
- *Iron:* Deficiency can cause anemia and make you tired and weak.
- *Magnesium:* Deficiency can cause nausea and vomiting and harm your bones over the long term.
- *Folate:*[27] Deficiency can cause anemia and increase your risk for heart disease.

Other Possible Complications

Additional complications that can occur after RYGB include the following:[28]

- Excessive bleeding: Intra-abdominal bleeding can happen not only during surgery but even when your surgery is over. About 1.9 to 4% of Roux-en-Y gastric bypass patients have excessive bleeding, and many of those need a another surgery.[29] A subphrenic hematoma is a type of internal bleeding that occurs below the diaphragm.

- Gallstones (cholelithiasis): Gallstones, also known as cholelithiasis, are painful, hard plaques that can block up your gallbladder duct. You are likely to get gallstones when you lose weight quickly, such as after getting RYGB. Chapter 3 already described gallstones and their symptoms and discussed the possibility of getting your gallbladder removed during your initial RYGB surgery. About one-third of patients develop gallstones within a few months. Most of them resolve themselves, so you can just wait them out.[30] If they do not go away on their own, your surgeon may need to do another surgery to remove them and/or remove your gallbladder.

- Gastric fistula: This is a hole or opening between your stomach and your abdominal wall that allows your stomach contents to leak out. It occurs in as many of 6% of RYGB patients, with laparoscopic patients at greater risk.[31] Symptoms can include pain, vomiting, poor weight loss, and hemorrhage, and you may need laparoscopic or open surgery o resolve a fistula.

- Marginal ulceration: An ulcer develops in between one and 16% of RYGB patients.[32] The main symptom is severe pain, and nausea and vomiting can also occur. Proton pump inhibitor medication prescribed by your doctor can usually help.

- Conversion to open surgery: Your surgeon may convert your laparoscopic procedure to an open one if something unexpected happens during surgery. Possible reasons include a minor injury or an inability to manipulate the laparoscopic instruments as needed to complete the RYGB. About 2%[33] to 3%[34] of laparoscopic RYGB surgeries are converted to open.

Many complications of RYGB require medical attention. Call your physician or surgeon if you have any of the following:

- Nausea that prevents you from drinking fluids for more than 12 hours
- Vomiting that lasts for more than 12 hours
- Unexplained severe abdominal pain or cramping
- Inability to swallow food or a suspicion that the food is stuck in your digestive tract
- Fever
- Anything you are unsure about

In addition to keeping your surgeon's and physician's numbers on hand, find out the phone number you should call after hours and on weekends.

- Food intolerances: Food intolerances occur when you do not digest your food very well or they are distasteful to you. Foods that you do not tolerate can cause unpleasant symptoms like diarrhea, bloating, and stomach pain after you eat. You might develop one or more food intolerances after RYGB because of minor changes to your digestive system. Dairy products[35] and protein foods, especially red meat,[36] are commonly not tolerated well after RYGB, especially in the first year. Fruits and vegetables, which are high-fiber, can also be troublesome. Your risk of intolerance decreases if you have a comprehensive aftercare program and follow your diet very carefully. If you develop intolerances, you may eventually be able to overcome them by taking smaller portions and chewing your food slowly.

- General gastrointestinal symptoms: Almost all RYGB patients get them at some point, but their frequency and severity decrease if you stick to your diet. Symptoms include the following:
  - Abdominal pain and cramping
  - Vomiting
  - Nausea
  - Diarrhea

You can lower your risk for many of the above complications by being especially careful to follow your gastric bypass diet. Only eat the allowed foods instead of high-sugar or high-fat foods, and stick to small portions so you do not stretch your pouch or cause nausea, heartburn, or pain. You are at higher risk for developing complications if before the surgery you already have certain conditions, such as type 2 diabetes, GERD, or sleep apnea. However, do not let that fact alone persuade you not to get surgery, since these conditions likely appeared in the first place because of your obesity.

The Need for Another Surgical Procedure

About 12% of gastric bypass patients, or one in eight, need some type of second surgery.[37] This may be to treat a complication, such as some of those described above. Another reason for a second surgery is if your weight loss is not satisfactory even though you are following the RYGB diet. A second surgery might make a stretched stomach pouch smaller, convert a short-limb RYGB to a long-limb RYGB, or put an adjustable gastric band over your stomach pouch in a "band-over-bypass" procedure. About 2% of RYGB patients end up converting their surgeries to a different procedure.[38]

Reducing Your Risk of Complicaions

You can reduce your risk of developing complications from the RYGB:

- Choose a good surgeon.

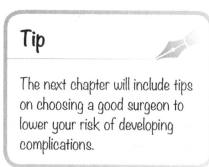

Tip

The next chapter will include tips on choosing a good surgeon to lower your risk of developing complications.

- Follow pre-surgery and post-surgery instructions from your surgeon and other members of your healthcare team.
- Do not cheat on your diet or recovery program.

Your risk of developing complications does not just depend on your own post-surgery behavior.[39] Your risk is also affected by things you cannot control. Your pre-surgery BMI and pre-surgery obesity-related diseases, or comorbidities, such as type 2 diabetes, sleep apnea, gastroesophageal reflux, and high cholesterol, raise your risk of complications.[40]

How Does Roux-en-Y Gastric Bypass Compare to Your Other Weight Loss Options?

Comparing RYGB to other weight loss options can help you decide whether to get the gastric bypass. As discussed in Chapter 1, your alternatives include:

- Doing nothing
- Dieting, exercising, or both
- Using weight loss drugs, probably in combination with a diet
- Choosing a different kind of weight loss surgery, such as the adjustable gastric band (lap-band), vertical sleeve gastrectomy, or complete biliopancreatic diversion with duodenal switch (BPD-DS)

Alternative Weight Loss Approach	Benefits of the Alternative Approach	Benefits of the Sleeve
Doing Nothing *Doing nothing gets you... nothing.*	• Do not have to pay for surgery • Easy • No risk of complications • Keep your natural stomach	• Can help you lose weight • Save money on obesity-related medical costs • Much greater chance of treating your obesity than doing nothing
Dieting, Exercising, or Both *It did not work before; will it work now?*	• Look and feel better • Will see health benefits if you follow a healthy diet and exercise regularly • No risk of surgery-related complications or side effects • Do not have to pay for surgery • Some people do lose weight and keep it off by committing to a healthy lifestyle.	• More likely to keep the weight off long term • Will see health benefits if you follow a healthy diet and exercise regularly • May save money by not purchasing expensive diet plans and foods • Diets and exercise have not worked for you in the past.

Alternative Weight Loss Approach	Benefits of the Alternative Approach	Benefits of the Sleeve
Weight Loss Drugs *There is no evidence to show that they are a long-term solution.*	• Everyone wants to take a pill to solve their problems because it seems like an easy solution! • Can help you lose a few pounds, which can be enough weight loss to improve your blood sugar control, blood pressure, and cholesterol levels.[41] • Need to follow a low-fat diet, which can be healthy. • Easy and convenient to take • Can take over-the-counter or prescription weight loss drugs • Do not need extensive planning and preparation	• Lower risk of fatty diarrhea and other side effects, such as nausea, vomiting, and dizziness with a careful diet • Will not damage your liver • A permanent change to your body and possible long-term obesity solution, while weight loss drugs are only for a few months or a year • Extensive pre- and post-surgery support from your surgeon and medical team if you choose them well • Can lose about 12 BMI points within a year—much higher than with weight loss drugs[42]
Alternative Weight Loss Surgeries *Each has its pros and cons.*	• The adjustable gastric band (lap-band) is fully reversible. • The lap-band can be adjusted for when your needs change, such as during illness or pregnancy. • The lap-band and vertical sleeve gastrectomy (VSG) are less likely to cause nutritional deficiencies. • Developed specifically to make weight loss surgery safer for super obesity for very high BMIs • The lap-band, gastric bypass, and biliopancreatic diversion with duodenal switch (BPD-DS) have been more extensively studied for a longer time. • Gastric sleeve reduces hunger by removing your stomach, which is a main source of a hunger hormone called ghrelin.	• The Roux-en-Y gastric bypass helps you lose weight through malabsorption, not just restriction. • Is a good middle ground between the lap-band and gastric bypass with complications[43] • Has the biggest benefits for high blood sugar levels • More weight loss expected within the first year than the lap-band or gastric sleeve, which has an average loss of 7 BMI points.[44, 45,46, 47] • High risk of dumping syndrome, making it a potentially good solution for obese individuals with a sweet tooth • Extensively studied surgery with a long history

Table 12: Comparing RYGB to other weight loss options

From *Table* 12, you can see that you do not have many choices. Doing nothing is not an option if you are not happy with where you are now. If diet and exercise attempts have failed for you in the past—probably numerous times—there is no reason to think they will work for you in the future unless you or something in your life changes. Weight loss drugs are almost laughable at this point because they only help you lose a few pounds, and you cannot take them for long. Bariatric surgery has helped thousands of patients lose weight and keep it off, and 200,000 weight loss surgeries were performed in the U.S. in 2007.[48]

✍ Summary

☞ This chapter was intended to help you continue to form a complete picture of RYGB. After reading this chapter and the previous one, you are aware of the potential benefits and risks of this surgery. Now you can think logically about whether the Roux-en-Y gastric bypass sounds like something you want to use in order to treat your obesity.

☞ The next chapter goes over some of the personal considerations of the RYGB, such as whether you are eligible. By the end of that chapter, you will be about ready to make your decision.

Time to Take Action: Are the Risks Worth Taking?

This chapter described some of the risks of the RYGB and side effects that can happen after the surgery. For some people, the risks are not worth the benefits. For others, the chance of having complications is small compared to the potential benefits for your weight loss and health.

Where do you stand? Do you feel that the benefits outweigh the risks?

....

....

....

What do you intend to accomplish by getting the Roux-en-Y gastric bypass? In addition to weight loss, you might, for example, answer that you intend to gain control of your eating and make healthy choices.

....

....

....

What are the biggest problems in your life? For each, what role, if any, do you see RYGB playing in solving them? Follow the examples as you add your own.

- Obesity: The RYGB can be a tool to help me lose weight.

- Low self-esteem: Now I feel ashamed to go out with my family. The gastric bypass can help me lose weight so I can go out with my family and keep up with my friends instead of saying no to their invitations.

- Anxiety: That I will not be there for my family. Losing weight after surgery can help me be healthier and not have diabetes.

- *Add your own*

....

....

....

....

....

....

....

1   Lee J. Vertical sleeve gastrectomy. Healthline Web site. http://www.healthline.com/adamcontent/vertical-sleeve-gastrectomy. Updated 2009, November 4. Accessed September 3, 2012.

2   Bhimji S, Zieve D. General anesthesia. Medline Plus Web site. http://www.nlm.nih.gov/medlineplus/ency/article/007410.htm. Updated 2011, January 26. Accessed September 3, 2012.

3   Griffith PS, Birch DW, Sharma AM, Karmali S. Managing complications associated with laparoscopic Roux-en-Y gastric bypass for morbid obesity. Can J Surg. 2012 Oct;55(5):329-36.

4   Gagnon L, Sheff Karwacki EJ. Outcomes and complications after bariatric surgery. AJN. 2012;112(9):26-36.

5   Hutter MM, Schimer BD, Jones DB, Ko CY, Cohen ME, Merkow RP, Nguyen NT. First report from the American College of Surgeons – Bariatric Surgery Center Network laparoscopic sleeve gastrectomy has morbidity and effectiveness positioned between the band and the bypass. Ann Surg. 2012;254(3):410-422.

6   Omalu BI, et al. Death rates and causes of death after bariatric surgery for Pennsylvania residents, 1995 to 2004. Arch Surg, 2007;142(10):923-928.

7   Yu J, Turner MA, Cho SR, Fulcher AS, DeMaria E, Kellum J, Sugerman H. Normal anatomy and complications after gastric bypass surgery: helical CT findings. Radiology, 2004;231:753-760.

8   Griffith PS, Birch DW, Sharma AM, Karmali S. Managing complications associated with laparoscopic Roux-en-Y gastric bypass for morbid obesity. Can J Surg. 2012 Oct;55(5):329-36.

9   Griffith PS, Birch DW, Sharma AM, Karmali S. Managing complications associated with laparoscopic Roux-en-Y gastric bypass for morbid obesity. Can J Surg. 2012 Oct;55(5):329-36.

10 Griffith PS, Birch DW, Sharma AM, Karmali S. Managing complications associated with laparoscopic Roux-en-Y gastric bypass for morbid obesity. Can J Surg. 2012 Oct;55(5):329-36.

11 Gagnon L, Sheff Karwacki EJ. Outcomes and complications after bariatric surgery. AJN. 2012;112(9):26-36.

12 Heller JL, Zieve D. Peritonitis – secondary. Web site. http://www.nlm.nih.gov/medlineplus/ency/article/000651.htm. Updated 2010, June 28. Accessed September 7, 2012.

13 Vorvick L, Storck S, Zieve, D. Adhesion. http://www.nlm.nih.gov/medlineplus/ency/article/001493.htm. Updated 2012, February 26. Accessed September 7, 2012.

14 Rosenthal RJ, International Sleeve Gastrectomy Expert Panel. International Sleeve Gastrectomy Expert Panel Consensus Statement: Best practice guidelines based on experience of ⃞ 12,000 cases. Surgery for Obesity and Related Diseases, 2012;8(1):8-19.

15 National Heart Lung and Blood Institute. What is a stent? Web site. http://www.nhlbi.nih.gov/health/health-topics/topics/stents/. 2011, November 8. Accessed September 7, 2012.

16 Rosenthal RJ, International Sleeve Gastrectomy Expert Panel. International Sleeve Gastrectomy Expert Panel Consensus Statement: Best practice guidelines based on experience of ⃞ 12,000 cases. Surgery for Obesity and Related Diseases, 2012;8(1):8-19.

17 Griffith PS, Birch DW, Sharma AM, Karmali S. Managing complications associated with laparoscopic Roux-en-Y gastric bypass for morbid obesity. Can J Surg. 2012 Oct;55(5):329-36.

18 Yu J, Turner MA, Cho SR, Fulcher AS, DeMaria E, Kellum J, Sugerman H. Normal anatomy and complications after gastric bypass surgery: helical CT findings. Radiology, 2004;231:753-760.

19 Yu J, Turner MA, Cho SR, Fulcher AS, DeMaria E, Kellum J, Sugerman H. Normal anatomy and complications after gastric bypass surgery: helical CT findings. Radiology, 2004;231:753-760.

20 Griffith PS, Birch DW, Sharma AM, Karmali S. Managing complications associated with laparoscopic Roux-en-Y gastric bypass for morbid obesity. Can J Surg. 2012 Oct;55(5):329-36.

21 Mechanick MD, Kushner RF…Dixon J. American Association of Clinical Endocrinologists, The Obesity Society, and American Society for Metabolic & Bariatric Surgery medical guidelines for clinical practice for the perioperative nutritional, metabolic, and nonsurgical support of the bariatric surgery patient. Obesity, 2009;17(S1):S3-72.

22 Laurenius A, Olbers T, Näslund I, Karlsson J. Dumping syndrome following gastric bypass: validation of the Dumping Symptom Rating Scale. Obes Surg. 2013.

23 Zieve D, Rogers A. Dumping syndrome. Medline Plus. Web site. http://www.nlm.nih.gov/medlineplus/ency/imagepages/19830.htm. Updated 2012, June 4. Accessed September 9, 2012.

24 Gagnon L, Sheff Karwacki EJ. Outcomes and complications after bariatric surgery. AJN. 2012;112(9):26-36.

25 Xanthakos SA. Nutritional deficiencies in obesity and after bariatric surgery. Pediatr Clin North Am, 2009;56(5):1105-1121.

26 Gagnon L, Sheff Karwacki EJ. Outcomes and complications after bariatric surgery. AJN. 2012;112(9):26-36.

27 Aarts EO, Janssen, IM, Berends, FJ. The gastric sleeve: losing weight as fast as micronutrients? Obes Surg. 2011;21(2):207-211.

28 Gagnon L, Sheff Karwacki EJ. Outcomes and complications after bariatric surgery. AJN. 2012;112(9):26-36.

29 Griffith PS, Birch DW, Sharma AM, Karmali S. Managing complications associated with laparoscopic Roux-en-Y gastric bypass for morbid obesity. Can J Surg. 2012 Oct;55(5):329-36.

30 Gagnon L, Sheff Karwacki EJ. Outcomes and complications after bariatric surgery. AJN. 2012;112(9):26-36.

31 Griffith PS, Birch DW, Sharma AM, Karmali S. Managing complications associated with laparoscopic Roux-en-Y gastric bypass for morbid obesity. Can J Surg. 2012 Oct;55(5):329-36.

32 Griffith PS, Birch DW, Sharma AM, Karmali S. Managing complications associated with laparoscopic Roux-en-Y gastric bypass for morbid obesity. Can J Surg. 2012 Oct;55(5):329-36.

33 Shin JH, Worni M, Castleberry AW, Pietrobon R, Omotosho PA, Silberberg M, Ostbye T. The application of comorbidity indices to predict early postoperative outcomes after laparoscopic Roux-en-Y gastric bypass: a nationwide comparative analysis of over 70,000 cases. Obes Surg, 2013;23(5):638-49. doi: 10.1007/s11695-012-0853-3

34 Gonzalez Valverde FM, Cifuentes AS, Marin MR, Rodriguez MT, Moncada JR, Marin-Blazquez AA. Frequency and causes of conversion from laparoscopic to open Roux-en-Y gastric bypass for morbid obesity: the experience in our service. Obes Surg, 2013;23(3):391-2. doi: 10.1007/s11695-012-0837-3.

35 Xanthakos SA. Nutritional deficiencies in obesity and after bariatric surgery. Pediatr Clin North Am, 2009;56(5):1105-1121.

36 Aills L, Blankenship J, Buffington C, Furtado M, Parrott, J. ASMBS Integrated health nutritional guidelines for the surgical weight loss patient. Surgery for Obesity and Related Diseases, 2008;S73-S108.

37 Leitman IM, Virk CS, Avgerinos DV, Patel R, Lavarias V, Surick B, Holup JL, Goodman ER, Karpeh MS Jr. Early results of trans-oral endoscopic plication and revision of the gastric pouch and stoma following Roux-en-Y Gastric Bypass Surgery. JSLS. 2010 Apr-Jun; 14(2): 217–220.

38 Edholm D, Svensson F, Naslund I, Karlsson FA, Rask E, Sundborn M. Long-term results 11 years after the primary gastric bypass in 384 patients. Surg Obes Related Dis. 2012.

39 Kaplan LM, Seeley RJ, Harris JL. Myths associated with obesity and bariatric surgery – myth 5: patient behavior is the primary determinant of outcomes after bariatric surgery. 2012;9(8):8-10.

40 Gagnon L, Sheff Karwacki EJ. Outcomes and complications after bariatric surgery. AJN. 2012;112(9):26-36.

41 Mayo Clinic Staff. Prescription weight loss drugs: can they help you? Web site. http://www.mayoclinic.com/health/weight-loss-drugs/WT00013/METHOD=print Updated 2012, July 27. Accessed September 15, 2012.

42 Hutter MM, Schirmer BD, Jones DB, Ko CY, Cohen ME, Merdow RP, Nguyen NT. First report from the American College of Surgeons Bariatric Surgery Center Network: laparoscopic sleeve gastrectomy has morbidity and effectiveness positioned between the band and the bypass. Annals of Surgery. 2011;254:410-420.

43 Jackson TD, Hutter MM. Morbidity and effectiveness of laparoscopic sleeve gastrectomy, adjustable gastric band and gastric bypass for morbid obesity. Advances in Surgery, 2012;46:255-68.

44 Jackson TD, Hutter MM. Morbidity and effectiveness of laparoscopic sleeve gastrectomy, adjustable gastric band and gastric bypass for morbid obesity. Advances in Surgery, 2012;46:255-68.

45 Jackson TD, Hutter MM. Morbidity and effectiveness of laparoscopic sleeve gastrectomy, adjustable gastric band and gastric bypass for morbid obesity. Advances in Surgery, 2012;46:255-68.

46 Hutter MM, Schirmer BD, Jones DB, Ko CY, Cohen ME, Merdow RP, Nguyen NT. First report from the American College of Surgeons Bariatric Surgery Center Network: laparoscopic sleeve gastrectomy has morbidity and effectiveness positioned between the band and the bypass. Annals of Surgery. 2011;254:410-420.

47 Jackson TD, Hutter MM. Morbidity and effectiveness of laparoscopic sleeve gastrectomy, adjustable gastric band and gastric bypass for morbid obesity. Advances in Surgery, 2012;46:255-68.

48 Gagnon L, Sheff Karwacki EJ. Outcomes and complications after bariatric surgery. AJN. 2012;112(9):26-36.

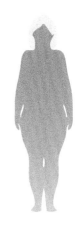

6

Considering Roux-En-Y Gastric Bypass? ....What You Need To Know

Chapters 4 and 5 introduced the pros and cons of Roux-en-Y gastric bypass. Before surgery, you should weigh its potential benefits, such as substantial weight loss and better health, against risks ranging from mild side effects to more dangerous complications.

Next to consider is whether you are a good fit for RYGB. Not everyone that is obese is eligible to get the gastric bypass surgery, and not everyone that is technically eligible *should* get the surgery. This chapter helps you figure out whether RYGB really is the right choice for you. This is what you will find in the following pages:

- Criteria for getting Roux-en-Y gastric bypass
- Conditions (known as contraindications) that may prevent you from getting RYGB
- Pregnancy and gastric bypass
- Getting bypass as a revisional surgery
- Special considerations for adolescents considering RYGB

By the end of this chapter, you will be ready to review again whether RYGB is for you.

Eligibility Criteria for Roux-En-Y Gastric Bypass

You need to meet certain requirements, known as eligibility criteria, before you can get Roux-en-Y gastric bypass. This section will cover the eligibility criteria as well as the contraindications, or potential reasons that would prevent you from being a good candidate even if you meet the other criteria.

Eligibility Criteria

The first requirement to get Roux-en-Y gastric bypass is that you have a lot of weight to lose. Chapter 1 explains BMI and can help you find yours.

- BMI over 40: To give you an example, a BMI of 40 is a weight of 233 pounds for someone that is 5 feet, 4 inches tall or 278 pounds for someone that is 5 feet, 10 inches tall.
- At least 100 pounds over a recommended BMI of 25: That is 245 pounds for someone that is 5 feet, 4 inches tall and 275 pounds for someone that is 5 feet, 10 inches tall.
- BMI over 35 with an obesity-related comorbidity, such as type 2 diabetes, high cholesterol, or osteoarthritis: That is a weight of 204 pounds for someone that is 5 feet, 4 inches tall and 244 pounds for someone that is 5 feet, 10 inches tall.

In addition to meeting one of the above weight criteria, you will probably need to meet these standard requirements:

- You have a history of failed diet attempts. You might have lost and regained the same weight or failed to lose significant amounts of weight while making serious diet attempts.
- Your obesity is not caused by a metabolic disorder, such as hypothyroidism

- You are between 18 and 60 years old[1]
- You understand that you play a major role in your own weight loss after getting the gastric bypass
- You are willing to attend post-surgery care appointments and support group sessions

These criteria may differ between surgeons. For example, some surgeons may be willing to perform the surgery if your BMI is between 30 and 35 and you have a serious comorbidity related to your obesity. Other surgeons might accept older adults or adolescents under age 18. Meeting additional eligibility criteria, such as following a six-month pre-surgery diet, may be necessary to get insurance reimbursement.

Contraindications

Contraindications prevent you from being a good candidate for Roux-en-Y gastric bypass. They may be health conditions that make the surgical procedure dangerous or that make you less likely to succeed with RYGB. These are some examples of contraindications:[2]

- *Advanced congestive heart failure*: It puts you at very high risk during surgery.
- *Substance abuse*: Surgeons argue that if you cannot get over your alcohol or drug addictions, you might not have the mental strength to stick to the RYGB diet.
- *Untreated depression or other psychological disorders*: Adapting the RYGB lifestyle requires mental strength. Struggling with mental health issues while you should be focusing on your new healthy lifestyle can make your mental condition worse or prevent successful weight loss.
- *A compromised immune system*: If you have an infectious disease or weak immune system, you are more susceptible to surgery infections. They can become serious and even lead to organ failure.
- *A very low pain tolerance*: You will be in pain as your surgical wounds heal after surgery. If you know that you are not as good at dealing with pain as some people, you might want to consider another option for weight loss.

Not all health conditions are automatically contraindications. Even though they may increase some of your risks with the gastric bypass, they are not considered to be contraindications, because the benefits of losing significant amounts of weight with RYGB may outweigh their risks. These are some examples:

- Patients at high risk for obesity-related health complications, such as type 2 diabetes
- Individuals with coronary heart disease that is likely to be improved with significant weight loss
- Individuals with cirrhosis or fatty liver disease[3]
- Lack of understanding about RYGB. Continue to do your research on the RYGB until you feel confident that you know enough about the procedure to make the right decision for yourself.

Who Gets RYGB?

108,000 patients got RYGB in 2003, or more than one in 3,000 Americans. Here is a snapshot of who they were:

- 84% were female.

- 82% were between 25 and 54 years old at the time of surgery.

- Before surgery, 44% of patients had high blood pressure, 33% had joint pain, and 10 to 28% had esophageal reflux (GERD), diabetes, and/or respiratory conditions such as asthma and sleep apnea.

- Patients were equally likely to be from the Northeast, Midwest, South, and West.

Source:[4]

Gastric Bypass and Pregnancy

Obesity is one of the most common causes of infertility in the U.S. Losing a significant amount of extra body fat can help you conceive a child. If you are a woman, having a healthy body weight during pregnancy can make your pregnancy easier and less risky for you.[5] Your child can benefit too. When you are at a healthy weight during pregnancy, your baby is less likely to be:

- Low birth weight
- Premature
- Prone to diabetes
- Overweight or obese as a child or adult

If you are hoping to become a parent, be sure to discuss pregnancy with your primary care physician and surgeon as you decide whether to get the gastric bypass. In general, you should wait at least 12 to 18 months following your surgery before getting pregnant.[6] You will need to consider the following factors as you plan your pregnancy:[7]

- Your focus after RYGB should be on weight loss. This means that you are restricting calories and do not have enough energy to support a healthy baby.

- The RYGB puts you at some risk for nutrient deficiencies, including folate deficiency. It is best to wait until your nutrients are under control before getting pregnant to reduce the risk of having a baby with a neural tube birth defect due to your low levels of folate.

- Iron, vitamin B12, and calcium are additional nutrients required for a healthy baby but whose levels can be low after surgery.

- Gastric bypass restricts the amount of food you can eat, but you need to get enough nutrients to support a growing fetus. You may need supplements, such as protein shakes.

Roux-en-Y Gastric Bypass as a Revisional Surgery

For most RYGB patients, the RYGB is an original surgery. For others, RYGB is a revisional surgery; that is, it is a second bariatric procedure performed to convert the original bariatric surgery into RYGB. These are the main reasons why you might choose to get RYGB as a second bariatric procedure:[8]

- Unsatisfactory weight loss after the first bariatric surgery even though you followed the diet
- Serious complications from the first bariatric surgery
- Severe nutritional deficiencies that you cannot overcome without another surgery

Types of Conversions to Roux-en-Y Gastric Bypass

These are some of the more common situations for considering a revisional RYGB surgery.

Short-Limb to Long-Limb RYGB

In Roux-en-Y gastric bypass, your small stomach pouch is attached to your small intestine. With a short-limbed RYGB, the pouch is attached higher up on the small intestine than with a long-limbed RYGB. In both procedures, food that you eat goes into your small stomach pouch and then to the small intestine, therefore skipping most of your original large stomach and at least part of the upper part of your small intestine. After short-limbed RYGB, less of your small intestine is bypassed, so food gets better digested and absorbed than after long-limbed RYGB, when food bypasses a larger portion of your small intestine. As discussed in Chapter 3, long-limbed RYGB typically leads to decreased nutrient absorption and faster weight loss than after short-limbed RYGB. Your surgeon might recommend conversion to a long-limbed RYGB if your weight loss is not satisfactory after short-limbed.

RYGB after Stomach Pouch Stretching

Gastric bypass helps you lose weight because of the small stomach pouch. If the stomach pouch stretches, you will not feel as much restriction. Compared to immediately after surgery, when your stomach pouch was tiny, filling up your stomach pouch will take longer. Some surgeons will recommend a second RYGB to give you a smaller pouch again.

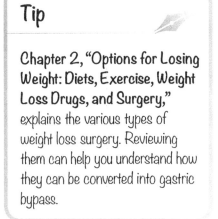

Tip

Chapter 2, "Options for Losing Weight: Diets, Exercise, Weight Loss Drugs, and Surgery," explains the various types of weight loss surgery. Reviewing them can help you understand how they can be converted into gastric bypass.

RYGB as a Conversion from the Gastric Band

Some patients consider RYGB if they are unhappy with results from the adjustable gastric band, whose brand names include Lap-Band and Realize Band. The band is fully reversible; your surgeon just needs to take it out and make sure your stomach and throat are fully healed before proceeding with your RYGB.

Why might you consider gastric bypass after the band? The band might not be the right tool to meet your weight loss goals. Some patients report that they never feel any restriction with the gastric band, so it does not help them with their weight loss. Another reason is that the band is only restrictive. The gastric bypass is not only restrictive but also malabsorptive, so you absorb fewer nutrients and lose weight faster. In addition, RYGB can cause dumping syndrome when you eat high-fat, high-sugar foods. The gastric bypass can be better at motivating you to avoid these high-calorie foods than the gastric band.

Another reason why some patients choose to remove the band and get the bypass is that some foods can cause complications. The gastric band can prevent you from eating these foods:[9]

- Stringy foods like broccoli, pineapple, and asparagus can get stuck in the band.
- Doughy bread and sticky foods, such as dried fruit and peanut butter, can cause obstructions.
- Seeds, nuts, and popcorn can get stuck in the band.

Considerations Surrounding RYGB as a Revisional Surgery

A revisional Roux-en-Y gastric bypass can be successful.[10] However, if you are getting RYGB as a conversion from another type of surgery, your weight loss is likely to be less than getting RYGB as a primary procedure.[11] Second surgeries also have higher complication rates than first surgeries.

A critical factor to consider when you are thinking about RYGB as a revisional surgery is why your first bariatric surgery did not work for you. RYGB will *not* help you lose weight if you do not follow the RYGB diet. If your first bariatric surgery failed because you did not follow the prescribed diet, you are not going to lose weight with RYGB unless you start to follow the proper diet. If you developed complications with your adjustable gastric band or first gastric bypass because you did not follow the proper post-surgery eating patterns, you are likely to face the same troubles after the revisional RYGB unless you have a new dedication.

For the RYGB to be a successful weight loss tool, you must be committed to the required diet for the long term.

What about RYGB and Adolescents?

Adolescent obesity is just as big of a public health concern as obesity among adults. Adolescent obesity rates are increasing at a frightening rate, and more than one-third of children and adolescents are overweight or obese.[12] Four percent of children and adolescents, or one out of 25, has extreme obesity.[13] These children and adolescents are more likely to become obese adults. And just like adults, many of them are already suffering the consequences of their excess weight. These include the following:

- High cholesterol and other risk factors for heart disease
- Type 2 diabetes or poorly controlled blood sugar

- Osteoarthritis
- Sleep apnea
- Higher risk for some kinds of cancer later in life
- Social stigma
- Low self-esteem
- Poorer performance in school

Eligibility for Weight Loss Surgery in Adolescence: Weight Criteria

As with adults, weight loss surgery can be an effective treatment for adolescent obesity. However, the weight criteria for the surgery are different for adolescents than for adults.[14] That is to be extra careful to prevent adolescents from getting the surgery when they do not truly need it.

- A BMI over 50
- A BMI over 40 and a less serious comorbidity, or obesity-related condition, such as high blood pressure, depression, or high cholesterol
- A BMI over 35 and a serious comorbidity, such as sleep apnea, type 2 diabetes, increased pressure within the skull, or liver disease

Eligibility for Weight Loss Surgery in Adolescence: Maturity

Maturity is the greatest difference between adults and adolescents when considering medical treatments such as weight loss surgery. Insufficient physical and/or psychological maturity can make RYGB an ineffective or dangerous procedure. Surgeons are likely to ask these questions before recommending RYGB for teenagers:

- Has the teenager already tried regular diets while being supported by the family?
- Does the adolescent have enough family support? Most adolescents are still living at home and depending on their parents for food and emotional support. Adolescents are more likely to succeed after surgery if their families are willing to show their support and commit to the lifestyle required for weight loss with gastric bypass.
- How old is the adolescent and at what point in his or her physical development? Adolescents should not get the surgery if they are still early in their growth spurt.
- How psychologically mature is the adolescent? Adolescence, especially early and mid-adolescence, is a time of emotional turmoil for some. RYGB presents challenges that can be difficult even for the most stable adult to take in stride. Adolescents are more likely to be able to overcome those challenges when they are closer to adulthood than earlier on.
- Does the adolescent fully understand the procedure, its risks, and its permanence?
- Does the adolescent understand and accept his or her role and responsibility for success with Roux-en-Y gastric bypass?

Best Practice Guidelines: Opinions from the Forefront of the Field

Sometimes a group of medical experts come together to discuss a certain medical issue. In this case, experts from hospitals and university medical centers discussed bariatric surgery for adolescents. Their purpose was to come up with recommendations, known as best practice guidelines, based on the latest scientific research. The group of experts provided suggestions for:

- When weight loss surgery should be considered for adolescents.
- When it is not a good idea.
- The pros and cons of different procedures.
- Expected results.
- Special considerations for planning for and taking advantage of weight loss surgery at this age.

Basically, these experts did the research so you do not have to! This section of the chapter summarizes their recommendations for RYGB and adolescents.

RYGB in Adolescence: Further Consideration

About 1,000 adolescents 10 to 19 years old got weight loss surgery in 2009. Most were over 17 years old, and as with adults, the majority were female. Fifty-eight percent had an obesity-related comparability, such as type 2 diabetes.[15]

When done for the right reasons and under the right conditions, Roux-en-Y gastric bypass in adolescents can be successful. One study found an average weight loss of 37% of starting BMI after one year; for someone with a starting BMI of 50, that translates to a BMI of 32 one year after surgery.[16]

Another study followed patients for 5 to 10 years after surgery. Their surgery was at the age of 14 to 18 years old. By the end of 5 to 10 years patients had lost, on average, 78% of excess body weight. The average BMI dropped from 45 to 28.[17]

The risks are similar to those in adults, which are covered in Chapter 5.

Here are some best practice guidelines, or standard recommendations, for adolescents that choose to get the surgery. Considering each of these factors when planning the surgery gives you (or your adolescent, if you are a parent) the best chances of success:[18]

- If you are a parent, do not force your child into having the surgery. Adolescents that are forced into getting weight loss surgery are not likely to succeed.
- When possible, the procedure should be done in a bariatric hospital with healthcare team members that have special training in pediatrics or adolescent health.

- A healthcare team that works together is even more important for adolescents than adults. Team members should include a qualified surgeon, pediatrician, dietitian, mental health professional, and a team coordinator, who is often a nurse.

- Adolescents need to be especially careful to get enough iron, vitamin B12, and calcium to prevent deficiencies. Osteopenia, or poor bone mineral density related to inadequate calcium or vitamin D, and thiamine or vitamin B1 deficiency are also threats.

- Female adolescents should understand that they should not get pregnant within at least 18 months of having the surgery.

Weight loss surgery is a serious decision for anyone, and adolescents have even more things to think about. It is a very individual decision that should not be taken lightly. To succeed with gastric bypass, adolescents must be close to physical maturity, mentally and emotionally capable, and supported at home. Adolescents need to understand the long-term commitment necessary—not only to lose weight and keep it off but also to prevent complications for life.

A Brief Overview: Review of RYGB's Effects

With so much information over the last few chapters, you might be feeling a little confused. Picking out the parts that matter most to *you* when you are learning so much information for the first time can be difficult. *Table 13* summarizes some of the likely effects of RYGB.

Measure	Likely Effects of the Sleeve
Weight Loss	The Roux-en-Y gastric bypass can provide hope for long-term successful weight loss even if you have not been able to overcome your obesity with serious diet attempts. It can lead to a hundred or more pounds of weight loss, far more than with any current weight loss drugs.[19] The average first-year weight loss after RYGB is more than the lap-band and gastric sleeve.
Likely Side Effects	You will be in pain for at least a week after surgery. If you go off of the bypass diet, you can get diarrhea, vomiting, nausea, and cramping. These are comparable to the side effects from weight loss drugs, which can cause dizziness, sweating, nausea, dry mouth, diarrhea, and constipation. However, these weight loss drug effects are largely unavoidable. Other possibilities of side effects from RYGB are gallstones resulting from rapid weight loss and food intolerances.
Possible complications	As discussed in Chapter 5, any surgery can cause: • Death • Excessive bleeding • An embolism or blood clot Other complications with gastric bypass can include: • Stricture • Leakage • Dumping syndrome

Measure	Likely Effects of the Sleeve
Nutrition	Your current diet is supporting obesity and may still be making you gain weight. The diet likely has these characteristics:[20] • High in calories • High in saturated (unhealthy) fat and sugar • Low in nutrient-rich foods, such as fruits, vegetables, and whole grains The gastric bypass diet is more likely to have these characteristics:[21] • Calorie-controlled • Emphasis on lean protein • Low in sugar and saturated fat • Contains fruits and vegetables Gastric bypass puts you at nutritional risk because of the low amount of food you will be eating and the nutrient malabsorption, but you can lower your risk for nutrient deficiencies by choosing nutrient-dense foods and taking dietary supplements as recommended by your dietitian. Overdosing on supplements can also be harmful.
Health	Maybe your mother, father, sister, or brother had or has an obesity-related health condition, and maybe you have had your own scare. These are some common conditions that can be improved after gastric bypass and losing weight: • Type 2 diabetes • High cholesterol or blood pressure • Osteoarthritis and joint pain • Sleep apnea and asthma
Quality of Life	The bottom line is that your quality life is the most important reason to get the gastric bypass. There is no reason to undergo surgery and put in the effort needed for success if your life does not get better. Everyone is different, but these are some ways that your life could be affected: • Better self-esteem • Lower risk for depression • More social confidence • More mobility and stamina so you can participate in fun activities • Better ability to get pregnant and more likely to have a healthy pregnancy and baby

Table 13: Review of RYGB's Effects

Summary

☛ This chapter was an opportunity for gastric bypass to become more real to you. By now you have a good idea of whether you are eligible and a good candidate for the surgery. You have the information you need about whether to pursue the Roux-en-Y gastric bypass to treat your obesity.

☛ The next chapter will help you move forward if you think you are going to go for the surgery. You have a lot of planning to do, so let's get going!

Time to Take Action: Do You Meet the Requirements for Getting the RYGB?

Are you ready and able to take the first steps toward getting RYGB? *Table 14* is a quick checklist of some factors to consider when thinking about the surgery. For each consideration in the left column, highlight or circle the middle box or the right box depending on the accurate answer. Then take a look and see whether you think you are eligible for the surgery.

Consideration	Candidate for the Roux-en-Y Gastric Bypass	Possible Contraindication
Age	Over 18 years old	Under 18 years old
BMI		
	Over 40	Under 40 with no comorbidity
	35 to 40 with a comorbidity	Under 35
Other medical conditions	none	Heart or lung conditions; bleeding disorders
Pregnancy	No, and not planning to become pregnant within a year	Yes, or planning to soon
Readiness to commit	Yes, completely ready to commit to drastic, long-term dietary changes	No, not sure about commitment or ability to follow the necessary diet
Understand the process	Yes, recognize my role in weight loss	No, would prefer to depend on a weight loss treatment that will do everything for me
Average ability to tolerate pain	Yes, at least average pain tolerance	No, cannot imagine recovering from a surgery without high doses of pain medications for a long time
Alcohol or drug addictions	No, none	Yes, abuse alcohol or drugs
Mental conditions	No, none; or, I am under treatment, and they are well-controlled.	Yes, and they are severe and not always under control.

Table 14: Checklist of factors to consider when thinking about the sleeve

1   Gagnon L, Sheff Karwacki EJ. Outcomes and complications after bariatric surgery. AJN. 2012;112(9):26-36.

2   Gagnon L, Sheff Karwacki EJ. Outcomes and complications after bariatric surgery. AJN. 2012;112(9):26-36.

3   Barreto CJ, Sarr MG, Swain JM. Bariatric surgery in patients with liver cirrhosis and portal hypertension. Bariatric Times. 2009, July 14. http://bariatrictimes.com/bariatric-surgery-in-patients-with-liver-cirrhosis-and-portal-hypertension/ Accessed September 13, 2012.

4   Shinogle JA, Owings MF, Kozak LJ. Gastric bypass as a treatment for obesity: trends, characteristics and complications. Obesity Research, 2005;13(12):2202-2209.

5   National Heart, Lung and Blood Institute. High blood pressure in pregnancy. National Institutes of Health. Website. http://www.nhlbi.nih.gov/health/public/heart/hbp/hbp_preg.htm. Accessed September 13, 2012.

6   Ziegler O, Sirveaux MA, Brunaud L, Reibel N, Quillot D. Medical follow-up after bariatric surgery: nutritional and drug issues. General recommendations for the prevention and treatment of nutritional deficiencies. Diabetes Metab. 2009;35(6 Pt 2):544-547.

7   Delamont K. Clinical considerations and recommendations for pregnancy after bariatric surgery. Bariatric Times. 2011;8(10):12-14.

8   Nesset EM, Kendrick ML, Houghton SG et al. A two-decade spectrum of revisional bariatric surgery at a tertiary referral center. Surg Obes Relat Dis 2007; 3: 25–30

9   Bioenterics Corporation. (ND). Information for patients, a surgical aid in the treatment for morbid obesity: a decision guide for adults. Inamed. Accessed September 12 2012 from http://www.lapband.com/local/files/Surgical_Aid_Booklet.pdf.

10   Kelly JJ, Shikora S, Jones DB, Hutter M, Robinson MK, Romanelli J, Buckley F, Lederman A, Blackburn GL, Lautz D. Best practice updates for surgical care in weight loss surgery. Obesity, 2009;17(5):863-870.

11   Mor A, Keenan E, Portenier D, Torquati A. Case-matched analysis comparing outcomes of revisional versus primary laparoscopic Roux-en-Y gastric bypass. Surg Endoscop, 2012.

12   Centers for Disease Control and Prevention. Childhood obesity facts. Web site. http://www.cdc.gov/HealthyYouth/obesity/facts.htm. 2012, June 7. Accessed September 13, 2012.

13   Xanthakos SA. Bariatric surgery for extreme adolescent obesity: indications, outcomes and physiologic effects on the gut-brain axis. Pathophysiology. 2008;15(2):135-46.

14   Nagle A, Zieve D. Weight-loss surgery and children. Web site. http://www.nlm.nih.gov/medlineplus/ency/patientinstructions/000356.htm. Updated 2011, July 1. Accessed September 13, 2012.

15   Kelleher DC, Merrill CT, Cottrell LT, Nadler EP, Burd RS. Recent National Trends in the Use of Adolescent Inpatient Bariatric Surgery: 2000 Through 2009. Arch Pedatr Adolesc Med, 2012;17:1-7.

16   Inge TH, Jenkins TM, Zeller M, Dolan L, Daniels SR, Garcia VF et al. Baseline BMI is a strong predictor of nadir BMI after adolescent gastric bypass. J Pediatr, 2010;156(1):103-108.

17   Nijhawan S, Martinez T, Wittgrove AC. Laparoscopic gastric bypass for the adolescent patient: long-term results. Obes Surg, 2010;22(9):1445-9.

18   Pratt JSA, Lenders CM, Dionne EA, Hoppin AG, Hsu GLK., Inge, TH, …, & Sanchez VM. Best practice updates for pediatric/adolescent weight loss surgery. Obesity (Silver Spring). 2009;17(5):901-910.

19   Mayo Clinic Staff. Prescription weight loss drugs: can they help you? Web site. http://www.mayoclinic.com/health/weight-loss-drugs/WT00013/METHOD=print Updated 2012, July 27. Accessed September 15, 2012.

20   Martinez-Gomez, MA, Garcia-Arellano A, et al. A 14-item Mediterranean diet assessment tool and obesity indices among high-risk subjects: the PREDIMED trial. PLoS One. 2012;7(8):e431-34.

21   Snyder-Marlow G, Tayle D, Lenhard MJ. Nutrition care for patients undergoing laparoscopic sleeve gastrectomy for weight loss. J Am Diet Ass. 2010;110(4):600-607

7

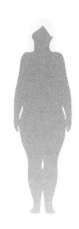

Planning for the Gastric Bypass

So, you have decided to get the Roux-en-Y gastric bypass! Congratulations on making your choice. Now you can focus on moving forward, and this chapter will help you do just that, assuming the following:

- You fully understand RYGB and how it works.
- You have a realistic idea of the amount of weight that RYGB can help you lose.
- You realize and accept the risks of surgery.
- You understand your role and responsibility in losing weight after RYGB and are willing to make the long-term commitment to success.

You are excited about this life-changing experience, but where do you even begin? How do you go from being interested to being a patient? And how do you make sure you get the best possible care? This chapter will explain these topics so you can build a solid foundation for success after gastric bypass:

- Continuing to learn about RYGB
- Choosing a surgeon and facility
- Gathering the rest of your healthcare team
- Paying for surgery: insurance and other options
- Medical tourism: getting the bypass in another country

This chapter is full of actions for you to take, and you will be much further in your path toward surgery by the end of this chapter. Ready to get started? Let's go!

Doing More Research on RYGB

Regardless of how much you already know about gastric bypass, more research can always be helpful. Being well-informed improves your chances of successful weight loss with minimal side effects and complications.

What should you be learning about? These are a few questions to start you off:

- How do I choose the best surgeon?
- How can I finance my surgery?
- How do I prepare for surgery?
- What will the recovery be like? How will I feel?
- What dietary changes can I expect?
- Where do most people get the support they need to get through this experience?
- How do I know if I am emotionally prepared for this change in my life?

You might get new insights or perspectives from different people and different sources. You are more likely to get better care and have better health when you stay involved in your care. You cannot prevent all the risks or guarantee a certain amount of weight loss, but you can definitely increase your chances of the results you want by staying informed.

Possible Sources of Information

Where do you go to get information? Getting started can be tough, but you will find that you are able to come up with resources more easily with a little practice. Many sources will lead you to one or more additional sources and you will soon have a wealth of trusty possibilities. BariatricPal.com is a great starting point and a source to carry you through surgery and beyond, no matter how much you know!

Reading Material

What can you read besides this book? Other RYGB and weight loss surgery books can offer fresh perspectives. You can get additional tips on topics such as:

- Qualifying for surgery
- Paying for surgery with insurance or yourself
- The pre-surgery and post-surgery diets
- How to set goals and work through challenges
- Which side effects and complications can occur
- How other RYGB patients describe their experiences
- How to prepare for the surgery and what to take to the hospital

You do not literally have to set foot in the library or a bookstore if that is just not your style. The point is to read everything you can get your hands on. Beside books and eBooks, magazines can be excellent sources of information. Weight loss-focused or lifestyle-focused magazines may have in-depth articles on specific weight loss patients, procedures, surgeons, or facilities.

Surprisingly, newspapers can be a great starting point for research. Pay close attention each time you see an article about weight loss surgery in general or RYGB in particular. You can use the article to help you think through your own decisions. For example, you might see a news article, such as one published in April of 2013, describing the new bariatric surgery guidelines from the American Association of Clinical Endocrinologists, The Obesity Society, and American Society for Metabolic & Bariatric Surgery.[1] This article might make you think about what changes have been made to the recommendations and why and whether you are still a good candidate for the procedure.

The News

The news can be a great conversation starter when you are trying to get information about the bypass. You can ask about an issue that you read about in the newspaper, a magazine, or online; see on TV; or hear about on the radio. Paying attention to the news gives you a good starting point when you are calling around to find a surgeon or you are talking to RYGB patients who you do not know that well. Ask their opinions and find out their reasoning to help you get an inside scoop and another perspective—the news media do not always tell the whole story.

The Internet

The Internet is a great resource for research at any point during your gastric bypass journey. It is an unlimited source of information covering pretty much everything. Start with basic searches, using keywords such as "roux-en-y gastric bypass" or "weight loss surgery diet." You will probably soon find that the search engines repeatedly direct you to a few sites, and these are often the most complete and useful. You will develop your own favorite sources as you get familiar with the options.

Sites for Fact-Finding

Not everything you read on the Internet is true. Anyone can post statements and advice online without any verification. You cannot always be certain about whether your source is accurate or not, but a few general guidelines can help you make good decisions:[2]

- *Check the website domain, which is the three letters at the end of the web address.* Sites ending in ".edu" and ".gov" are typically credible; they are sponsored respectively by educational institutions and the government.

- *Company sites ending in ".com" and organizations' sites ending in ".org" can have good information.* Just be aware of their possible causes. Companies are probably going to push a product or service. Organizations may be pushing certain causes, such as pro-weight loss surgery or anti-insurance coverage for RYGB.

- *Think about potential bias.* Does the owner of the website have an obvious interest in trying to persuade you one way or another? A surgeon that specializes in the lap-band, for example, might paint a rosy picture of the band while portraying the other weight loss surgeries—such as the gastric bypass—as particularly dangerous. Or a company that offers weight loss surgery packages to Mexico might emphasize the high cost of the surgery in the U.S. and the ease of getting the surgery done in Mexico.

- *Check other sites.* Any information that you find on one site is probably going to be findable on other sites if it is accurate information. Unfortunately, though, this method is not foolproof, since misinformation is often repeated.

- *Use common sense.* Sometimes you just have to use your best judgment. A good rule of thumb is to avoid making serious decisions based on what you find online if you are not certain about its truth. Instead, pose your questions to a surgeon or another qualified professional, such as a dietitian if you have diet questions.

Online Communities

Others' Personal Experiences and Asking Your Own Questions

Online communities, such as discussion boards and social networks, can be valuable research resources. Members of communities are often willing to share their experiences and advice for each stage of your gastric bypass process from making the decision to getting the procedure to learning how to live with it. You can ask detailed questions about your particular situation and concerns and get more personalized answers to your questions than when you stick to solely informational sites.

Online communities are abundant, but some have unique features that make them more attractive than others. BariatricPal.com is one of those. It is specifically geared toward weight loss surgery patients and individuals that are considering surgery or are scheduled to get it. BariatricPal.com has some other advantages too:

- It has an entire set of forums dedicated specifically to Roux-en-Y gastric bypass patients.
- It has a high standard of courtesy, and its moderators are constantly looking out for anyone who violates the zero-tolerance policy.
- It is absolutely free to join and to use all the features.
- There are separate discussion boards dedicated to different topics and audiences, so you can find what you need easily, whether you are looking for diet information, post-surgery recovery tips, or stories from moms who got gastric bypass.
- You can use it to find a surgeon (more about that later in this chapter).

Talking to People to Gather Information

People are among your best resources. In general, people are very willing to share their own experiences, especially if they think they can help you out. It can be tough to get started if you feel shy about gastric bypass. Also, chances are that you do not know—or do not *think* you know—anyone with the weight loss surgery. Once you start to ask around, however, you may realize that more people have it than you thought. A great way to find RYGB patients is through bariatric surgeons. They might invite you to a weight loss surgery support group meeting so you can meet gastric bypass patients. Surgeons and clinical staff may also have lists of gastric bypass patients who have said they are willing to talk to people like you who need information.

These are some of the unique perspectives that you can get from gastric bypass patients:

- Things they wish they had known before the surgery
- What they would have changed if they could do it over again
- Some of the hardest parts about the surgery and lifestyle changes
- Whether they are glad that they got the surgery

Medical Professionals

Who better to go to for learning about weight loss surgery than medical professionals who have dedicated their lives to it? These healthcare professionals should be able to answer your questions about the procedure, preparation for and recovery from surgery, the diet, the risks, and what to expect throughout your experience:

- Bariatric surgeons
- Dietitians with experience in working with gastric bypass patients
- Mental health care professionals
- Bariatric center staff members, such as nurses and receptionists

You can call their offices, contact them via website contact forms, or even try walking in off the street if you prefer to make face-to-face contact. They should be well equipped to answer your questions and offer additional facts that you might not have even thought about since they take care of patients like you every day. Surgeons can show you diagrams of the surgical process and explain the post-surgical care that you will receive; dietitians can go over sample meal plans; psychologists can talk to you about strategies for overcoming your concerns; and nurses can describe your in-clinic experience.

Weight Loss Surgery Seminar

Weight loss surgery seminars are excellent opportunities to learn more about gastric bypass. Seminars usually last a few hours. They are typically free, but they may require telephone or online administration days or weeks in advance. Because seminars can get pretty crowded, you might only be allowed to bring one single guest. Usually, the seminar's main speaker is a surgeon; there may be multiple surgeons if the seminar is hosted by a larger facility. Roux-en-Y gastric bypass and other weight loss surgery patients may be on hand to share their experiences and answer your questions about personal experiences.

Many bariatric surgery seminars cover the other types of surgeries too. The seminars may be sponsored by hospital bariatric centers or other clinics specializing in bariatric surgery and they will probably include a presentation on each type of weight loss surgery that they offer. This is a good chance for you to learn more about RYGB and also to reconsider—and possibly reaffirm—your choice of the gastric bypass over the other weight loss surgeries.

A benefit of attending seminars is that they give you the chance to get to know the presenting surgeon in person. If you like that surgeon, you might end up selecting him or her for your surgery. That is not always practical, since the surgeon may be located too far away from your home to be practical or may not accept your insurance. Still, you can ask the surgeon for his or her recommendations to get a lead on some other possibilities.

The seminar will answer many of your questions and provide additional information too. The seminar may be your first opportunity to ask a professional about your specific situation, so take a list of questions with you and bring a pencil and paper to jot down notes.

To summarize, these are some things to think about when you are at a seminar:

- Do you understand enough about the RYGB process and life after getting surgery to be confident in your decision?
- Are you clear about the risks and benefits of RYGB, especially as compared to other weight loss surgery options?
- Did the seminar bring up any new concerns about the process?
- Do you like the surgeon who gave the seminar enough to consider choosing him or her for your own procedure?
- Do you now have a list of questions and criteria that can guide you when you are selecting a surgeon?
- Do you know the contact information of a few RYGB patients who are willing to answer your questions along the way?

You can find a seminar by searching online. Another option is to call around to a few local bariatric center clinics and ask them for information about their seminars and other seminars in the region.

Do not despair if the seminar schedule does not fit with yours or there are no upcoming seminars. Some seminars are offered as live webcasts. That means you can watch them live online from your computer. This type of seminar is often set up to let you participate by typing in your questions and comments. Pre-recorded seminars are options if you just cannot make a live or webcast seminar in real-time. Save your questions to ask a surgeon when you get a chance.

Learn Your Terms

Your research is not helpful if you do not understand what you are reading. Be sure to look up medical terms and other RYGB-related words that you do not know. Many of them are located in this book's glossary, but some will not be. That is okay; we have left space for your new terms in the glossary. Just write each new term in the table along with the definition and where you saw it. If you do this, all of your new words and definitions will be in the same easy-to-find place.

Choosing a Surgeon

Now we are really getting to the exciting part of your Roux-en-Y gastric bypass experience. In the next part of this chapter, we will go over the process of selecting a surgeon and figuring out where you will get your surgery done and who the other members of your healthcare team are. It is a challenging job, but we will give you tips and guidelines to make it easier. You want to make the most you can out of this early stage of your gastric bypass experience.

First, why are choosing a surgeon, locating your clinic, and assembling the rest of your team so important? Despite your best intentions, deep commitment, and in-depth research, your own actions are not the only factor in your success.[3] You are more likely to have better weight loss, fewer complications, and a better overall experience if your surgeon is competent, your hospital or clinic has the right amenities, and your healthcare team members are experienced in treating bariatric patients. In addition, a comprehensive post-surgery care program contributes to your success, so it is better to make sure that your surgeon leads one or has provisions for you to be enrolled in one.[4]

If the process is so critical, how can it be fun too? Here is why. At this point in your life, *you* get to be in charge. *You* are hand-picking the group of experts who will take care of you over the coming months and years. In fact, you might even want to approach the process as though it were a series of interviews. The truth is that each member of your team is applying for the privilege of working with you.

These are some of the basic questions that you need to have answered and should keep in mind when gathering information and making your decision:

- Do you have a formal gastric bypass or bariatric surgery patient support program that starts before surgery and goes through surgery and for years afterward?

- How much experience do you have with the Roux-en-Y gastric bypass? How many bypasses have you done, and how many procedures do you perform in an average month?

- Do you primarily perform RYGB? What other bariatric surgeries do you do and how many? How do you choose which procedure to perform on a patient? Do you do any other types of surgeries?

- Is your facility (clinic or department) dedicated to bariatric patients? Do you treat patients for conditions unrelated to obesity?

- What percent of your patients need to undergo a second surgery, such as a conversion to a long-limbed RYGB or the addition of an adjustable gastric band (lap-band)? Why does this happen?

- What is the average weight loss of your patients after a year and after five years?

- What percent of your patients are not hitting their weight loss goals? Why does that happen?

These are just a few questions to keep in mind when you are looking around. We will go through some more specific tips to consider when choosing each of the members of your team. As you go through this section, you will understand how to evaluate these questions and what the "right" answers are.

Find Possible Surgeons

Where do you even start when you want to choose a surgeon? Online searches are a good place to start. You can use a search engine or online directory just as you would when you are trying to find any other kind of service. Most surgeons are findable online, and you can narrow searches by location and ratings.

Personal Recommendations

It is hard to know which ratings and reviews are trustworthy when you are browsing online. They can be posted by paid reviewers that may not have even truly seen the surgeon they are reviewing. A better option than relying strictly on online ratings is to gather opinions directly from real, live gastric bypass patients online or in person.

Ask all the RYGB patients you know how they would rate their surgeon and the overall experience and whether they have any tips for you as you choose your own surgeon. Be sure to find out why they did or did not like their surgeon. You may not be able to use the same surgeon for reasons such as lack of insurance coverage or a bad location for you, but their recommendations are still valuable. They will help you figure out your own preferences.

BariatricPal.com

You may not personally know anyone with gastric bypass. Even after you go to a seminar or two, you still might not be confident that you have all the information that you need to make the right surgeon choice. BariatricPal.com is a resource that can help by offering the following features:

- Thousands of members that are gastric bypass patients that are willing to offer advice
- A surgeon directory complete with member ratings and reviews—and you can be confident that they are honest, not paid, reviews.
- Honest discussions that may bring up important points about choosing a surgeon that you had not even considered before

Verifying Surgeon Qualifications

In the U.S., all surgeons are full medical doctors.[5] They completed medical school, went through residency trainings in the area of surgery. Each state has its own requirements for licensure for practicing surgeons, and you can ask your surgeon about current credential. So far, these requirements are pretty broad and easy to meet. Additional criteria can help you select the best surgeon from the rest.

Specific and Recent Training

A surgeon can perform Roux-en-Y gastric bypass without much formal education in bariatric surgery, gastric bypass, or laparoscopy. However, checking on a few optional criteria can help you choose a highly qualified surgeon. Do not be shy about asking, it is *your* body.

- *Membership, or Fellowship, in the American College of Surgeons, or ACS.* It is easy to tell if your surgeon is a fellow because surgeons that have fellowship are allowed to place the letters FACS after their name, next to their M.D. for medical doctor. The ACS publishes regular scientific journals and newsletters so that fellows can learn about things such as new techniques and updates on guidelines for better patient care for bariatric surgery patients.[6]
- *Participation in ongoing educational opportunities.* Years or even decades may have passed since surgeons completed medical school and got their licenses to practice surgery. There are a variety of ways that surgeons can choose to enhance their skills and stay updated with the latest developments in bariatric surgery, laparoscopic surgery, and Roux-en-Y gastric bypass. New information is constantly emerging to help surgeons and patients achieve better outcomes. Ask what your potential surgeon is doing to stay current.
- *Surgeons with the PALSS certification have demonstrated their skills in laparoscopic surgery.* The PALSS, or Peer Review of Laparoscopic Surgical Proficiency, certification is from the American Society of General Surgeons[7].

- This certification from the American Society of General Surgeons requires surgeons to be at Level I, or advanced laparoscopic surgeon. That is the top level that the ASGS recognizes.

- To be certified, surgeons must be evaluated while doing surgery. They can send in a video of themselves doing a surgery, or they can have an evaluator in the operating room to watch. The surgeon gets evaluated on a variety of specific technical skills and procedures that are important for the gastric bypass.

- *Membership in the American Society for Metabolic and Bariatric Surgery.*[8] Again, this is not a requirement, but it is a way to feel more confident in your choice of surgeons.

  - Regular members are certified by the American Board of Surgery or the American Osteopathic Board of Surgery and/or are fellows in the American College of Surgeons, or FACS, or one of the Royal Colleges of Surgeons in United Kingdom or Ireland. They also have completed at least 25 bariatric surgeries within the past two years.

  - Affiliate members are bariatric surgeons that have not met the above requirements but have a letter of recommendation from a current regular member.

  - International members have completed at least 25 bariatric surgeries within the past two years and have recommendation letters of support.

Experience and Current Focus

You do not just want a doctor; you do not just want a surgeon; and you do not just want a weight loss surgery expert. You want an expert in the Roux-en-Y gastric bypass. It does not matter how many other skills your surgeon has; you want your surgeon to be the best possible surgeon for your own procedure. Ask whether the gastric bypass is one of the main procedures that your surgeon does. It is only reasonable to expect that he or she performs other bariatric surgeries too, but your surgeon should focus on bariatric patients and regularly perform gastric bypass procedures.

In general, more experience is better. You are less likely to have complications when your surgeon has had plenty of practice with other patients. Ask potential surgeons when they started doing Roux-en-Y gastric bypass and how many patients they have had. Also ask how many of these surgeries they do per week or month. You want to be sure that they are comfortable doing gastric bypass.

Asking the Tough Questions

Healthcare professionals, especially your own physician, surgeon, and healthcare members, are ethically obligated to provide you with the information you need to make the best decisions for your health.[9] Despite this, the majority of patients have unrealistic expectations about the amount of weight they are likely to lose and may not fully understand the risks they take with the procedure.[10] Physicians need to be prepared to tell you about the procedure and the potential benefits and the risks. It is safest to rule out surgeons that will not be open about this information.

Patient Records

It is perfectly legitimate to ask potential surgeons about how their patients do after surgery. These questions can be uncomfortable if you are shy, but you have every right to know this information. Surgeons who are hesitant to answer your questions or who act offended by them are raising red flags. They should be proud, not embarrassed, to talk about their role in their patients' success and safety. At a minimum, you should ask about the following:

- Average patient weight loss at a few months, a year, and several years after surgery
- Percent of laparoscopic procedures that are converted into open surgeries during surgery
- Percent of patients that require a second surgery due to complications
- Rate of complications and which types are most common

Once you get these answers, compare the numbers to the numbers you saw in Chapters 4 and 5 of this book in the discussions on expected weight loss. Of course, you want the weight loss numbers to be among the higher values seen in Chapter 4, *"RYGB & It's Potential Benefits."*

Think twice about trusting surgeons that will not or cannot tell you how their patients do long term. Surgeons with good follow-up care programs know how their patients are doing.

You want a surgeon whose patients have a low rate of complications is a pretty good indicator of a surgeon's ability to perform RYGB. If the surgeon has a relatively high rate of complications, be sure to dig deeper into the possible reasons. Some demographic groups,

Red Flags

The best surgeon for you might not have the "right" answers to every single one of your questions. That is okay as long as you are comfortable with the surgeon and you get the "right" answers to the questions that are most important to you. However, it may be time to rule out surgeons if they show any of these red flags:

- Acting offended when you ask about personal RYGB training and experience and patient history of weight loss and complications
- Lack of knowledge about patient weight loss after a few years — a good follow-up program keeps in touch with patients for years.
- Unwillingness to discuss what happens if you have complications
- Not treating you as an individual with your own legitimate concerns
- Not well acquainted with each member of the healthcare team
- Inability to answer questions regarding care that is not strictly related to the surgery procedure. This shows that the surgeon is only actively involved in the surgical procedure and not your pre-operative and post-operative care as well.

such as patients with a higher pre-surgery BMI, males, and older adults, have complication rates as much as 20 times higher—and the complications are due to patient characteristics. They are not the surgeon's fault.[11]

Post-Surgery Care or Aftercare Program

Once you are convinced that a surgeon is well qualified and has good technical expertise, your next step is to really dig into the surgeon's aftercare, or post-surgery care, program. All gastric bypass surgeons should be able to describe the surgery to you in their sleep. A more revealing test is whether the surgeon can clearly explain the aftercare program. The aftercare experience may be inadequate if your surgeon does not know all the details of a comprehensive post-surgery care plan. This can be devastating, since post-surgery follow-up care improves your chances of success.[12]

Basics of an Aftercare Program

The surgery is only an early step in your weight loss journey. A post-operative care plan needs to be comprehensive and mandatory to maximize your chances of good weight loss and minimal complications after RYGB. A comprehensive plan includes input from your surgeon and provides support for your physical and psychological health, as well as dietary support. Depending on your surgeon's preferences and/or the facility's procedure, the program may be mandatory for just a few months, a year or two, or even life.

Getting the Scoop on Post-Surgery Care

Ask specific questions as you are trying to choose a surgeon. You should be concerned if the surgeon or patient care specialist is unable or unwilling to clarify each component of the post-op care program. It may mean that the program is not well-structured and that some patients slip through the cracks. You do not want to be one of those patients! Following are some questions that you might want to ask when you are trying to find out about aftercare. Always feel free to ask different people multiple times within one clinic to be sure that you are getting an accurate picture of the program. You might also want to ask patients that you see about their experiences.

- After the surgery, how often are patients required to have appointments with the surgeon?
  - If everything is going well, you should see your physician 1, 3, and 6 to 12 months after surgery.[13]
- How often and for how long do you meet with the other members of your medical team?
  - Ideally, you should meet weekly or biweekly with your dietitian right after RYGB as your diet is rapidly changing. Continue to meet regularly for months after the procedure and as needed for meal plans, recipes, and tips. You should also have ongoing meetings with a mental health professional to make sure that you are doing well. If possible, find a program with a physical therapist that can design a customized program for you.
- What happens if you miss your appointments?

- The clinic might ask you to sign a contract that you will follow through with your aftercare. If you need to miss appointments due to scheduling conflicts and you notify the clinic ahead of time, the clinic should be accommodating and reschedule you as soon as possible.
- When and how often are support groups meetings held? What happens if you cannot make those meetings because of your schedule? For how long are you required to attend?
  - If you can, choose a surgeon that will connect you with patient peer-to-peer support groups that are convenient for you. Many clinics ask you to attend weekly meetings right after surgery and monthly meetings for years or for life.
- How does the clinic help patients who are not meeting their target weight loss goals?
  - You want to be sure that if you start to falter, the surgeon will reach out to you and make the effort to figure out what kind of extra help you need. This is your time to be successful, so choose a surgeon who will be there for you when you need it most.
- Why do some patients not make their target weight loss goals?
  - You want to be sure that you are not going to become one of them. Some reasons that patients might get off track is if they were not good candidates in the first place or did not want to commit to the dietary changes. You need to be cautious if the clinic staff do not seem to know why some patients do not get the success they want.
- What happens in the case of an emergency if your surgeon is out of town and you need urgent help with a problem such as slippage or obstruction?
  - There should always be an available surgeon who is on call at the same or a nearby facility to cover for your surgeon if you have an emergency.
- How experienced are the nurses?
  - A CBN is a Certified Bariatric Nurse. Nurses with this qualification have at least two years of experience caring for morbidly obese patients.[14] CBNs need to take a recertification exam every four years to maintain their status as a CBN.

Chapter 10, *"Final Preparation for RYGB,"* is devoted to recovering from surgery and your post-op care plan. You can find more details about follow-up care in that chapter.

Choosing a Surgeon Based on Insurance Coverage

Often your choice of surgeons will be partly or completely determined by your insurance plan. If your insurance plan will only reimburse you if you go to a specific surgeon, you still need do your background research and find out whether you are comfortable with that surgeon. Chances are that you will be comfortable with the surgeon that you are offered. If not, continue to explore other options. This is a big step in your life, and you want to be sure that you are going to work well with your surgeon now and in the future.

Choosing a Location for Your Surgery

Choosing a location for your surgery often goes hand in hand with choosing a surgeon. The surgeon you decide on may determine the location of your surgery. Or you may only be near one or two facilities that offer bariatric surgery, so your location will partially determine your surgeon choice. If you are able to have some input in your choice of facility, there are a few criteria you can look for to improve your chances of a safe and successful experience.

Certified Weight Loss Surgery Centers

In the U.S., the American College of Surgeons Bariatric Surgery Center Network Program, or ACS/BSCNP, and ASMBS have certain criteria for hospitals to become accredited bariatric surgery centers.[15] The Bariatric Surgery Center of Excellence, or BSCOE, program was formerly part of the Surgical Review Corporation. Now it is a joint program of the ACS and ASMBS.[16] Medicare and many other insurance programs require facilities to be certified to qualify for insurance reimbursement.

Here is a list of some features to look for when you are choosing a facility for your RYGB. Having these amenities will make your surgery safer and your entire experience more pleasant.[17] We will talk in more detail about some of these next.

- Large and stable wheelchairs, stretchers, and walkers for heavy patients
- Large-sized monitoring devices, such as blood pressure cuffs
- Wide, heavy-duty beds
- Wide commodes and toilets
- Wide doorways, halls, and chairs
- Emergency equipment for large people
- Large scales
- Wide operating table with high weight capacity
- Open MRI and CT scan with high weight capacity
- Specially-trained personnel and appropriate lifting equipment

A Few More Considerations

Other considerations when choosing a clinic are its size, comfort, and convenience.

Size: The idea of a small clinic with a single bariatric surgeon might be appealing because it seems more personal, but it is not always the best choice. In fact, on average, you are more likely to do better if you get your surgery done at a larger facility that treats a lot of patients like you. Hospitals and large medical centers are examples. These high-volume facilities are typically safer and more effective for a few reasons:[18]

- They have entire departments that are more focused on bariatric surgery. In addition to your bariatric surgeon, these departments may have nurses, mental health professionals, and other staff members with special training in bariatric surgery.[19] Bariatric centers should also have special equipment and procedures for lifting patients when necessary.

- They have established protocols. The entire program, from surgery planning through aftercare, is very well planned and clear. You walk in and there is no hesitation because they know what works and what does not. Their experience comes from treating many, many patients just like you, and you will benefit from this expertise.

- They may have more than one surgeon that is an expert in RYGB. That means that if your surgeon is away, you can get care immediately and prevent more serious complications if you have a small problem. Even if your own surgeon is the only one at your clinic, a large clinic is more likely to be able to get you an appointment quickly with another partner clinic.

- The post-operative care program is probably more developed. With so many patients, there are probably more opportunities to attend peer-to-peer support groups compared to smaller facilities. There is probably an established schedule of post-surgery follow-up care so that there is no uncertainty about which appointments you will have with whom.

- There are more support staff, such as dietitians, nurses, exercise physiologists, and psychologists. This makes it easier for you to get appointments and increases the chances of getting all of your appointments scheduled on a single day.

Physical and Emotional Comfort: Between the pre-surgery preparation, the surgery itself, and the post-surgery care, you will be spending a lot of time at the clinic. You will do better if you are physically and emotionally comfortable. If you have been obese for years, you already know the huge importance of things such as chairs that are wide enough to sit in, toilets that are easier to sit down on, beds that are big enough for you, scales that can weigh you, hospital gowns that you can fit into, and doorways that you can actually get through. Wider wheelchairs and operating tables for obese patients are just a couple examples of amenities that facilities with a lot of experience with obese patients will have for you.

The other part of comfort is your mental comfort. You want to feel comfortable throughout the whole process, from when you walk in the door and the receptionist greets you, to being cared for by nurses, to communicating well with your surgeon, to feeling secure talking to your dietitian and other members. You do not ever want to feel embarrassed to bring up your issues or feel like your healthcare team is not listening. That can lead to problems for your health.

Convenience: When all other things are equal, choose a facility that is close to your house. Getting the actual surgery done in a place that requires a long drive or overnight stay is one thing. Making frequent travel arrangements or taking some time off work every time you have to see a distant surgeon is quite another. In most cases, you will have to see your surgeon several times from the time of your first pre-surgery appointment until you reach your goal weight. It is most convenient to be treated at a clinic that is located near you.

Choosing a large clinic for your gastric bypass care can be more convenient because you can often get all of your appointments and medical tests done in one trip and in one facility when possible. Think about the other services you will probably be using regularly:

- Dietitian consults
- Blood tests in a lab
- X-rays or MRI or CT scans in a radiology department
- Group support meetings

In a large facility where everything is located on-site, you can get two or three tasks done in one trip. But if your surgeon is from a small clinic, you might have to go to appointments at different locations. You might not be able to get more than one appointment or service done at once.

Where Should Adolescents Go?

If you are an adolescent or a parent of one who is going to get RYGB, you may be wondering whether to opt for a pediatric center or a bariatric center in a regular hospital. The ideal scenario would be for adolescents to go to a pediatric bariatric center. That way, they would get the best of both worlds with age-appropriate treatment and bariatric medical expertise. A children's bariatric center probably is not available, and experts recommend that adolescents get their procedures done in an adult center to take advantage of the better facilities.[20] The same criteria for adults apply to adolescents: choose a surgeon who is competent and qualified and who makes you feel comfortable.

It Is Too Confusing!

The whole process of choosing a surgeon, building the rest of your healthcare team, and figuring out insurance can be confusing. Often the information you need to make your decision is in complicated medical or legal jargon. BariatricPal.com is a good resource for translating some of this information into language that you can understand. It is a huge community of Roux-en-Y gastric bypass patients and individuals who are considering weight loss surgery. Many of them are willing to help you out by explaining the process and letting you know what is important and what is not when you are choosing your surgeon and trying to fund the surgery.

Summary

☛ This chapter is pivotal. Now you know how to choose a surgeon. Once you make the decision about a surgeon and where you will get your surgery done, you have professionals to guide you. From now on, they will be your main sources of instruction.

☛ In the next chapter, we will continue with the preparation for surgery. You will learn about paying for your surgery using insurance or with other options. Let's get going!

Time to Take Action: Choosing a Surgeon

This chapter covered some of the things you should look for when you are choosing a surgeon and a facility for your weight loss. Every RYGB patient has slightly different wants and needs, though. In this worksheet, you will say how important each of the following characteristics is to you. When you are done, you will have a better idea of how to evaluate your own potential surgeons when you are trying to choose.

On a scale from 1 (not important) to 5 (extremely important), how important to you are the following?

Your surgeon has good user reviews and ratings.

1   2   3   4   5

Your surgeon was recommended to you by someone you know and trust, such as a family member or friend.

1   2   3   4   5

Your surgery is done in a facility (or department of a hospital) that is dedicated to obese patients.

1   2   3   4   5

Your surgeon runs his or her own support group meetings.

1   2   3   4   5

A dietitian is on site at the clinic or hospital where your surgeon works.

1   2   3   4   5

Knowing that you are going to need to visit your surgeon several times before and after surgery, how far are you willing to travel to see your surgeon? Miles

1   Newswise. New evidence prompts update to metabolic and bariatric surgery clinical guidelines. PR Newswire. http://www.newswise.com/articles/view/601305/?sc=rsmn. 2013, April 13. Accessed April 27, 2013.

2   Evaluating web-based health resources. National Center for Complementary and Alternative Medicine, National Institutes of Health. Web site. http://nccam.nih.gov/health/webresources Modified January 2011. Accessed September 18, 2012.

3   Kaplan LM, Seeley RJ, Harris JL. Myths associated with obesity and bariatric surgery – myth 5: patient behavior is the primary determinant of outcomes after bariatric surgery. 2012;9(8):8-10.

4   Mechanick MD, Kushner RF…Dixon J. Clinical practice guidelines for clinical practice for the perioperative nutritional, metabolic, and nonsurgical support of the bariatric surgery patient – 2013 update: cosponsored by the American Association of Clinical Endocrinologists, The Obesity Society, and American Society for Metabolic & Bariatric Surgery. Obesity, 2013;9:159-191

5   Bureau of Labor Statistics. Physicians and surgeons. http://www.bls.gov/ooh/healthcare/physicians-and-surgeons.htm. Published 2012, March 29. Accessed September 20, 2012.

6   American College of Surgeons (n.d.). Retrieved from http://www.facs.org/index.html

7   Education: Peer review of laparoscopic surgical proficiency. (n.d.) American Society of General Surgeons. Retrieved from http://www.theasgs.org/education/education1.html

8   Become a member. American Society for Metabolic and Bariatric Surgery. Web site. http://asmbs.org/become-a-member/ Accessed September 21, 2012.

9   Wee CC, Pratt JS, Fanelli R, Samour PQ, Trainer LS, Paasche-Orlow MK. Best practice updates for informed consent and patient education in weight loss surgery. Obesity (Silver Spring). 2009;17(5):885-888.

10 Wee CC, Pratt JS, Fanelli R, Samour PQ, Trainer LS, Paasche-Orlow MK. Best practice updates for informed consent and patient education in weight loss surgery. Obesity (Silver Spring). 2009;17(5):885-888.

11 Wee CC, Pratt JS, Fanelli R, Samour PQ, Trainer LS, Paasche-Orlow MK. Best practice updates for informed consent and patient education in weight loss surgery. Obesity (Silver Spring). 2009;17(5):885-888.

12 Mechanick MD, Kushner RF…Dixon J. Clinical practice guidelines for clinical practice for the perioperative nutritional, metabolic, and nonsurgical support of the bariatric surgery patient – 2013 update: cosponsored by the American Association of Clinical Endocrinologists, The Obesity Society, and American Society for Metabolic & Bariatric Surgery. Obesity, 2013;9:159-191.

13 Mechanick MD, Kushner RF…Dixon J. Clinical practice guidelines for clinical practice for the perioperative nutritional, metabolic, and nonsurgical support of the bariatric surgery patient – 2013 update: cosponsored by the American Association of Clinical Endocrinologists, The Obesity Society, and American Society for Metabolic & Bariatric Surgery. Obesity, 2013;9:159-191.

14 American Society for Metabolic and Bariatric Surgery. CBN Certification FAQ. Web site. http://asmbs.org/cbn-certification/. Accessed September 22, 2012.

15 Lautz DB, Jiser ME, Kelly JJ, Shikora SA, Partridge SK, Romanelli JR, Cella RJ, Ryan JP. An update on best practice guidelines for specialized facilities and resources necessary for weight loss surgical programs. Obesity (Silver Spring). 2009;17(5):8911-917.

16 American Society for Metabolic and Bariatric Surgery. Unified national accreditation program for bariatric surgery announced by American College of Surgeons and American Society for Metabolic and Bariatric Surgery. Web site. http://asmbs.org/2012/03/unified-national-accreditation-program-for-bariatric-surgery-centers-announced-by-american-college-of-surgeons-and-american-society-for-metabolic-and-bariatric-surgery/. 2012, March 9. Accessed September 20, 2012.

17 Lautz DB, Jiser ME, Kelly JJ, Shikora SA, Partridge SK, Romanelli JR, Cella RJ, Ryan JP. An update on best practice guidelines for specialized facilities and resources necessary for weight loss surgical programs. Obesity (Silver Spring). 2009;17(5):8911-917.

18 Agency for Healthcare Research and Quality. (January 2011). Outcomes/effectiveness research: serious complications from bariatric surgery are fewer when done by high-volume hospitals and surgeons. *United States Department of Health and Human Services*. Retrieved from http://www.ahrq.gov/research/jan11/0111RA9.htm

19 Lautz DB, Jiser ME, Kelly JJ, Shikora SA, Partridge SK, Romanelli JR, Cella RJ, Ryan JP. An update on best practice guidelines for specialized facilities and resources necessary for weight loss surgical programs. Obesity (Silver Spring). 2009;17(5):8911-917.

20 Pratt JSA, Lenders CM, Dionne EA, Hoppin AG, Hsu GLK., Inge, TH, …, & Sanchez VM. Best practice updates for pediatric/adolescent weight loss surgery. Obesity (Silver Spring). 2009;17(5):901-910.

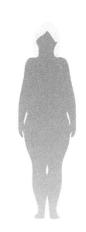

8

Roux-En-Y Gastric Bypass Costs, Insurance and More

The last chapter provided some guidelines on choosing a surgeon, a facility, and the rest of your medical team. You may have a few options in mind. Maybe you already know who is going to do your surgery. Now that the surgery seems as though it is in the not-so-distant future, it is time to cover one of the least exciting but nonetheless necessary topics related to your surgery: payment. Your payment options can be a little confusing, so this chapter will explain the most common scenarios and serve as a guide. We also discuss these topics:

- Investigating whether your health insurance covers the gastric bypass
- How to get your insurance company's pre-approval for reimbursement for the gastric bypass
- Self-pay and financing options for the RYGB
- Medical tourism: getting the bypass in another country to lower costs

This chapter takes a giant leap toward making your surgery a reality. By the end of the chapter, you will know how to pay for it, so the surgery will seem much closer than it was before. Let's plow ahead!

Paying for the Bypass

After deciding that you want the RYGB, you need to figure out how to pay for it. Your insurance plan, if you have one, may cover part or all of the costs of the bypass and related expenses. If your insurance does not cover all of the RYGB, you will need to pay for part or all of it yourself either with cash or a financing plan.

Cost of the RYGB

How much does the gastric bypass cost? As with any medical procedure, patients' final charges can vary quite a bit. You can get the most accurate prices by asking each facility to estimate how much they charge.

Many factors affect the cost of the RYGB:

- Different surgeons and clinics that charge different prices for their services
- Whether you have health insurance
- The state and zip code where you live
- Complications during or after the surgery that require extra medical care
- A health condition that requires special care during, before, or after surgery
- Which services are included in this estimate

Online searches can help you gather information on the cost of the gastric bypass. Numerous sites provide estimates of the cost:

- Fair Health Consumer Cost Lookup provides estimates based on your zip code and health insurance.[1]

- Consumer Health Ratings has several links to sites that provide estimates of RYGB costs. The link is at the end of this chapter.[2]
- Many state government sites provide useful information on medical costs. For example, the California Office of Statewide Health Planning and Development, lets you look up the average cost of the bypass, as well as average length of hospital stay, in facilities throughout the state.[3] You can find California's and many other states' medical cost sites at Consumer Health Ratings.

The RNY gastric bypass may cost about $8,000,[4] but this amount can vary by thousands of dollars. This figure is an estimate for the LRYGB procedure and a three-day hospital stay. By the time you add in the costs of pre-surgery and post-surgery care, not to mention any unexpected medical costs from complications, the number can be several times higher, in the range of $10,000 to 20,000. You also need to consider that your quoted figure may not include all of your expected costs related to surgery. When a bariatric facility gives you an estimated cost, specifically ask whether the figure includes:

- The surgery itself
- Pre-surgery tests to make sure you are a good candidate for surgery
- Pre-surgery preparation, such as diet counseling
- Cost of anesthesia and pain medications if you use them
- Expected care in the hospital if you have no complications
- Regular post-surgery follow-up appointments with your surgeon

When you are gathering cost estimates, looking up your healthcare coverage, and doing your budget, do not forget to consider other likely costs, such as:

- Ongoing post-surgery appointments with a dietitian
- Regular medical tests, such as laboratory blood tests for your nutritional status
- Extra care in the hospital if your surgery leads to a longer hospital stay than expected
- Further procedures, such as a revisional procedure, if you have complications
- The cost of diagnostic tests, such as x-rays or MRIs, if you have complications
- Extra appointments with your physician or surgeon to troubleshoot side effects

When you are adding up the costs of the RYGB, do not forget about potential savings too. Bariatric surgery may end up saving you money if it truly helps you lose weight and get healthier. You will not have to pay for any more fad diets, and you may save money on doctor's visits, medical tests, and prescription drugs if Roux-en-Y gastric bypass works for you. Along with economic concerns, there is also the issue of your health and quality of life. Do you expect your weight loss, health, and general quality of life to improve enough to be worth the investment in gastric bypass?

Insurance

- Health coverage is becoming more common for bariatric surgery.[5] The government's largest plans, Medicare and Medicaid, have covered the Roux-en-Y gastric bypass for eligible patients since 2006.[6]
- Aetna Inc.[7] and United Healthcare[8] are examples of large private medical insurance providers that cover the RYGB.

If you have been considering weight loss surgery for a few years and your healthcare coverage did not cover it before, it is probably worth checking again. More insurance providers are deciding to cover weight loss surgery, especially the RYGB, because it makes good business sense. Covering the procedure ends up saving them money.[9]

Figuring out your insurance coverage can be tough, and we will try to guide you through it over the next few pages. Some of the main sources of information on whether the procedure is covered or whether a specific surgeon takes your insurances include:

- The specific surgeon or his or her office
- Your healthcare coverage insurance customer service representative
- The human resources department at your workplace
- The insurance coverage map from ASMBS, which is a work in progress and should be a valuable resource when it is complete[10]

Identifying Which Type of Insurance Plan You Have and Getting Information about RYGB Coverage

The first step is to figure out what kind of insurance plan you have. Then you need to figure out how to get information about your specific benefits. You might already be familiar with all of these aspects, especially if you have medical problems that you have to deal with on a regular basis. Your experience will help you now!

But if you are lucky enough to have good insurance and you have never had to worry about your medical costs because you have never asked for anything extra, you might not have ever really thought about health insurance. For many of us, health insurance is a blurry concept that does not really come into focus until we need something specific—right now, it is the gastric bypass and the other costs that come along with it. This section will walk you through getting any reimbursement that you are entitled to. This section will include this information:

- Types of private insurance plans and how they work
- National health insurance coverage: Medicare and Medicaid and how they work
- Getting information about what is covered by your insurance plan
- Asking for pre-approval for reimbursement and appealing a denied claim

Private Insurance: HMOs and PPOs

Private health insurance is insurance that you or your employer pays for. You need to know what kind of insurance plan you have so that you know how to get the benefits you are entitled to and where to find information.

HMOs and PPOs: The most common systems of private health insurance are health management organizations, or HMOs, and preferred provider organizations, or PPOs.

- In an HMO, you typically get all of your medical care done by healthcare providers within the network. You need a referral from your primary care physician in order to get reimbursed for care by specialists such as the RYGB surgeon. An HMO will most likely only reimburse you for the gastric bypass if you go to a surgeon within the network. If the entire network only has a few RYGB surgeons, you may need to travel out of town to get your surgery done by an approved surgeon. This can make aftercare difficult and inconvenient as you will need to see your surgeon multiple times in the weeks and months after surgery. However, you may be allowed to see a more local doctor within the HMO for your post-surgery follow-up.

- If you are part of a PPO, you are usually covered for care when you see any provider in the network. Depending on which PPO you belong to, you might need a referral for seeing a specialist. Relatively expensive and major procedures, such as the RYGB, are more likely to require referrals before you can get reimbursed.

Coverage with Fully-Insured and Self-Insured Insurance Plans: A *fully-insured* insurance plan is one that you pay for directly to the insurance company or your employer pays part or all of it for you. A *self-insured* insurance plan is one that your employer has negotiated with the insurance company; the exact list of services that are covered may be different than what the insurance company offers to other companies and individuals. Either plan can be an HMO or PPO.

Why does it matter whether you have a fully-insured or self-insured plan? This information is a clue to where you can find information about the coverage. On a fully-insured plan, the information you need is in the *Summary of Benefits* (SOB) or *Certificate of Coverage*. With a self-insured insurance plan, you will need the *Summary Plan Description (SPD)*. There is not a big difference between these two items, but knowing the proper terms will help you track down the documents you need.

Once you have those documents, look through them carefully for information about weight loss surgery coverage. This can take a while because the documents are not usually very easy to read. They are full of jargon that is tough to wade through. These are a few key words to look for as you skim through your policy:

- *Exclusion clauses*: These sections list services that *are not* covered by the policy. An exclusion clause might list all obesity treatments, including weight loss surgery, as excluded services — they are not covered at all by your policy.

- *Inclusion clauses*: These sections list services that *are* covered by the policy. Your policy might state that the open or laparoscopic gastric bypass is covered, or it might state nonspecifically that some types of bariatric surgery are covered. It might be as general as stating that many types of obesity treatment are covered. If the policy does not specifically state the RYGB as an included procedure, you will need to call your representative.

- *Expenses Covered* or *Expenses Not Covered*: These might come in the middle of an exclusion clause or an inclusion clause, or they might come in their own separate lists elsewhere in the policy. Again, if you do not see the RYGB mentioned anywhere, it is time to call an insurance representative. Be sure to ask whether it is covered when it is *medically necessary* because some insurance representatives will answer "no" when you simply ask whether it is covered. Often the RYGB is covered *only when medically necessary*.

Do your best with the dense, legal-style language and medical terminology. Whether you think you understand it or not, it is a good idea to check with a representative from the insurance company (if you have a fully-insured plan) or with an insurance expert in your human resources department (if you have self-insured insurance coverage). Ask them to explain anything that you do not understand. Also ask them to mail you a copy of everything related to obesity treatment so you can read it at your leisure.

A Few Tips to Make the Insurance Process Easier

Dealing with health insurance companies is challenging. Getting information from them can take hours. You can feel as though you are going around in circles because of so many phone calls with so many different representatives. These are a few tips that can help prepare you for possibly frustrating encounters with the company:

- *Take notes.* That includes having a pen and paper in hand so you can take notes whenever you make a phone call or look something up online. Keep records of all your phone calls, noting the time and date.

- *Be patient and persistent.* You might be on hold, you might get a rude representative, and you might get an answer that you are sure is wrong. Take a deep breath and try again. Keep your eye on the prize, which could be as much as several thousand dollars for a life-changing medical procedure.

- *Be prepared with the following information.* Insurance provider's contact information (name, fax number, phone number, email address, website).

- *Make sure everything is verifiable.* Get all promises in writing and ask for your customer service rep's name each time you make a call. Do not depend on your memory or on a spoken promise.

- *Do not give up.* Keep trying until you are satisfied with the answer and you have any promises for reimbursement in writing.

As you investigate reimbursement for the RYGB, do not forget about the other treatments that you will need—and that cost money. You will need to have multiple pre-surgery and post-surgery appointments with your surgeon, as well as the dietitian, psychiatrist, and other members of the medical team.

- Each service may require a pre-approval separate from the pre-approval for the bypass.
- Some services may not be covered even if the gastric bypass is.
- These other services may be covered even if the actual gastric bypass is not. This can make the entire procedure affordable for you.

Be especially careful to read the fine print if you are looking into the gastric bypass as a revisional surgery. For example, you might have already gotten the adjustable gastric band (lap-band) or the vertical banded gastroplasty and you are now interested in getting the bypass because your first procedure is not working for you. Many plans have an exclusion policy for all bariatric surgeries that are not your first. That means that insurance companies will only reimburse you for your first weight loss surgery, even if your previous surgery was with another insurance company or you paid for it yourself.

Some plans, however, do cover revisional surgeries when they are considered necessary. This may occur when:[11]

- You did not lose at least 50 percent of your excess body weight within the first two years of your gastric band, vertical banded gastroplasty, or first gastric bypass procedure even though you followed your prescribed diet and exercise program.
- You were losing weight successfully until your gastric pouch dilated, or expanded, and you need a second procedure to make the pouch smaller.

Your insurance may provide complete coverage, but it may limit the total cost or type of services that you can receive in a year. If this is the case, you can find out your out-of-pocket fees, which is the amount you will be paying yourself.

- Add up the total cost of the RYGB surgical procedure and related costs of pre-surgery and post-surgery care.
- Find out the maximum amount of reimbursement.
- Then subtract the amount of reimbursement from the total cost to find out your out-of-pocket fees.

Getting Pre-Approval from Your Insurance Provider

Getting pre-approval in writing is critical! Without getting the promise of reimbursement in writing, you could end up with the gastric bypass and no way to pay for it.

The pre-approval process often is straightforward. Usually, someone at your surgeon's office will fill out the paperwork for you requesting coverage for the surgery. They will send it to your insurance carrier, who should approve it if it is part of your plan.

If your surgeon does not take care of the paperwork for you, you can do it yourself. Write a letter explaining the procedure, the amount you are asking for, and the surgeon and other health professionals that you will be purchasing services from. Explain the gastric bypass procedure and the reasons why it is a medically necessary procedure. Use the official codes for the best chances of getting approved on your first try.

- *Current Procedural Terminology, or CPT, Code*: The CPT Code is an official designation published by the American Medical Association.[12] There is a different CPT for each medical procedure. The CPTs get updated often, so check the AMA's website for the CPT code for the gastric bypass when you are ready to write your letter.

- *The RYGB may have a different code from the laparoscopic RYGB, or LRYGB.* Ask your surgeon which to include in your letter.

- *International Classification of Diseases, 9th Edition, or ICD-9*: Each ICD-9 describes a health condition or disease that is a justification for asking for medical treatment. Most insurance companies use the ICD-9 to decide whether to provide reimbursement.

In your letter, request pre-approval in writing. Mail your letter using certified mail so that someone at the insurance company has to sign for delivery and you have proof that your letter arrived safely.

Appealing a Denied Claim

Your insurance company might refuse to grant pre-approval, or prior approval, for your bariatric surgery the first time you or your surgeon's office submits the request. This happens pretty often, and you should not panic or lose hope if you get denied after your first try. What you can do is appeal the denial. Your surgeon's office might automatically resubmit the claim for you and try to get the denial overturned. Or you might need to submit the appeal yourself. In that case, call your insurance representative and request an explanation in writing so that you can address each point. You are legally entitled to an explanation in writing.

Look carefully at the reason for the denial to increase your chances of getting the denial overturned:

- If your insurance company denied your request claiming that you did not give a sufficient reason for the RYGB, make sure that you filled in the ICD-9 number correctly and that you submitted a letter from your physician recommending that you get the bypass.

- If the company claims that the procedure is experimental and therefore not covered, you can use existing research on the history, safety, and effectiveness of the RYGB. Your surgeon should be able to provide a letter backing you up.

- If the insurance company says that the procedure is excluded but you are certain that your policy covers the gastric bypass, double-check to make sure that the CPT Code you entered was correct.

- If you are under a self-insured plan from your employer, you can ask your employer to add the bypass to the list of covered procedures. Remember, a self-insured plan includes only those services that your employer chooses, and your employer has the ability to change the service plans.

These are a few tips for composing a letter to your insurance company or insurance representative in your employer's human resources department:

- If you filled out the initial pre-approval form incorrectly or you believe you were denied because of an error, specifically point out which parts were mistakes. It may be that you filled in the wrong ICD-9 or CPT Code or that the insurance company wrongly interpreted your entitlement or request.

- Most insurance companies will only cover bariatric surgery if it is a medical necessity. In your letter, include specific information about the health consequences of obesity. Chapter 1 of this book is a good place to start when you are gathering your data. You do not have to make it too long, but you can point out that obesity can cause a high risk of diabetes and cardiovascular disease, a shorter life expectancy, and more than $1,000 per year in extra medical costs.. You can also mention any health conditions you have because of your obesity. Your surgeon can help with this part.

- Describe the data showing that weight loss surgery can be more effective than diet and exercise and that the bypass has been successful for many patients who have not been able to lose weight through dieting.[13] Again, your surgeon can help.

- Briefly describe your personal situation. State how long you have struggled with obesity and describe your obesity-related health conditions. Explain that you feel that the Roux-en-Y gastric bypass surgery is medically necessary because you have already tried diets and have not been able to find a successful long-term solution for your weight. Just demonstrate that you have exhausted other options and the gastric bypass is the most promising option that is left.

- Keep your letter as short as possible. You are sending it to someone who does not know you personally and who may receive hundreds of similar letters each day. The person reading your letter may take only seconds to decide whether to pursue your appeal. You do not want your letter tossed in the garbage (or placed in the pile of rejected queries) just because it is too long. Do your best to balance the necessary information while keeping the letter short.

The Obesity Action Coalition (OAC), a good resource: The OAC is a non-profit organization whose purpose is to advocate for people with obesity. The OAC publishes a variety of educational materials that you can get for free from the OAC's website. One resource is an excellent brochure for when you are trying to figure out whether your insurance will reimburse the gastric bypass.[14] The brochure, called "Working with Your Insurance Provider: A Guide to Seeking Weight Loss Surgery," offers step-by-step guidance and tips for getting any reimbursement that your insurance plan entitles you to receive.

Medicare and Medicaid

In the U.S., the two main public health insurance systems are Medicare and Medicaid. They are run by the Centers for Medicare and Medicaid Services, or CMS, which is part of the Department of Health and Human Services. Both programs have covered bariatric surgery for years.[15] To be eligible, patients must have a BMI over 35, at least one obesity-related health condition, and a history of unsuccessful medical treatment for obesity.

Medicare is the national insurance coverage plan for individuals age 65 and older. It is designed to help with your medical bills after you retire if you have been paying into your Medicare plan during the years that you were working. Medicare also covers younger individuals with disabilities. Medicare coverage is consistent nationwide because the federal government has significant control over funding and administration.

Medicaid is a health insurance program for low-income individuals. It is a health insurance premium payment program, or HIPP, which is a type of managed care program. That means that the state government pays for you to enroll in a private insurance plan. Each state is responsible for paying for a high proportion of Medicaid to supplement the federal government's funds. Compared to Medicare, there is a lot of flexibility in each state's eligibility criteria and benefits with Medicaid. Each state has its own name for its Medicaid program. For example, California's Medicaid program is called Medi-Cal, Oregon's program is the Oregon Health Plan, Oklahoma has Soonercare, and Tennessee has TennCare. You can find the Medicaid program for your state from Medicaid's website at www.Medicaid.gov.[16]

You need to go to a qualified surgeon to receive coverage under Medicaid or Medicare. Only some surgeons meet CMS requirements for the procedure. To qualify, surgeon facilities need to have certification either as a Level 1 Bariatric Surgery Center as defined by the American College of Surgeons or as a Bariatric Surgery Center of Excellence as defined by the American Society for Bariatric Surgery. You can search for participating surgeons within your region at the CMS site.[17]

Extra Requirements for Surgery Reimbursement

You already saw the eligibility criteria for RYGB listed in Chapter 6, "*Considering Roux-En-Y Gastric Bypass? …What You Need To Know*." To qualify for reimbursement through your healthcare coverage, you may need to meet one or more of these additional requirements:

- Provide your insurance company with a Letter of Medical Necessity from your doctor.
- Lose a certain amount of weight before your surgery.
- Follow a pre-surgery diet under the supervision of your surgeon and dietitian.
- Have a psychological evaluation.
- Choose a facility with ASMBS BSCOE certification.[18]

Many of these requirements are the same as the ones that most surgeons would require you to do anyway before getting the RYB.

What Does "Cost-Effective" Mean, and How Does It Translate into Better Coverage for Bariatric Surgery?

Something that is cost-effective means that it is at least as valuable as its price. Insurance companies are interested in making profits, so they conduct cost-benefit analyses pretty much all the time to decide:

- Whether they should cover certain procedures
- Which of their customers should receive which procedures
- How much their patients' contributions should be

For example, most insurance companies cover regular physical exams. The cost-benefit analysis is likely to show that the cost to the insurance company for you to get regular blood cholesterol and blood pressure tests is way less than the cost of paying for your treatment for advanced heart disease or a stroke that might happen if you do not get the early screening tests. Therefore, screening for high cholesterol and high blood pressure is considered cost-effective.

The gastric bypass and other weight loss surgery procedures are generally considered to be cost-effective, especially as they become more common and we learn more about their effects. Researchers in one published study found that having RYGB saves thousands of dollars per patient. That is due to better overall health when you lose weight. You and your insurance company save money on so many doctor's appointments to monitor your health conditions; a bunch of medications to lower your blood pressure, cholesterol, and glucose; glucose testing kits if you had diabetes; and hospital stays if you had a serious obesity-related health condition like heart disease.

Sources:[19,20,21]

Paying Out-of-Pocket and Financing Options

Personal financing, paying out-of-pocket, and self-pay all mean the same thing: You need to pay for it yourself. You are going to have to pay a good chunk of money if:

- You do not have health insurance
- Your insurance does not cover the gastric bypass
- Your insurance only provides partial reimbursement, leaving you responsible for the rest
- Your insurance does not cover the related expenses, such as follow-up care or regular post-surgery medical tests

Is It Really That Expensive?

Now that you know how much money is going to be coming out of your own pocket, are you sure that it is worth it? It is worth it if the benefits and cost-savings are more than the cost. If you successfully lose weight with after gastric bypass, how will it save you money?

Obesity is an expensive condition, and the cost will only increase, as you remain obese. It is impossible to know the exact cost of obesity for each individual, but there are some estimates. On average, an obese person has medical costs of $1,723 per year.[22] Those are just the direct medical costs, but obesity is expensive in other ways too. Have you considered these costs:

- How much do you spend on food? If you get a lot of restaurant or prepared snacks and meals, it might be a lot more than you would like to admit.

- How much have you spent on diets? How much have you spent on diet plans, prepackaged diet food, special types of food, and diet supplements? How many times have you paid to lose the same 50 or 100 pounds? The bypass is designed to be a permanent solution if you use it well.

- How much have you spent on gym memberships and exercise equipment that you do not use?

- How much do you spend on clothing? How many times have you thrown away the larger clothes when you are dieting and thrown away the smaller clothes when you gain the weight back? How much have you spent on sets of clothing in various sizes?

- How many days of work do you have to take as vacation days because you are home sick and you have already used up all of your sick days? You may be sick so often because of your obesity.

- How much do you spend on medical bills, including trips to the doctor, medical tests, prescription medications, and other obesity-related health costs?

Life is not just about money. Even if you were not going to save money on healthcare and food costs, there is another reason to shell out a few thousand dollars for the VSG. It is your *quality of life*. Being obese is unpleasant. It makes you uncomfortable. It makes people think they have the right to look down on you. It makes you tired during the day and restless at night. You may be at the point where all you can think of is food and your body. You deserve better than that! Are you willing to pay cash for a procedure that may help you avoid these feelings and situations?

How much is being at a healthy weight worth to you? If nothing else has worked and you are willing to commit to following the healthy lifestyle changes that you will need in order to succeed with the bypass, self-pay might not seem so bad after all.

Financing Plans and Options

One self-pay option is to pay in cash or put the bypass on your credit card if you have a high enough credit limit. If this is not an option for you, there are other possibilities for payment. You can get a loan from a bank or another lending institution.

Another option is to do medical financing. This is similar to any other financing plan for a major purchase. You may have a down payment and monthly payments due for a few years until you have paid off the amount you agree on. These are a few examples of companies that offer financing plans for bariatric surgery:

- CareCredit
- Credit Medical
- Med Loan Finance
- My Medical Loan
- SurgeryLoans.com
- Surgical Services International/APF USA[23] (Advanced Patient Financing)

Some banks and credit card companies also have special programs for financing medical expenses. You can find more financing options by searching online. If you cannot tell whether they cover the gastric bypass or if you have other questions, just call them. Do not bother chasing down companies that are not easy to contact. Just go on to the next company on your list. You do not want to get started with a company that is not helpful!

Most medical facilities clinics accept one or more types of financing plans. Your surgeon's clinic may recommend a specific plan, or it may accept a variety of payment plans.

As you would whenever you sign up for financing, take personal responsibility for your money.

- Find out the upfront cost, the interest rate, and the total cost.
- Make each payment on time.
- Check how much each payment will be, and compare those amounts to your income. Do you have enough money to pay for it?
- Read the terms and conditions. Find out the interest rates and penalties for late payments.
- Consider what might happen if you have an unexpected complication with the Roux-en-Y gastric bypass. Will you be able to finance the medical care you may need *while still making* your original RYGB payments?

If you fully understand the terms of your loan plan and feel able to commit to them, the plan can be your ticket to getting bariatric surgery if you would not be able to afford it otherwise.

Medical Tourism: Going to Another Country for the RYGB

Medical tourism is what it is called when you go to another country to get a medical procedure done. Some bariatric patients from wealthier countries, such as the U.S., Canada, and European nations, choose to go to foreign nations where they can get the RYGB done cheaper. Mexico, Venezuela, and India are examples of destinations for medical tourism. Do not count on a lot of sightseeing when you go abroad for medical tourism. The whole time you are there, you will be prepping for surgery, at the hospital, and recovering from surgery.

Medical Tourism to Reduce Costs

The main reason to opt for medical tourism is to save money. You might consider it if you are not getting insurance coverage for the RYGB and you do not want to or cannot pay the price in the U.S. Mexico is an example of a nation that can offer cheaper medical services because of a lower per capita gross domestic product, or per capita GDP. The average Mexican makes less than one-third of that of the average American, and products and services tend to be cheaper in Mexico. The bypass can be thousands of dollars cheaper in Mexico than in the U.S.

All about Getting a Current Passport

If you are going abroad for your bypass, you should have a passport that is good for at least six months from the time you leave the U.S. and enter the other country. This is a recommendation for American visitors to Mexico. The U.S. Department of State provides information and instructions for renewing your old passport or getting your first one at travel.state.gov.

You need to apply in person if:

- Your previous passport was lost, stolen, or damaged.
- Your previous passport was issued more than 15 years ago.
- You have never had an American passport before.
- You are under age 16 (unlikely, but possible, for RYGB patients).

You can do the entire process by mail if *all* of these are true for you:

- Your previous passport is intact, and you still have it.
- Your previous passport is less than 15 years old.
- You are more than 16 years old.
- You have not legally changed your name since your last passport was issued.

Getting your passport takes approximately four to six weeks for regular service. You can pay for expedited service, including overnight shipping both ways, and shorten the time to two to three weeks. In either case, you can see that planning ahead is necessary to keep your RYGB surgery on schedule!

Sources:[24,25,26]

Package Deals to Make Planning Easier

Getting the Roux-en-Y gastric bypass is already a pretty big deal because it is such a life-changing event. Plus, it requires a lot of research and planning. As you have seen in this and previous chapters, for example, you need to select a surgeon and facility, get the rest of your medical team together, and figure out your financing situation. Medical tourism may be your best option, but making the necessary plans can be overwhelming. Some companies offer package deals so you do not have to make all the plans yourself.

Why Would You Get a Package Deal?

You might be interested in a package deal if one or more of these describe you:

- You do not know how to get started. Do you know what paperwork is necessary, whether your passport is current, which airport you will land at, where to stay, how you will get there, and how to get to and from the hospital—especially after surgery when you will be in no condition to start calling around for a taxi? Some people actually *do* know how to accomplish these things—but if you do not even know where to get started, a package deal might be your best bet.

- You are not an experienced traveler. Traveling on your own comfortably takes some practice. If you do not often travel, you may experience anxiety or stress at being in a foreign country with nobody to take care of things for you. This anxiety will not help your surgery go better!

- You are pretty sure you want to get your surgery done in another country, but you are not sure about how to choose a hospital that has an English-speaking staff and surgeon and performs up to American standards of care and cleanliness. A medical tourism company can act as a go-between between you and the hospital.

- You are traveling without your family but like the idea of having everything taken care of for you, from your pre-surgery and post-surgery food to having an assistant available so you are not alone.

- Your family is coming with you, and you are interested in having them entertained as part of the package deal.

Examples of Medical Tourism Bundles

You can get medical tourism bundles from a variety of private companies. Some of the more established clinics may have their own bundles that you can find out about by contacting them directly. Find a company that:

- Makes all travel arrangements for you, including to and from your destination city and within the city as you go to and from the hospital.

- Takes charge of necessary paperwork, including medical paperwork and tourist paperwork, such as passports.

- Includes all expected expenses, such as meals and regular medical tests and procedures.

MySurgeryOptions.com is an example of a medical tourism company that provides package deals for weight loss surgery in Mexico.[27] MySurgeryOptions.com will help you through the entire gastric bypass procedure.

- *Before surgery:* counsels you on surgery-related decisions, suggests surgeons for you, and makes your travel arrangements
- *During your trip to Mexico:* pre-surgery and post-surgery travel arrangements to and from the hospital
- *After your trip:* access to a support community and a trainer and nutritionist

Look for some additional features when choosing a company to help you plan your RYGB in Mexico. MySurgeryOptions.com, for example, has these benefits:

- A lowest-price guarantee for the package you choose
- Visits by the staff to each surgeon and facility in Mexico that belongs to the network
- 24/7 availability by phone or email during your trip
- Continued support after surgery

When you purchase a package deal for medical tourism, you will need to pay for any non-included expenses, such as the cost of medical care from unexpected complications. You will also need to pay extra if you stay in a hospital or a patient recovery house longer than the originally expected length of time.

Investigating International Locations for Your Surgery

If you are getting the bypass done outside the U.S., your facility will not be accredited by the ACS and ASMBS. Instead, to find a quality facility, check for International Centers of Excellence, or ICE, as designated by the Surgical Review Corporation[28]. International Centers of Excellence must meet 10 requirements:

1. *Institutional commitment to excellence:* Hospitals show their commitment to excellence and dedication to improvement by defining surgery guidelines for their programs.
2. *Surgical experience and volumes:* Surgeons that lead bariatric surgeries at the center must have completed at least 25 bariatric surgeries in their lifetimes.
3. *Designated medical director:* This ensures that there is always a specific person overseeing the bariatric program and maintaining standards.
4. *Responsive critical care support:* Hospitals need to be ready to respond to any medical emergency.
5. *Appropriate equipment and instruments:* This may mean purchasing new, larger-sized equipment and instruments to safely and accommodate extremely obese patients.
6. *Surgeon dedication and qualified call coverage*: Surgeons show their dedication by becoming certified by a respected organization.

7. *Clinical pathways and standardized operation procedures*: Hospitals should include programs such as pain management, patient instruction and evaluation, research, or pre-surgery workups.

8. *Bariatric nurses, physician extenders, and program coordinator:* These staff members ensure that the bariatric program remains focused on weight loss surgery and meets patient needs.

9. *Patient support groups:* These are almost indispensible for success. Support groups keep you motivated, provide information, and demonstrate the surgeon and facility's commitment to you.

10. *Long-term patient follow-up, including BOLD*: Long-term follow-up helps improve your weight loss by keeping you accountable for longer after the surgery. The Bariatric Outcomes Longitudinal Database is the world's largest database of bariatric surgery patients.[29] Publicly reporting patient results to BOLD gives hospitals and surgeons an extra incentive to work hard for your weight loss success.

Being unable to evaluate a facility's quality can make your RYGB in another country more stressful. The ICE designation can help you increase your confidence in your choice because you know that the facility is experienced, well-equipped, and well-staffed.

Similarly, you can check to see whether the surgeon you are considering has a Bariatric Surgeon of Excellence, or BSOE designation.[30] Surgeons who have this have completed 125 weight loss surgeries in their lifetime and at least 100 of these surgeries per year. They comply with the requirements of ICE hospitals too.

Additional Advice for Choosing a Surgeon and Clinic

If you are getting your RYGB in Mexico, you probably will not be able to meet your surgeon in person before arriving at your destination city, such as Baja, California, Mexico City, or Tijuana. Instead of being able to use your own instinct when choosing a surgeon, you will have to depend more heavily on the surgeon's qualifications and other people's recommendations. In addition to the guidelines listed above, here are a few more tips for choosing a surgeon without meeting him or her first:

- Ask all of your questions. This might take a lot of emailing back and forth, but your surgeon should be willing and able to clearly answer your questions without evading any of them.

- Ask about travel arrangements and what happens in case of unforeseen complications that force you to stay in the hospital a little longer than planned.

- Get recommendations from people who have had the bariatric surgery done during a medical tourism experience. They can provide names of medical tourism companies and surgeons.

- Once you have narrowed down your search to a few surgeons, ask them if you can contact some of their RYGB patients. They should be willing to do this for you.

BariatricPal.com: An Unbiased Source for Surgeon Information

Unbiased opinions are valuable when you are considering medical tourism and you are looking for a surgeon in another country. BariatricPal.com is a community dedicated to the weight loss surgery community. Many of its members have chosen to get bariatric surgery done in a foreign nation. Their experiences, surgeon reviews, and recommendations can help you make your own decisions with more confidence.

When you visit the site and look at the main page of discussion topics, you will notice an area that is dedicated to discussions among special groups. These discussions are open to the public, but they are more focused than the general discussions on the board. Among the special groups is an entire forum dedicated to self-pay and medical tourism RYGB patients. Everyone is welcome to join the conversations and ask their own questions.

Considerations with Medical Tourism

Medical tourism can be a great solution to high costs in the U.S., but there are some additional things to think about before you make your choice and as you plan your trip. Consider an English-speaking facility, your personal safety, what to pack, and how to choose a surgeon in another nation.

Potential for Language Barriers

If your Spanish is not fluent, you will be depending on your caregivers to speak English so that you can communicate. So many Americans go south for the bypass that this may not be a problem; many surgeons and their clinics promise that you will not encounter any language barriers during your entire experience because of their fluency in English. Furthermore, many surgeons that participate in medical tourism were originally Americans, so they and some of their staff may be native English speakers.

Do Not Depend on Your High School Spanish!

You may have been a star Spanish student in high school, but do not depend on those skills unless you have continually practiced speaking it since then. Even if you do remember as much as you think, you may have trouble being clear and understanding well when you are under a stressful situation, such as being in the hospital for the gastric bypass.

A simple step to make sure you will be able to communicate when you are at the clinic is to call the facility on the phone or use an inexpensive online service, such as Skype. The person answering the phone should have no trouble understanding you or speaking in English; if he or she does, you should be able to be connected within seconds to someone who is fluent. If not, it is probably not worth your while to consider that hospital or clinic for your surgery.

Even if the front desk sounds convincingly fluent, it can be a challenge to figure out exactly how great the language barrier will be. It is possible that everyone from the nurses to your surgeon to the driver of your shuttle to your hotel will speak perfect English. On the other hand, it is possible that only the surgeon and the receptionist, who might be your only contacts before you go to the clinic, are fluent in English. The other staff, such as the nurses and anesthesiologist, might not speak English. That can be a problem if you have urgent needs while you are under their care. To protect yourself, ask your contacts at the clinic whether everyone at the clinic speaks English. If not, ask whether there is always a translator available at a moment's notice.

Safety in Foreign Countries

Mexico has a high crime rate. Drugs and street crime in drug-ridden rural areas often make the news. Although big cities and regions with tourist attractions are generally safer, the U.S. Department of State warns travelers to be aware of their surroundings and the potential for crime. 31 A travel warning, inspired by increases in kidnappings, drug-related violence, and murders, was issued in November of 2012.[32]

Complication Rates and Medical Tourism

You always have a risk for complications when you get the gastric bypass. Your complications may be higher when you go abroad for your procedure in a nation that is not as wealthy as the U.S. Facilities might not be as up-to-date or hygienic as in the U.S., and that can increase your risk for complications during or after your procedure. Some research shows that there are more complications among patients that choose medical tourism for bariatric surgery, although there are certainly a high number of perfectly safe clinics abroad.[33]

Physical Challenges of Travel

Regardless of how easy the trip is or how nice the accommodations are, the truth is that traveling is tough on your body. Almost everyone sleeps better in their own beds compared to even the nicest of luxury hotels. You might have jet lag or extra anxiety making you tired and putting you at risk for getting infected. A minor infection, such as the common cold, makes your immune system work harder and can make your recovery from surgery more challenging.

Traveler's diarrhea is another challenge to your body when you are doing medical tourism. Between 30 and 70 percent of all tourists to foreign nations get some form of traveler's diarrhea.[34] Along with diarrhea, you might also have symptoms of vomiting, bloating, and stomach pain. These are especially unpleasant when your body is already fighting hard to recover from the RYGB and effects of anesthesia during surgery.

Post-Surgery Care and Medical Tourism

You will not likely be able to see your surgeon during your aftercare program if your surgeon lives in another country. Be sure that your post-surgery care is arranged before you get the bypass. You might end up participating in a local surgeon's care program that includes appointments and support group meetings. Your surgeon in Mexico or the company that you choose for your medical tourism package should be able to help you find a surgeon that will accept you as a patient and treat you as well as if you got your gastric bypass in the U.S. It is absolutely necessary that you have someone near your home to go to for emergencies.

What Is Montezuma's Revenge, and How You Can Protect Yourself from It?

You have probably heard of Montezuma's revenge to describe the severe traveler's diarrhea that many travelers to Mexico get. Montezuma's revenge is a reference to the Aztec emperor who was in power when the Spanish Conquistadors arrived in Mexico in the early sixteenth century. The Spanish conquered the Aztecs but came down with severe diarrhea, which was attributed to Mexican gods taking revenge on the Christian Spaniards.

In reality, Montezuma's revenge is a disease caused by bacteria in contaminated food or water. The most common bacteria to cause it are E. coli, Campylobacter jejuni, Shigella, and Salmonella. You can get Montezuma's revenge, or traveler's diarrhea, anywhere, not just in Mexico. It can prevent you from doing much of anything for a full 24 hours as you fight the nausea and other symptoms. It leaves you feeling exhausted. How can you prevent traveler's diarrhea, especially around the time of your important surgery:

- Choose your foods carefully. Most traveler's diarrhea comes from improper handling techniques in restaurants. You might be better off using your hotel's food service or the hospital cafeteria instead of eating the local cuisine at restaurants or from street vendors. Avoid fresh fruits and vegetables, which should not be much of a problem because they are not part of your post-surgery recovery diet.

- Avoid tap water. Since you will be on a liquid diet for much of your time in Mexico, this one is pretty important. Be sure to boil your water or use bottled water instead of tap water. Watch out for potential sources of tap water, such as ice cubes.

- Wash your hands. This simple trick can prevent a lot of infections. Wash your hands or use a sanitizer after going to the bathroom, before eating, and whenever you touch a surface that may be dirty. A hand sanitizer should contain at least 60 percent alcohol.

✍ Summary

☛ This chapter covered the cost of the Roux-en-Y gastric bypass. You may get reimbursed by your health insurance, or you may be stuck paying for the entire RYGB yourself. If you need a finance plan to be able to afford the bypass right now, many are available to choose from.

☛ Also, you can opt for medical tourism as a cheaper option to self-pay in the U.S. Now that you have been hit with some of the cold hard cash figures, it is another time to reconsider whether the cost of the RYGB seems worth it to you. If it is, full speed ahead! The next chapter covers your preparations for the actual surgery as the time get closer.

Time to Take Action: Paying for the Bypass

This chapter talked about paying for the bypass with or without the help of insurance coverage. This worksheet can guide you as you figure out your own payment options.

Will your insurance cover the sleeve? YES / NO

If yes, what other expenses remain? These might include things such as dietitian appointments and additional lab work.

If no, will your insurance cover any part related? YES / NO

How much will you need to pay out of pocket?

Is the surgery worth it to you? YES / NO

Can you afford cash or do you need financing?

How much can you afford to pay each month?

RYGB Patient Story: Aleysia

Aleysia is a single mother with a 16-year-old boy and a 10-year-old girl. She works as a registered nurse (RN) on a Women's Unit. She got Roux-en-Y gastric bypass at the age of 36 after being uncomfortable with her weight for 20 years. Down 50 pounds from her pre-surgery weight of 397 pounds, Aleysia is still towards the beginning of her weight loss journey. This is her story so far.

On Her Weight Gain and Decision to Get RYGB

I have been overweight since I hit puberty or shortly thereafter. In fact, I do not remember not being overweight, though my parents have pictures where I wasn't. The first time I actually felt "fat" was when we were at Disney World when I was 16. I saw a sign on one of the coasters that said, "May not accommodate persons of larger size." I suddenly got scared and refused to go on the coaster. I never rode one again until last summer. It seems crazy, because I wasn't "too fat" at that point.

I gained a bunch of weight with both of my pregnancies, and my weight has been on a roller coaster ever since. I gain and I lose. My weight hit a personal high after my daughter was born and skyrocketed further when my husband left. By the time my daughter was 7, I was 430 pounds – but it may have been higher, since I avoided scales. I used MyFitnessPal and lost at least 50 pounds. But I got lazy and went back to around 400. By this time, my blood pressure was out of control, and I was an insulin-dependent diabetic. Walking from my car to the elevator at work got me out of breath, and I was on a fast road to my grave. I decided that I needed gastric bypass or I wasn't going to see my kids grow up.

On Her Weight Loss and Challenges So Far

On surgery day I weighed in at 397 pounds. I am now 10 weeks out and 50 pounds down. This is the least I have weighed since the day my daughter was born, and I am ecstatic. I have passed my first goal of being under 350, and my goal at this point is to get below 300. I can't look at the long term. It is too daunting. Slow and steady will win my race.

That's not to say that it's been without issue. I had horrid pain issues; they were all muscular, not from the gas from surgery. I know that it wasn't a major complication, but for five weeks I was in pain that made me cry and yelp out when I had to be in a sitting position for even a second. I felt like I was going nuts, but all that is behind me. Even having suffered the pain, I would do it again in an instant.

On the Benefits She's Noticed

I know that I have made great strides already. I am off all my medications now. My blood sugars are within normal ranges, with the highest being 150 mg/dl right after I eat. I can walk very quickly from my car and into the hospital to get on the elevator to my nursing unit without getting winded. My crazy coworkers think I should take the stairs to the eleventh floor with them. Now, I'd be dead by the third floor, but maybe someday I will be able to go with them!

On Earning Her Father's Approval and Other "A-ha!" Moments

My dad was dead set against my surgery because he knew someone who died from complications of this surgery. Any time I would ask him to be more specific, he would get very angry and think I was belittling his friend's death. He has since come around, and "Mr. Against It" has even contributed to one of my three best "a-ha!" moments at this point after surgery. What happened was that he made me laugh when he told me that my butt was getting much smaller! My dad is a man of few words, and his presentation of his idea of a compliment was hysterical but very much appreciated.

Another "a-ha!" was my daughter laying in bed with me and telling me all the things on my body that had gotten smaller since surgery. The third "a-ha!" moment was yesterday at the hospital when my mom said, "I can't believe I'm saying these words, but Aleysia, you need to slow down. You're walking too fast for me."

Her Advice for Other RYGB Patients

Stick to your guns. Do what's best for you and not someone else. Don't let others' biases influence your outcomes. The journey may not always be easy or smooth, but in the end, it will all be worth it.

1   FAIR Health, Inc. Fair Health Consumer Cost Lookup. Web site. http://fairhealthconsumer.org/. Copyright 2012. Accessed February 6, 2013.

2   Compare inpatient hospital costs and prices – by hospital name. Consumer Health Ratings. Web site. http://www.consumerhealthratings.com/index.php?action=showSubCats&cat_id=233. Accessed February 6, 2013.

3   Common surgeries and charges comparison. California Office of Statewide Health Planning and Development. Web site. http://www.oshpd.ca.gov/commonsurgery/Default.aspx. Accessed February 6, 2013.

4   Mosti M, Dominequez , Herrerra MF. Calculating surgical costs: how accurate and predictable is the cost of a laparoscopic Roux-en-Y gastric bypass? Obes Surgery, 2007;17(12):1555-7.

5   Picot J, Jones J, Colquitt JL, Gospodarevskaya E, Loveman E, Baxter L, Clegg AJ. The clinical effectiveness and cost-effectiveness of bariatric (weight loss) surgery for obesity: a systematic review and economic evaluation. Health Technology Assessment, 2009;13:1-90.

6   National coverage determination (NCD) for bariatric surgery for treatment of morbid obesity (100.1). Centers for Medicare and Medicaid Services. Web site. http://www.cms.gov/medicare-coverage-database/details/ncd-details.aspx?NCDId=57&ncdver=4&bc=AAAAgAAAAQAAAA%3d%3d&. Reviewed 2012, June. Accessed February 6, 2013.

7   Clinical policy bulletin: obesity surgery. Aetna Inc. web site. http://www.aetna.com/cpb/medical/data/100_199/0157.html. Reviewed 2012, December 28. February 6, 2013.

8   Bariatric surgery. United Healthcare. https://www.unitedhealthcareonline.com/ccmcontent/ProviderII/UHC/en-US/Assets/ProviderStaticFiles/ProviderStaticFilesPdf/Tools%20and%20Resources/Policies%20and%20Protocols/Medical%20Policies/Medical%20Policies/Bariatric_Surgery.pdf. Effective 2012, December 1. Accessed February 6, 2013.

9   Faria GR, Preto JR, Costa-Maia J. Gastric bypass is a cost-saving procedure: results from a comprehensive Markov Model. Obes Surg, 2013.

10   American Society for Metabolic and Bariatric Surgery. National insurance coverage map. Web site. http://asmbs.org/2011/12/national-insurance-coverage-map/. 2011, December. Accessed September 26, 2012.

11   Clinical policy bulletin: obesity surgery. Aetna Inc. web site. http://www.aetna.com/cpb/medical/data/100_199/0157.html. Reviewed 2012, December 28. February 6, 2013.

12   American Medical Association. CPT – current procedural terminology. Web site. http://www.ama-assn.org/ama/pub/physician-resources/solutions-managing-your-practice/coding-billing-insurance/cpt.page. 2012. Accessed September 27, 2012.

13   Kaplan LM, Seeley RJ. Myths associated with obesity and bariatric surgery: myth 1: weight can be reliably controlled by voluntarily adjusting energy balance through diet and exercise. Bariatric Times. Mars Initiative Series. http://bariatrictimes.com/2012/04/18/myths-associated-with-obesity-and-bariatric-surgery/. 2012. 9(4):12-13. Accessed September 27, 2012.

14   Obesity Action Coalition. Working with your insurance provider: a guide to seeking weight loss surgery. Web site. http://www.obesityaction.org/educational-resources/brochures-and-guides/oac-insurance-guide/reviewing-your-insurance-policy-or-employer-sponsored-medical-benefits-plan. 2009. Accessed September 27, 2012.

15   National coverage determination (NCD) for bariatric surgery for treatment of morbid obesity (100.1). Centers for Medicare and Medicaid Services. Web site. http://www.cms.gov/medicare-coverage-database/details/ncd-details.aspx?NCDId=57&ncdver=4&bc=AAAAgAAAAQAAAA%3d%3d&. Reviewed 2012, June. Accessed February 6, 2013.

16   Medicaid. Medical enrollment by state. Centers for Medicare and Medicaid Services, Department of Health and Human Services. http://www.medicaid.gov/Medicaid-CHIP-Program-Information/By-State/By-State.html. Accessed September 27, 2012.

17   Centers for Medicare and Medicaid Services. Bariatric surgery. Department of Health and Human Services. http://www.cms.gov/Medicare/Medicare-General-Information/MedicareApprovedFacilitie/Bariatric-Surgery.html. 2012. Accessed September 27, 2012.

18   American Society for Metabolic and Bariatric Surgery. ASMBS BSCOE Benefits. Web site. http://asmbs.org/wp-content/uploads/asmbs_bscoe_benefits1.pdf. September 20, 2012.

19   Picot J, Jones J, Colquitt JL, Gospodarevskaya E, Loveman E, Baxter L., Clegg AJ. The clinical effectiveness and cost-effectiveness of bariatric (weight loss) surgery for obesity: a systematic review and economic evaluation. Health Technology Assessment, 2009;13:1-90.

20   Maklin S, Malmivaara A, Linna M, Victorzon M, Koivukangas V, Sintonen H. Cost-utility of bariatric surgery for morbid obesity in Finland. Br J Surg. 2011;98(1):1422-9.

21   Faria GR, Preto JR, Costa-Maia J. Gastric bypass is a cost-saving procedure: results from a comprehensive Markov Model. Obes Surg, 2013.

22   Tsai AG, Williamson DF, Glick HA. Direct medical cost of overweight and obesity in the USA: a quantitative systematic review. 2011;12(1):50-61.

23   Frequently asked questions. Surgical Services International, Inc. Web site. http://www.surgicalservicesinternational.com/faq.htm. 2005. Accessed September 17, 2012.

24   Renew passport. U.S. Department of State. Web site. http://www.travel.state.gov/passport/renew/renew_833.html. Accessed October 2, 2012.

25 First-time applicants. U.S. Department of State. Web site. http://www.travel.state.gov/passport/get/first/first_830.html. Accessed October 2, 2012.

26 Processing times. U.S. Department of State. Web site. http://www.travel.state.gov/passport/processing/processing_1740.html. Accessed October 2, 2012.

27 MySurgeryOptions.com. web site. http://mysurgeryoptions.com/. Accessed February 8, 2013.

28 Surgical Review Corporation. ICE designation requirements. Web site. http://www.surgicalreview.org/ice/requirements/. Accessed September 20, 2012.

29 Surgical Review Corporation. BOLD overview. Web site. http://www.surgicalreview.org/bold/overview/. Accessed September 22, 2012.

30 Surgical Review Corporation. Bariatric Surgeon of Excellence Program. Web site. http://www.surgicalreview.org/international/bsoe/. Accessed September 20, 2012.

31 Mexico: Country Specific Information. U.S. Department of State. Web site. http://travel.state.gov/travel/cis_pa_tw/cis/cis_970.html. Accessed September 17, 2012.

32 Travel Warning. Bureau of Consular Affairs, US Department of State. Web site. http://travel.state.gov/travel/cis_pa_tw/tw/tw_5815.html. 2012, November 20. Accessed February 8, 2013.

33 Birch, D.W., Vu, L., Karmali, S., Stoklassa, C.J., & Sharma, A.M. (2010). Medical tourism in bariatric surgery. *American Journal of Surgery*, 5: 604-8.

34 Connor, B.A. Chapter 2: The pre-travel consultation: self-treatable conditions: traveler's diarrhea. Yellow Book, Centers for Disease Control and Prevention: Atlanta, GA. Retrieved from http://wwwnc.cdc.gov/travel/yellowbook/2012/chapter-2-the-pre-travel-consultation/travelers-diarrhea.htm. Updated 2012, February 9. Accessed September 28, 2012.

9

Pre-Surgery Tips

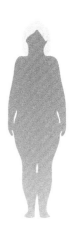

The last couple of chapters have taken you from considering the bypass to thinking about how you are going to make it a reality. You have your surgeon and medical team all picked out, and you know how you are going to pay for the surgery. You can really start to feel as though your life is changing as your surgery approaches.

This chapter will take you through the weeks or months of pre-surgery preparation that you will need. This is some of the information that is in the chapter:

- Medical appointments before your surgery: surgeon, dietitian, and psychologist
- Medical tests to determine that surgery is as safe as possible for you
- Getting your psychological evaluation
- Meeting with the dietitian and following the pre-surgery diet
- Scheduling your surgery within your busy schedule

By the end of the chapter, you will know what to expect in the weeks and months before the RYGB procedure. This information will keep you right on track with these early stages of your weight loss journey. It is time to get going!

How to Prepare For Your Pre-Op Appointment

Your surgery date is likely to be a few weeks or months from when you make the final decision about getting the gastric bypass. During this time, you will probably have one lengthy pre-surgery appointment with your surgeon. It is a chance for you to ask all of your additional questions and clarify anything you do not understand. Your surgeon will be able to verify that you are a good candidate for the procedure before setting a date for surgery. From now on, you will be working closely with your surgeon. It is critical to establish mutual trust and have good two-way communication.

Questions That Your Surgeon Might Ask

Your pre-surgery appointment should include a long conversation with your surgeon. The most likely questions that your surgeon will ask are about your medical history. This includes past doctor's visits, test results, and medical treatment, plus current health conditions and treatments, including prescription medications.

If you are in a managed care plan, such as an HMO, a PPO, or Medicare, your medical information should be available on electronic health records, also known as EHR or e-records.[1] That means your surgeon and any of your other caregivers who need to know your medical history can access it on the computer from a single, secure database.

You may be asked to fill out a medical history form before coming to the clinic or in the waiting room before your appointment. The form may ask questions that are designed specifically for weight loss surgery candidates. These are some examples:

- Do you tend to throw up easily?
- Do many tastes and smells make you feel nauseous?
- How high is your pain tolerance? Are you more or less sensitive to pain than other people?

These questions help predict your recovery from the RYGB and ongoing weight loss success.

Your surgeon might ask follow-up questions on any unexpected or unusual answers or information from your medical history. Answers that stand out from the rest don't automatically disqualify you from getting the bypass. Instead, they are more likely to give your surgeon and the rest of your medical team some guidance in personalizing your pre-surgery preparation program.

Tips for Preparing for Your Pre-Op Appointment

You do not want to run out of time or forget to ask your surgeon something important, so prepare for your appointment! Gather all that you can about your personal medical history and write it down so you can take it to your surgeon. A personal health record, or PHR, is a great way to store your medical information. It is like an EHR, but it is for your own personal use. Your healthcare provider likely offers one and can help you set it up.

Research your family's medical history. You cannot learn every detail about your parents and grandparents, but any information that you are able to find can be helpful for you and your surgeon.

Do not rely on your memory! Instead, write down everything you want to cover during your pre-op surgeon's appointment even if you are not usually a "list" person. You do not want to accidentally forget to ask your surgeon something just because you are feeling nervous, excited, pressured, or distracted at your appointment. These are some of the topics that you might want to ask your surgeon about:

- *A review of the Roux-en-Y gastric bypass:* You may know the physiology of the procedure pretty well by now from your research and from seeing a surgeon explain it using a lifelike model during a seminar. However, having your own surgeon explain the procedure can solidify the details in your mind. This explanation also lets you ask questions during the explanation, which may not have been possible at a large group seminar.

- *"What if…"* You can ask about the "what-ifs" that have been bothering you. What if something goes wrong during surgery? What if you have complications? What if you need care in the middle of the night? What if you have trouble while you are on vacation? Get all of your worries addressed so that you can be confident going into surgery. Your surgeon should be willing to patiently respond to all of your worries and be able to respond to your doubts. Keep asking until you are satisfied. If your surgeon is not able to respond sufficiently, you might want to consider switching to another surgeon.

- *Medical conditions:* Even if you have talked about them before, you want to be absolutely certain that you cover everything and give your surgeon time to consider each condition carefully.

- *Over-the-counter and prescription medications:* Your medications can interfere you're your nutritional status, and your surgeon should know about them. Another important point is that you will not be eating solid foods right after your surgery, so you will not be able to take your regular pills or capsules. Ask your doctor whether your medications are available in liquid, gel, or powder form. Another option is to grind up medications that are in hard pill forms and dissolve them in water so that you can absorb them. Your surgeon should be able to figure out how you will take your medications after surgery.

- *Dietary supplements, such as vitamins, minerals, and herbal supplements:* You are not going to be eating much during the first days, weeks, and even months after getting the RYGB. Dietary supplements help you meet your nutrient needs, but you will not be able to take whole pills or capsules right after surgery. As with medications, multivitamins in gel, powder, or liquid form are viable options. You also want to ask about herbal and other supplements to make sure they will not interfere with your surgery or recovery.

- *Birth control:* If you are currently taking oral contraceptives, now is a good time to discuss alternative methods. You might not be allowed to take oral contraceptives for the first few weeks or months after your gastric bypass. Your focus after getting weight loss surgery should be on weight loss, and most surgeons will recommend waiting for at least 12 to 18 months before trying to get pregnant.[2]

Setting the Date of Your Gastric Bypass

You and your surgeon might set the date of your gastric bypass at your pre-surgery appointment. The surgery needs to be at least a few weeks away to give you time to prepare, and it may be a few months away. These are some factor that can affect when your surgery will be:

- *Pre-surgery diet:* At a minimum, you will need to follow a liquid diet for a few days before surgery. Many patients follow a weight loss diet for a few weeks before surgery. The weight loss and liquid diet make your liver a little smaller to make it easier for your surgeon to see your stomach and esophagus during surgery; this reduces the risk of complications.[3] Your pre-surgery diet may be even longer if your health insurance requires it.

- *Your work schedule:* You may be able to return to work one to two days after your bypass procedure; you will have to wait longer if you have complications or if your job is physically demanding. If possible, schedule surgery for a time when your work schedule is expected to be a little less hectic than normal. Avoid scheduling your gastric bypass during or before conferences or important work events. In addition to missing work time for surgery and recovery, you will want to have the option, after returning to work, of taking an afternoon or day off of work without getting behind. The RYGB can make you miss work time when you feel nauseous or have surgeon appointments.

- *Your personal schedule:* Minimize the interference with your personal life. If you are a parent, you might want to get the gastric bypass during the school year so that your children are away for most of the day. If you are a schoolteacher or an adolescent, it is probably best to set your date at the end of the school year, right before your summer vacation. That will give you time to adjust to your new eating plan and get over the worst of the side effects before going back to school. Take a look at your calendar and make sure your surgery will not interfere with any big events, like a friend's wedding or a major anniversary party. Of course, these considerations with your personal schedule are not always practical, and that is okay. The RYGB is a medical procedure that you can fit into your life no matter what if necessary.

- *Facility availability:* Often hospitals and clinics fill up their bariatric surgery schedules months ahead of time. There is not much you can do about that, and you will just have to work with the appointment scheduling center to get the soonest possible appointment that works for you. As with other appointments and medical procedures, you might be able to get on a waiting list to be called in case there is a cancellation ahead of you and an appointment slot opens up.

- *Medical tourism:* There is a lot of planning to do if you are going to Mexico for your Roux-en-Y gastric bypass. Americans do not need a special visa to visit Mexico for the short time that you will need to stay to get the bypass and to recover,[4] but you do need a current passport. As you schedule your surgery date, keep in mind that your passport renewal can take several weeks. You will also have to plan for time off of work and schedule your transportation and hotel accommodations if you are making your own arrangements rather than purchasing an all-inclusive package deal for your surgery. Travel can be a lot cheaper during the off-season and when you make arrangements far in advance.

You might have to wait a few months to meet all of the requirements and get your RYGB surgery done. That can seem like a long time, but the long waiting period has its benefits:

- You have more time to try out the weight loss surgery diet and lifestyle.
- You have more time to do research on the bypass so you know what to expect.
- You can lose a little extra weight before surgery to reduce your risk for complications during and after surgery.

Reminder: It Is Not Too Late to Change Your Surgeon

We want to remind you that it is not too late to change your surgeon. You can change your surgeon at any point up until you go in for surgery. Even after surgery, you can change your surgeon if you feel you are not getting the right aftercare, and you can find another surgeon who will give you the post-surgery guidance you need.

Of course it is easier if you choose the right surgeon for you on your first try, but these are some reasons why you might want to change your surgeon:

- Your surgeon makes you feel uncomfortable when you are asking questions.
- Your surgeon does not give satisfactory answers to your questions.
- You simply do not have a good feeling about your surgeon.

- Your surgeon does not seem concerned about your personal success and individual concerns.

Do not worry about losing the time and effort that you have already put in toward the surgery. All of your research on RYGB is still useful. If you already got medical tests done under your old surgeon, your new surgeon will probably accept most or all of the medical tests, dietary assessments, and psychological evaluations that you have gone through.

We are not encouraging you to actively *look* for reasons to change your surgeon, but we do want to remind you that you are still in control of your own health and always should be. Some patients mistakenly think that they are stuck with a surgeon who does not turn out to be as good as hoped for based on their first impressions. That is absolutely not the case!

Why a Chest X-ray?

It is very important to make sure that your heart and lungs are healthy enough to undergo the laparoscopic or open gastric bypass gastrectomy. Chapter 3, "All About the Roux-En-Y Gastric Bypass (RYGB)," describes the pneumoperitonuem, or air pumped into your abdominal cavity. Chest and heart conditions, or cardiopulmonary diseases, can make a laparoscopic procedure dangerous, so you may need the open procedure instead. Certain conditions can make any surgery too high of a risk to be recommended.

Likely Medical Tests

It is a long list…but the tests are not as bad as they sound! They are necessary for making sure that you are a good candidate for surgery. A lot of them are routine tests that you have had before; they are just checks to make sure your body is working normally and can handle the surgery.

Some of the Medical Tests

These are some of the tests that you might have done:

- *Ultrasound of your gallbladder:* Rapid weight loss after surgery increases your risk of developing gallstones and makes existing gallstones worse. If the ultrasound detects that you already have gallstones, your surgeon might decide to remove your gallbladder during surgery to prevent the need for a second surgery to remove your gallbladder, known as a cholecystectomy.

- *Gastrointestinal x-rays:* This series of x-rays can verify that your gastrointestinal system has normal physiology; that is, that everything is in the right place. It is helpful for your surgeon to know whether everything is in the usual place before starting the surgery. If you have minor abnormalities, your surgeon can prepare for the surgery better and figure out whether to make different cuts on you compared to on other patients.

- *Electrocardiogram, or EKG, or ECG:* This test gives you a line graph of alternating peaks and valleys that may look familiar. Each cycle on an ECG graph represents a heartbeat, and it gives a cardiologist a lot of information about your heart function. You get an ECG when a technician sticks some stickers (called leads, or electrodes, if you are curious) onto the front and maybe back of your torso. Some wires are clipped to the stickers and placed in the ECG reader. The graph of your ECG shows up on the screen within minutes so the technician or doctor can look at them.

- *Chest x-ray:* An abnormal chest x-ray or sleep apnea, asthma, or shortness of breath can indicate trouble with your lungs. If you have these symptoms, you might be given additional lung tests, such as a chest CAT scan to give a more detailed image of your lungs, an oximetry or arterial blood oxygenation test to measure the amount of oxygen getting from your lungs to your blood, or a spirometry test, which assesses how much and how strongly you can breathe. You may need to see a pulmonologist, or lung specialist, for further testing. Lung function is important because your lungs need to work harder during the laparoscopic procedure.

Likely Blood Tests

You will have an extensive panel of blood tests, known as a metabolic panel. Almost everyone is used to getting these done—you just need to go to the lab and have your blood drawn. The doctor who orders the tests or a nurse will tell you whether you need to get the tests done in the morning after an overnight fast. If you forget what the instructions are, just call the lab the day before you are planning to get your blood drawn and ask whether you need to fast. The metabolic panel is a basic set of tests that you have probably had a million times before and probably never looked twice at the results. Chances are, you will not need to look twice at the results now either. Your tests will probably include some or all of the following:[5]

- *Blood sugar, or blood glucose, test:* If you get your blood sugar or glucose tested regularly, you might already know whether you are normal, pre-diabetic, or diabetic. If this test shows that your blood sugar is higher than you thought, you will be especially motivated to lose weight if you have diabetes. That way, you can start treatment for it with a better diet and possibly medications.

- *Carbon dioxide (CO_2)[6] and/or calcium test:* These tests measure acid-base balance in your body. Abnormal results can mean that you are having trouble with your kidneys, that you have uncontrolled diabetes, or that your lungs are not functioning well.

Tip

What about Calcium?

A blood calcium test does not reflect the amount of calcium you get from your diet. No simple blood test can measure that. The best way to make sure that your calcium intake is adequate is to count up the amount of calcium you are getting from your diet and supplements. We will go over your daily calcium requirements and good sources of calcium in **Chapter 14, "RYGB Diet 101."**

- *Serum electrolytes:* Electrolytes maintain fluid balance in your body and include sodium, chloride, and potassium.[7] If your electrolytes are out of whack, you could be dehydrated, have high blood pressure, or have trouble with your liver, kidneys, lungs, or heart.

- Kidney tests: Blood urea nitrogen, or BUN, and creatinine tests are common for checking kidney health.[8,9] Your kidneys act as filters for your blood, and one of their jobs is to make sure that you do not have too much protein (estimated by measuring creatinine or nitrogen) staying in your blood. BUN is related to protein in your body, and the test does not tell you how much protein you get in your diet.

- *Liver function tests:* Your blood levels of aspartate aminotranferase, or AST, and alanine transaminase, or ALT, tell your doctor how well your liver is working.[10,11]

- *Nutrient status:* Your surgeon might order a few tests to see whether you are eating enough of key nutrients. These may include thiamin, or vitamin B-1, iron, folic acid, vitamin B-12, and vitamin D. These tests will probably become part of your regular routine after your gastric bypass surgery because you are at higher risk for deficiencies of those nutrients.[12]

You will have the tests done before your pre-op appointment so that you can go over the results with your surgeon. Do not be alarmed if one or more of your values comes back abnormal. It probably does not indicate a serious health problem, and it does not necessarily mean you cannot get the bypass. Often your surgeon or primary care physician should figure out the cause of the out-of-range values and tailor your care if necessary.

Psychological Evaluation

Most surgeons require a psychological evaluation before doing bariatric surgeries. If your healthcare coverage covers the RYGB, your insurance company may require the evaluation as a condition for reimbursement, especially if you have a history of psychiatric disorders.13 The psychologist and your health team want to be sure that you are mentally and emotionally ready for surgery and beyond since you are going to have to make drastic, long-term changes to achieve and maintain weight loss.

A lot of us naturally fear psychological evaluations because it conjures up thoughts of a mysterious person reading your mind and uncovering deep, dark secrets that you did not even know you had. That is not even close to the truth! In fact, psych evaluations are not that scary, and getting them done does not mean you are weird. The tests are nothing to worry about, and you might even find them kind of fun.

What Are Mental Health Professionals Looking for During Your Evaluation?

These are some of the things that the psych evaluation checks:

- *Your mental preparedness:* The bypass is just a tool, and weight loss requires changes in your diet. Furthermore, you should be prepared to make a lifelong commitment.

- *Your support system:* To make sure that you have a support system in place, your psychologist may ask you about the role that your friends and family members play in your life and where else you go for support. If you have gotten involved on BariatricPal. com, you will have plenty to talk about when the psychologist asks about your support system!

- *Your mental stability:* Untreated mood disorders and other uncontrolled psychological disorders can make it more difficult to cope with changes in your life, such as getting the bypass and making dramatic lifestyle changes. Losing weight brings its own set of changes, such as how you feel and how others treat you. Mental stability helps you overcome the challenges that you will almost certainly encounter.

- *Your maturity:* Adolescents are still gaining emotional maturity. Only adolescents who are mature for their ages are good candidates for RYGB. You need to understand that the procedure will change your life. You will always have to be careful about what you eat. You will not be able to eat the same things as your friends; there will be days when you do not feel well and may need to skip school, and every day of your life you will probably have to face forbidden foods at school, home and, when you are older, at work.

- *Binge eating disorder and emotional eating:*[14] Binge eating is when you eat abnormally large amounts of food in short periods of time. You may feel out of control. Emotional eating, or compulsive eating, is when you eat to comfort yourself or cope, not to reduce hunger. Emotional eating may lead to binge eating, but it does not always. Binge eating and emotional eating can interfere with your weight loss because they show that you are not in control of your food intake. Your food intake needs to be very controlled for the RYGB to help you to lose weight without complications.

- *Night eating syndrome:*[15] You may have night eating syndrome if you eat more than one-quarter of your daily calories late at night, you skip breakfast and are starving by the end of the day, and/or you wake up at night and eat so you can get back to sleep. Night eating is associated with weight gain, and bariatric surgery candidates have higher rates of night eating than normal-weight individuals. Night eating is associated with depression and anxiety too.[16] Behavioral counseling and/or medications may be treatment options if you and your psychologist determine that you have night eating syndrome. You will be more likely to succeed with the Roux-en-Y gastric bypass if you are able to get over night eating syndrome before surgery.

- *Drug or alcohol abuse:*[17] An inability to stop abusing drugs or alcohol shows that you may not have the self-discipline that you will need to stick to the weight loss surgery diet. Surgeons may require you to get over your addiction before agreeing to do the operation.

- *Untreated depression:* Getting RYGB can improve your life and mood, but it will not cure depression. The large amount of weight loss and sudden changes in your life can even make depression worse. If you have major depressive disorder, it is best to get it under control and understand the reasons for it before going ahead with the gastric bypass. You may need medications to correct a chemical imbalance in your brain, or you may need counseling to resolve underlying emotional issues. Once your depression is under control, you are a much better candidate for surgery.

What to Expect in the Psychologist's Office

There is no standard protocol to determine your psychological eligibility for the bariatric surgery.18 The experience varies depending on the specific psychologist or psychiatrist that you see. You might even see a social worker to give you all or part of the psychological evaluation.

Face-to-Face Interview

You will probably start by talking with your mental health professional. The conversation may be free flowing or might involve a list of questions that your psychologist asks one by one. Most likely there will be a bit of both in what is called a Structured Clinical Interview. You will have a lot of open-ended questions to answer, and the doctor will take some notes. The face-to-face interview can be very brief or it can take more than an hour.

Written Evaluation

Your psychological evaluation may include a written portion. This part may have many or just a few questions. The questions are usually multiple choice, so they are not too tiring for you to answer.

Answer Truthfully!

What is the right answer to each question? The truth! Seriously, answer honestly without trying to cheat the test and give the psychologist the answer you think he or she is looking for. There are two main reasons for this:

- *Cheating the test is really only cheating yourself.* Yes, it is cliché, and yes, it is true — way truer than it was in grade school when your dog ate your homework or you "borrowed" your buddy's exam answers. These psych tests are designed to guess whether the RYGB is going to work for you. You do not want to undergo the RYGB and spend the rest of your life with altered insides if being truthful now can prevent it. Do not lie to try to get the GB. If it is not right for you, another treatment for obesity is better for you.

- *You might not even know what the "right" answers are.* There are so many scoring systems and different ways of looking at the results that you might accidentally give some answers that make your evaluations come out unfavorable. If you lie on the tests and your psychologist tells you that you are ineligible for the RYGB because of your answers, you will feel pretty embarrassed when you try to explain that you

What Kind of Tests Might You See?

Anything is fair game! Each clinic has its own set of favorite assessments designed to test different aspects of your psychological readiness for surgery. These are a few of the more widely used tests:

- Minnesota Multiphasic Personality Inventory (MMPI) for depression
- Beck Depression Inventory (BDI)
- The Moorehead-Ardelt Quality of Life Questionnaire is a short test for the evaluation of possible mood disorders
- Beck Anxiety Inventory (BAI)
- Mini International Neuropsychiatric Interview (MINI)
- Internalized Shame Scale (ISS)
- University Rhode Island Change Assessment to estimate your readiness to change or how prepared you are to change your lifestyle.
- Revised Master Questionnaire (RMQ) for the "psychological evaluation of cognitive and behavioral difficulties related to weight management." It aims to uncover reasons why you have had trouble managing your weight and evaluate whether surgery will be helpful for you or whether you will likely fall into the same patterns.

Psychological testing is a bit tricky because every individual patient is, of course, an individual. Plus, many aspects of mental health can affect success with the RYGB. That makes it hard to develop a single test or set of tests to predict success with the GB.

- For example, the University of Rhode Island Change Assessment test sounds pretty useful, but research has found that it might not do a good job predicting your total weight loss or whether you will have complications.
- A single test does not tell the whole story, which is why psychologists need to use a bunch of different tests before they are confident that you are ready for surgery.

It is not as simple as throwing a few tests at you and scoring them on a standard scale. That is where the education and experience of your psychologist comes in. Your psychologist chooses the set of tests that you will get and looks carefully at the results. You should be asked specifically about anything that looks unusual so that you and your psychologist can make the best decision.

Sources:[19, 20, 21, 22, 23]

lied on some answers because you were trying to cheat the system but could not figure it ou!

Changing Your Diet

You will start working on your dietary changes before surgery. You can lose a few pounds during your pre-surgery preparation period. You may meet with a dietitian one or more times to:

- Assess your current diet.
- Go over the RYGB diet more specifically to clear up the details.
- Point out changes that you will need to make to follow the RYGB diet.
- Develop your pre-surgery weight loss diet meal plan if your surgeon or insurance company requires you to lose weight before surgery.
- Get the instructions for the liquid diet that you will follow before surgery.

Working with a Dietitian

Working with a dietitian can seem intimidating at first. You may feel embarrassed about your diet because your diet made you obese. However, just like when you see the psychologist, it is important for you to remember that the dietitian is on your side. The dietitian wants to you succeed in losing weight and living a healthy lifestyle. You and your dietitian both know that your past diet was not very good and that you are working toward getting the GB, so be honest about your diet and be open to your dietitian's advice on improving it.

Purpose of a Dietary Assessment

Your first appointment with a dietitian will probably include a dietary assessment. This lets your dietitian learn a bit about your current diet. The purpose is to be helpful, not to make you feel bad about your current choices. A dietary assessment can be helpful at this point in your RYGB journey in these ways:

- It gets you out of denial so you can think about your true diet. You probably spend a lot of time focusing on food and your diet, but many of us tend to "forget" the parts that we are not proud of, like the extra scoop of ice cream or the drive-through order at McDonald's on your way home from work. It is hard to improve your habits when you do not realize or admit what you have been eating.
- It is a starting point. A diet assessment gets everything down on paper so you can see where you are now and where you need to be to follow the gastric bypass diet. When your diet is written out on paper, your dietitian can make specific, achievable suggestions for changing your food choices, serving sizes, and meal and snack patterns to improve your diet.

- It makes you think. When you are forced to do a dietary assessment with a nutrition professional like a dietitian, you start to think about each bite that goes into your mouth. That is also what you need to do after weight loss surgery. It is best to start practicing now when you have the dietitian guiding you through the process of remembering the "extra" foods, such as snacks, condiments, beverages with calories, and fat used in cooking.

- It brings up the question of portion sizes. As the dietitian asks about how much you eat, you might start to realize that you are not always sure. Once you actually measure your foods, you might be surprised at how many "servings" you actually eat at one time just because you did not realize how small a serving was. Just cutting back on your serving sizes will really help you lower your calorie intake and speed up weight loss.

Dietary Assessment Using a 24-Hour Recall

How does a diet assessment work? The most common choice for clinical dietitians is a 24-hour recall. Why?

- You do not have to prepare for it.
- It is pretty accurate at estimating your nutrient intake.
- It lets you practice monitoring your diet under the guidance of a dietitian.

A 24-hour recall is just like it sounds. In the recall, you identify each food and beverage that you have consumed in the past 24 hours. If you are doing the recall in a 10:00 a.m. dietitian appointment, for example, you would tell the dietitian everything you have eaten starting from 10:00 a.m. the day before and going up through breakfast this morning.

The dietitian will write each item down and ask you for details, such as serving size, how you prepared it, and what else you ate with it. He or she will also ask you if you have eaten normally over the past day or if whether, for some reason, your meal patterns and food choices were different from your normal diet over the past day.

You will also tell the dietitian about any nutritional dietary supplements that you take so that your dietitian will have a better idea of your average nutrient intake. These might include the following:

- Individual or combined vitamins and/or minerals, such as iron, calcium and vitamin D, or vitamin B-12
- Multivitamin and mineral supplements, such as a daily tablet or capsule with a variety of vitamins and minerals
- Omega-three fatty acid supplements, such as fish oil supplements, DHA and EPA, or linolenic acid supplements

Why Does My Dietitian Repeat So Many Questions?

The 24-hour recall can feel repetitive. The dietitian asks you to go over your food and beverage intake a few times, not just once. It is not because your dietitian is not listening or thinks you are lying. In reality, the dietitian is following a standard method of doing a 24-hour recall. A common choice is the USDA's Multiple-Pass Method, which has you go over your intake five times. Each of the following steps, or "passes," of the Multiple Pass Method is slightly different from the others:

1. *Quick list:* The dietitian listens without interrupting to each food and beverage you list starting exactly 24 hours ago. This is to get your memory working.

2. *Forgotten foods:* In this pass, or go-through, your dietitian prompts you to remember items that you might have forgotten. These might include snacks, side dishes, and condiments. The dietitian might ask, for example, whether you had jam on the toast that you listed for breakfast; another question might be whether you had an evening snack after dinner last night.

3. *Time and occasion:* You go over when, what time, and with whom you ate each meal or snack. This step helps you remember any snacks that you might have forgotten; for example, you might realize that you ate such an early lunch yesterday that you had an extra afternoon snack. Remembering the occasion might help you remember more foods; for example, you might suddenly remember that you had a glass of wine last night to celebrate your wife's birthday. Recording the time and occasion can also help you identify your meal and snack patterns so that you know how you will need to change your patterns to follow the weight loss surgery diet.

4. *Detail cycle:* This is when you try to get the details set. The goal for each food is to know what you had with it and how much you had. The dietitian might ask how you prepared each item to see whether you added anything. For example, if you listed fried fish, you probably also had oil or salt and might have had some sort of batter on it. This is the time to provide details about brand names, if you remember them from food packages. This is also when you estimate your portion sizes. It can be surprisingly tough to remember and try to figure exactly how big your portions were! Now is a good time to start practicing because you will definitely be using and developing these skills over the next months and years in your gastric bypass diet! The dietitian might provide various tools to help you with portions as you do your 24-hour recall.

   • Food models are usually made of plastic, and they are very lifelike, three-dimensional models of different kinds of foods and beverages in standard serving sizes and realistic shapes. For example, you might see one cup of plastic cereal sitting in one half-cup of plastic milk in a plastic bowl.

- Pictures of food, plates, and utensils. These are usually life-sized photographs of different foods. They often have rulers and other familiar objects, like pennies, golf balls, and decks of cards, in the photos to give you some perspective. Photos are only two-dimensional, but they can help you visualize and figure the amount of each food that you ate.

- Measuring cups and tablespoons. These are a little more abstract than actual models, but they are, of course, very accurate for quantities. You will definitely be practicing using measuring cups and tablespoons, so you might as well get their sizes in your head now.

5. *Final probe:* This is like the proofreading part of the process. You and the dietitian take one last look at the list of foods and beverages to make sure it is as accurate and complete as you can make it. If you have not already talked about them, this is also when your dietitian will ask about any dietary supplements that you are taking.

You can see that the 24-hour recall has a lot of repetition because you cover the same 24 hours over and over and over again. But each step has a specific purpose, and research studies show that this type of approach is relatively accurate.

Source: [24]

Other Diet Assessment Methods

The dietitian might choose one of these common methods in addition to or instead of a 24-hour recall:

- *Food frequency questionnaire:* A purpose of a food frequency questionnaire, or FFQ, is to get a general picture of what you have typically eaten over the past year or so. You do an FFQ by filling out multiple-choice forms that ask you to choose how often you eat different types of foods. There are a few variations of FFQs.[25] The difference between the different kinds of questionnaires is the specific foods and quantities that are listed on them and how many different foods there are. For example, one FFQ might ask how often you eat fruit, while another might offer distinct choices for apples, oranges, bananas, and other types of fruits. More food choices make an FFQ more accurate but also make it take longer for you to fill out. FFQs are good because they give a nice general picture of your regular diet and you do not have to remember every detail. They are really good at pointing out general patterns, such as eating a lot of sweets or rarely eating whole grain foods.

- *Food record:* Before your first appointment, at your first appointment, or sometime later on your weight loss journey, your dietitian might ask you to fill out a food record, food journal, or food log. That is when you write down everything you eat or drink right as you are eating it or just after the meal. You will try to write down the same information that your dietitian collects during a 24-hour recall: what you ate, when you ate it, how much you ate, whom you were with, and how you prepared it. Usually food records last for three days, and your dietitian might ask you to complete your record during two weekdays and one day on the weekend. A benefit of a food record is that you are less likely to forget foods compared to doing a 24-hour recall. That is because you can write them down as soon as you eat them. Also, you will not have to be trying to remember your diet while you are on the spot as you are during an appointment with the dietitian doing a recall. They are kind of annoying at first because you have to remember to write things down and it can feel like a waste of time, but keeping a food journal will probably become a part of your life for at least a few months following surgery. People that keep food journals tend to have better success with weight control, so it is a great idea to get used to keeping a food diary now. It will get easier pretty soon and will not feel like such a chore.

Figuring Out Your Nutrient Intake

After gathering information about your food intake from a 24-hour recall, an FFQ, and/or a food record, your dietitian needs to analyze your diet. That just means figuring out the calories and nutrients in your food. The dietitian can use an online database, such as one provided by the USDA, to calculate your nutrient intake and compare it to your recommendations. Many dietitians use specialized nutritional software to make their jobs easier.

The dietitian will discuss the results with you and may suggest a few foods or supplements to add to your diet to improve your nutrient intake if you are low in certain nutrients. More than 60 percent of RYGB patients are low in vitamin D before surgery, and pre-surgery patients are also often deficient in vitamin B12 and iron.[26] These deficiencies can cause fatigue, infections, and other complications and long-term health problems.

Talking about the Gastric Bypass Diet with Your Dietitian

Success after the RYGB will depend largely on how closely you follow the right diet. What better time to talk about the diet than before the surgery when you meet with the dietitian? These are some topics you might want to discuss:

- A sample menu showing a few days of RYGB-appropriate eating
- How you will plan the timing of meals, snacks, and fluids
- Which foods you will and will not be able to eat with the bypass
- Concerns about real-life situations, such as holiday parties, late nights at work, and having company for dinner

Pre-Op Weight Loss and Liquid Diets

Many bariatric patients go on a weight loss diet for several weeks or a few months before surgery. Your surgeon might require this for safety and to demonstrate your ability to follow the post-surgery diet. Your insurance company might require you to follow a pre-surgery weight loss diet to show your commitment to the RYGB lifestyle and convince the insurance company that the cost of surgery is a good investment.

Benefits of the Pre-Surgery Weight Loss Diet

This diet will be similar to the diet that you will follow for weight loss and maintenance in the months and years following the RYGB procedure. The diet will probably include about 800 to 1,200 calories per day and will emphasize healthy choices and controlled portion sizes. These are some of the reasons why you may be asked follow this diet:[27,28]

- *It helps you lose weight.* Losing at least five percent of your total body weight before bariatric surgery shortens recovery time and reduces your risk of complications.[29] That is a loss of at least 12 if your starting weight is 250 pounds or 15 to 30 pounds if your initial weight is 300 pounds.

- *It is proof that you can follow this diet.* Following the bypass diet before surgery tests your commitment to the RYGB lifestyle and shows that you have the discipline and motivation to change your dietary habits. This gives you confidence in yourself, convinces your surgeon that you are a good candidate for the gastric bypass, and fulfills the requirements for reimbursement that your health insurance provider might set.

- *It makes your post-surgery transition easier.* The pre-op diet lets you practice for the post-surgery diet. Making mistakes before surgery is better because you are in a low-pressure situation. After surgery, something as simple as eating the wrong amount or type of food can lead to stomach pain or more serious complications.

The pre-surgery diet is low-calorie, but it is nutritious enough to follow for as long as your surgeon recommends. Make sure to follow your surgeon's and dietitian's recommendations for healthy food choices so that you can get enough protein, vitamins, and minerals. You may need supplements.

The diet may be challenging. You might feel hungry and cranky, but you will get through it with persistence. Within a few days, the diet will become a habit. You will figure out some mental coping techniques, and you might start to realize that you are not really as hungry as you thought you were; at least you will learn that you can handle being hungry. Keep your eye on the prize—a hard-earned RYGB and the chance to achieve your goal weight for life.

The Pre-Surgery Liquid Diet

The diet that you follow for the final few days or couple of weeks before surgery will be even stricter than the longer-term weight loss diet that may have lasted for months. The pre-surgery diet is very low-calorie and unlikely to meet your daily nutrient needs. It is only safe for a short period before risking health problems, and you should only follow it under physician supervision. The diet makes your liver smaller by about 8 to 14 percent, so it is easier for your surgeon to perform surgery.[30]

The preoperative diet is usually a liquid diet, but your surgeon may allow selected other foods. Many hospitals and dietitians have a prepared flier or brochure that describes the diet, lists what you can and cannot have, and suggests a sample meal plan. You might see your dietitian specifically to discuss the liquid diet, or you might just rely on the handout and telephone calls with your surgeon or dietitian to guide you through the diet. Call your surgeon or dietitian if you have questions. Another option is to log onto BariatricPal.com to ask post-surgery members about their pre-surgery diet experiences.

Foods on a Liquid Diet[31]

Allowed - Liquids	Depends on Surgeon – Pureed Foods	Not Allowed – Solid Foods
• Milk	• Cream of wheat	• Bread, pasta, rice
• Tea, Water, Coffee	• Applesauce	• Nuts, beans, seeds
• Protein shakes	• Pureed potatoes	• Meats, poultry, fish
• Gelatin	• Oatmeal	• Cheese
• Popsicles	• Other cooked cereals	• Raw fruit
• Ice cream and sherbet	• Strained meats	• Raw vegetables

Table 15: Foods on a Liquid Diet

High-Nutrient, Low-Sugar Choices on Your Liquid Diet

You will probably exchange each of your regular meals for a diet or high-protein meal-replacement beverage, such as a can of regular or high-protein Slim-Fast, a Medifast shake, or a protein shake that is fortified with vitamins and minerals.[32] You can reduce your hunger while following the very low-calorie liquid diet by choosing high-protein and high-fiber options. Also, choose ones that are lower in added sugars so you avoid sugar spikes and crashes.

Be sure to read the nutrition facts label to find out how many calories it contains. Some brands have 100 to 200 calories in a serving, while others have 300 or more calories. You do not want to be eating way more calories than you think and prevent weight loss while on a liquid diet. Avoiding full-sized shakes between meals will also help you limit your calorie intake. Instead, choose calorie-free beverages, such as water, tea, and coffee, and low-calorie beverages, such as diet juice drinks and low-calorie flavored waters, such as Crystal Light and sugar-free Kool-Aid.[33] You can also have sugar-free gelatin and popsicles between meals.

Your liquid diet will not allow sugary liquids, such as

> **Tip**
>
> Chapter 15, "The RYGB Diet & Nutrition," will cover nutrition labels and ingredients lists on foods and beverages. We will go over what information you can find on them, how to read them, and what to look for when you are choosing your food. You can find out about more about added sugars in **Chapter 13, "Post-Surgery Diet: From Liquid Diet to Solid Foods."** That chapter also has much more detail on a standard liquid diet, which you will also be following for a few weeks after your procedure.

fruit punch, sports drinks, energy drinks, soft drinks, or sweetened ice coffee or tea. These do not provide important nutrients; they give you a lot of calories, and they can make you feel shaky when you are not eating solid foods with them. You will also need to avoid carbonated beverages to prevent an upset stomach.

The Liquid Diet and Diabetes

Any special diet is an extra challenge if you have pre-diabetes or diabetes because your body has trouble keeping your blood sugar levels constant. Your blood glucose levels can skyrocket, which is hyperglycemia, when you get too many calories or too much sugar, such as from a high-carbohydrate meal replacement beverage.

The other consideration is hypoglycemia. This can occur between meals when you have not eaten any carbohydrates for a while. Before starting your liquid diet, it is especially important to discuss your diabetes and strategies for controlling your blood sugar with your dietitian. You will need to monitor the amount of carbohydrates that you have, and be sure to spread out your intake throughout the day to avoid high and low blood sugar levels.

Pre-Surgery Exercise Program

Some patients can start exercising before surgery. Activity burns extra calories so you lose weight faster, it helps stabilize your blood sugar levels, and it gets you stronger before surgery. Up until now, your obesity can be preventing you from exercising because of embarrassment, pain, asthma, or discomfort while moving.

After you lose weight on the pre-operative diet, you may be able to do light exercise more easily than before. If your physician gives you the go-ahead, you might try gentle stretching, water aerobics, water jogging, or slow walking, either on your own or hanging onto the rails of a treadmill for support.

An exercise program might not be possible if your obesity is still causing too many problems. That is okay. For now, just focus on your eating and on your other preparations for surgery. There will be plenty of time later for getting into an exercise program and using physical activity as another tool in your weight loss journey with the gastric bypass.

> **Tip**
>
> Chapter 2, "Options for Losing Weight: Diets, Exercise, Weight Loss Drugs, and Surgery," has a discussion of the health benefits of exercise. Chapter 16, "Physical Activity to Control Weight Loss," lets you know what to expect and how to stay safe when you are starting an exercise program and some ways to stay motivated to exercise regularly.

Summary

☛ Surgery is no longer a vague idea in your mind — it is a real event that is about to take place in your life! After this chapter, you know what the typical patient goes through before having RYGB. Your role is to follow your medical team's directions and to ask all of your questions so that you have the best chances for success.

☛ This chapter covers the months and weeks before surgery; the next chapter goes through the final crucial days and hours before you go in for surgery. The chapter's goal is to prevent you from worrying about overlooking things so you can have peace of mind. Let's get to it!

Time to Take Action: Getting Ready for Your Surgeon Visits

The chapter talks a lot about visits to your surgeon or other members of your healthcare team. You will get the most out of each one if you do your homework beforehand. This worksheet should help.

Write down the name, address, telephone number and email address of your surgeon.

Do the same for each other member of your medical team.

Dietitian

Psychologist

Reception desk of clinic or front desk of hospital

Look up everything you can find about your family medical history. Write down any important information here. Try to get at least your parents' information, as well as that of your siblings and any grandparents whose information you can track down.

Name

Relationship to you

Medical conditions

Name

Relationship to you

Medical conditions

———•———

Name

Relationship to you

Medical conditions

———•———

Name

Relationship to you

Medical conditions

———•———

Write down your own medical information.

Prescription medications

Name brand and generic name

Purpose (why are you taking it: what health condition is it treating?)

Dosage and frequency

———————•———————

Name brand and generic name

Purpose (why are you taking it: what health condition is it treating?)

Dosage and frequency

———————•———————

Name brand and generic name

Purpose (why are you taking it: what health condition is it treating?)

Dosage and frequency

Write down any other relevant medical history. What conditions do you have? Have you had any medical conditions or major medical procedures in the past?

Do you take dietary supplements? This includes vitamins, minerals, herbals, and natural supplements. YES/NO

Write them down here. Include the dosage and how often you take it.

Supplement 1

....

....

....

Supplement 2

....

....

....

Supplement 3

....

....

....

Supplement 4

....

....

....

1   Medicare. Managing your personal health information online. Centers for Medicare and Medicaid Services. U.S. Department of Health and Human Services. Web site. http://www.medicare.gov/navigation/manage-your-health/personal-health-records/personal-health-records-overview.aspx. Accessed October 6, 2012.

2   Apovian CM, Cummings S, Anderson W, Borud L, Boyer K, Day K, Hatchigian E, Hodges B, Patti ME, Pettus M, Perna F, Rooks D, Saltzman E, Skoropowski J, Tantillo MB, Thomason P. Best practice updates for multidisciplinary care in weight loss surgery. Obesity (Silver Spring). 2009;17(5):871-879.

3   Apovian CM, Cummings S, Anderson W, Borud L, Boyer K, Day K, Hatchigian E, Hodges B, Patti ME, Pettus M, Perna F, Rooks D, Saltzman E, Skoropowski J, Tantillo MB, Thomason P. Best practice updates for multidisciplinary care in weight loss surgery. Obesity (Silver Spring). 2009;17(5):871-879.

4   Mexico country specific information. Bureau of Consular Affairs, U.S. Department of State. Web site. http://travel.state.gov/travel/cis_pa_tw/cis/cis_970.html. Accessed October 2, 2012.

5   Basic metabolic panel. Pubmed Health, U.S. National Library of Medicine. Web site. http://www.ncbi.nlm.nih.gov/pubmedhealth/PMH0003934/. Reviewed 2011, May 30. Accessed October 2, 2012.

6   CO2 blood test. Pubmed Health, U.S. National Library of Medicine. Web site. http://www.ncbi.nlm.nih.gov/pubmedhealth/PMH0003940/. Reviewed 2011, May 30. Accessed October 2, 2012.

7   Chloride test - blood. Pubmed Health, U.S. National Library of Medicine. Web site. http://www.ncbi.nlm.nih.gov/pubmedhealth/PMH0003956/. Reviewed 2011, June 1. Accessed October 2, 2012.

8   Creatinine - blood. Pubmed Health, U.S. National Library of Medicine. Web site. http://www.ncbi.nlm.nih.gov/pubmedhealth/PMH0003946/. Reviewed 2011, June 1. Accessed October 2, 2012.

9   Blood urea nitrogen – BUN test. Pubmed Health, U.S. National Library of Medicine. Web site. http://www.ncbi.nlm.nih.gov/pubmedhealth/PMH0003945/. Reviewed 2011, May 30. Accessed October 2, 2012.

10   .Dugdale DC. Zieve D. AST. MedlinePlus, U.S. National Library of Medicine. Web site. http://www.nlm.nih.gov/medlineplus/ency/article/003472.htm. Reviewed 2011, February 20. Accessed October 2, 2012.

11   Dugdale DC, Zieve D. ALT. MedlinePlus, U.S. National Library of Medicine. Web site. http://www.nlm.nih.gov/medlineplus/ency/article/003473.htm. Updated 2011, February 20. Accessed October 2, 2012.

12   Apovian CM, Cummings S, Anderson W, Borud L, Boyer K, Day K, Hatchigian E, Hodges B, Patti ME, Pettus M, Perna F, Rooks D, Saltzman E, Skoropowski J, Tantillo MB, Thomason P. Best practice updates for multidisciplinary care in weight loss surgery. Obesity (Silver Spring). 2009;17(5):871-879.

13   Clinical policy bulletin: obesity surgery. Aetna Inc. web site. http://www.aetna.com/cpb/medical/data/100_199/0157.html. Reviewed 2012, December 28. February 6, 2013.

14   Apovian CM, Cummings S, Anderson W, Borud L, Boyer K, Day K, Hatchigian E, Hodges B, Patti ME, Pettus M, Perna F, Rooks D, Saltzman E, Skoropowski J, Tantillo MB, Thomason P. Best practice updates for multidisciplinary care in weight loss surgery. Obesity (Silver Spring). 2009;17(5):871-879.

15   Apovian CM, Cummings S, Anderson W, Borud L, Boyer K, Day K, Hatchigian E, Hodges B, Patti ME, Pettus M, Perna F, Rooks D, Saltzman E, Skoropowski J, Tantillo MB, Thomason P. Best practice updates for multidisciplinary care in weight loss surgery. Obesity (Silver Spring). 2009;17(5):871-879.

16   Striegel-Moore RH, Rosselli F, Wilson GT, Perrin N, Harvey K, DeBar L. Nocturnal eating: association with binge eating, obesity and psychological distress. Int J Eat Disord. 2010;43(6):520-526.

17   Apovian CM, Cummings S, Anderson W, Borud L, Boyer K, Day K, Hatchigian E, Hodges B, Patti ME, Pettus M, Perna F, Rooks D, Saltzman E, Skoropowski J, Tantillo MB, Thomason P. Best practice updates for multidisciplinary care in weight loss surgery. Obesity (Silver Spring). 2009;17(5):871-879.

18   Sogg S, Mori DL. The Boston Interview for gastric bypass: determining the psychological suitability of surgical candidates. Obesity Surgery.14(3):2004.

19   Moorehead AK, Ardelt-Gattinger E, Lechner H, Oria HE. The validation of the Moorehead-Ardelt Quality of Life Questionnaire II. Obesity Surgery. 2003;13:684-92.

20   Nicolai A, Ippoliti C, Petrelli MD. Laparoscopic adjustable banding: essential role of psychological support. Obesity Surgery. 2002;12:857-63.

21   Hayden MJ, Brown WA, Brennan L, O'Brien PE. Validation of the Beck Depression Inventory as a screening tool for a clinical mood disorder in bariatric surgery candidates. Obesity Surgery. 2012. epub ahead of print.

22   Lier HQ, Biringer E, Stubhaug B, Tangen T. Prevalence of psychiatric disorders before and one year after bariatric surgery: the role of shame in maintenance of psychiatric disorders in patients undergoing bariatric surgery. Nordic Journal of Psychiatry. 2012. epub ahead of print.

23   Corsica JA, Hood MM, Azarbad L, Ivan I. Revisiting the Revised Master Questionnaire for the psychological evaluation of bariatric surgery candidates. Obesity Surgery. 2012;22: 381-8.

195

24   USDA Automated Multiple-Pass Method. Agricultural Research Services, United States Department of Agriculture. Web site. http://www.ars.usda.gov/Services/docs.htm?docid=7710. Modified 2010, September 29. Accessed October 3, 2012.

25   Thompson FE, Subar AF. Chapter 1: Dietary Assessment Methodology. Nutrition in the Prevention and Treatment of Chronic Disease, 2nd ed. National Cancer Institute: Bethesda, Maryland.

26   Aills L, Blankenship J, Buffington C, Furtado M, Parrott, J. ASMBS Integrated health nutritional guidelines for the surgical weight loss patient. Surgery for Obesity and Related Diseases, 2008;S73-S108.

27   Pre-surgery bariatric diet. Bariatric Choice: The Leading Source of Bariatric Nutrition. Retrieved from http://www.bariatricchoice.com/pre-op-bariatric-diet-for-bariatric-gastric-bypass-surgery-patients.aspx. 2011. Accessed October 4, 2012.

28   Snyder-Marlow G, Tayle D, Lenhard MJ. Nutrition care for patients undergoing laparoscopic sleeve gastrectomy for weight loss. J Am Diet Ass. 2010;110(4):600-607

29   Apovian CM, Cummings S, Anderson W, Borud L, Boyer K, Day K, Hatchigian E, Hodges B, Patti ME, Pettus M, Perna F, Rooks D, Saltzman E, Skoropowski J, Tantillo MB, Thomason P. Best practice updates for multidisciplinary care in weight loss surgery. Obesity (Silver Spring). 2009;17(5):871-879.

30   Goldenberg L. Weight loss before weight loss surgery: what do we know about dropping those preoperative pounds? Bariatric Times. 2010;7(7):18-20.

31   Dugdale DC, Zieve D. Liquid diet – full. Medline Plus, National Institutes of Health. Web site. http://www.nlm.nih.gov/medlineplus/ency/patientinstructions/000206.htm. Updated 2010, November 21. Accessed October 4, 2012.

32   Slim-Fast and Medifast are trademarked names, and this book is not affiliated with Slim-Fast or Medifast.

33   Crystal Light and Kool-Aid are trademarked and are not affiliated with this book.

10

Final Preparation for RYGB

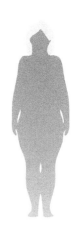

Surgery is quickly approaching, and this chapter will get you up to speed so you know exactly what to do to get ready and what to expect at the hospital on your surgery day. This is some of the information that is in the chapter:

- Planning your home for your post-surgery recovery time
- Packing for the hospital
- Following an overnight fast and adjusting your medications the night before surgery
- Checking into the hospital and going into surgery

This chapter will take you up until you lose consciousness and go into the operating room for surgery. It is a time for excitement and probably a few nerves, but knowing what to expect can calm your nerves and make everything go better than you would have hoped.

Preparing Ahead Of Time

Your big day is approaching. You have met the surgeon and other members of your medical team and you are medically cleared for the gastric bypass procedure; you know what to expect during and after surgery. Now is a good time to take care of some practical matters to make surgery day less stressful and your recovery easier. Planning ahead can prevent you from forgetting things in the excitement of finally getting to have weight loss surgery.

Time off from Work

Make sure that you arrange for time off work if you have not already done so. You will need to take at off least one to two weeks. You need to plan for longer if you have an active job, and you will need extra time if you have complications during or after surgery. If you feel comfortable doing so, let your supervisor know about the possibility of taking off extra time so that it does not come as a surprise. Of course, you have the right to choose whether to tell your supervisor the entire truth about your surgery. A lot of patients choose not to tell their employers about bariatric surgery.

> **Tip**
>
> Chapter 18, "The Benefits of a Strong Support System," talks about whether to tell people about your surgery and how to decide. It is entirely up to you whom to tell or not to tell and how many details you choose to give.

Getting Your Home Ready

You will be feeling sick and tired when you get home from the hospital after surgery. You will not be in any mood for household chores or grocery shopping. Prepare your house ahead of time to make your post-op recovery easier.

Pain Medications

You are going to have pain after surgery. Your abdominal area will be hurting from the skin to the places that the surgeon had to make cuts during surgery. You may also have shoulder pain from gas that remains in your body from the pneumoperitoneum portion of the laparoscopic procedure. Before surgery, possibly in your pre-surgery appointment, get your surgeon to advise you in stocking up on the pain medications that you are likely to need. Your surgeon may prescribe some strong painkillers. Even if you only plan to use over-the-counter painkillers, make sure you purchase enough so that they are on hand when you need them after surgery.

Non-Steroidal Anti-Inflammatory Drugs (NSAIDs)

Pain medications known as non-steroidal anti-inflammatory drugs, or NSAIDs, are familiar to most of us. You probably have some in your medicine cabinet already. Some of the many common over-the-counter and prescription pain medications that are NSAIDs are aspirin, ibuprofen, tolfenamic acid, and celecoxib. Using certain prescription NSAIDs after surgery can reduce your need to use opioid painkillers, which can be addictive. Limiting or avoiding opioids is especially beneficial if you have obstructive sleep apnea.[1]

Acetaminophen (Tylenol)

Acetaminophen, whose most common name brand is Tylenol, is an over-the-counter pain medication that is not an NSAID. It can be a good option for post-operative pain management, although you never want to overdose on any pain medication.[2]

Narcotics (Opioids)

Prescription narcotics, or opioids, include codeine, morphine, and oxycodone.[3] Follow your doctor's instructions carefully for use; in most cases, you will be told to take them only when you need them and not necessarily on a set schedule. Narcotics are strong painkillers that are available by prescription only. Your surgeon will probably write you a prescription in advance so that you can pick up your medications before going into surgery.

It may be a little scary when you start thinking about the pain that you might have after your surgery, but in reality, you will be fine. It is not a big deal—it is just something to expect and plan for so that it does not take you by surprise. If you do not want to think about it, don't. Just know that you may have pain and that you will deal with it. Following your surgeon's instructions should be enough to manage the pain safely through the pain.

Why Can NSAIDs Be Dangerous after RYGB?

You will probably need some kind of pain relief after the gastric bypass, taking too much medication can increase your risk of side effects. Let's look more closely at NSAIDs and talk about another class of painkillers, steroids, that are not recommended after surgery.

The U.S. consumes billions of doses of NSAIDs each year. They are available over the counter and by prescription. They are so common because they relieve pain and, compared to other drugs, have few serious side effects. So why should you limit your use of NSAIDs after the RYGB?

Many NSAIDs are cox-2 inhibitors. They prevent your body from producing cyclooxygenase 2, or cox-2. That is good because cox-2 causes pain and inflammation. However, cox-2 inhibitors that also inhibit cox-1 can increase your risk for stomach ulcers. Cox-1 is necessary for keeping your gastrointestinal tract and stomach lining strong and healthy. You do not want to mess with your stomach any more than necessary when you have just had surgery on it!

Aspirin is a type of NSAID with an additional potential danger. In addition to being an anti-inflammatory cox-2-inhibitor and a pain killer, aspirin is a blood thinner. It reduces blood clotting and helps prevent strokes and heart attacks. Normally that is a good thing, and you might even take aspirin regularly to prevent heart attacks. However, aspirin can increase your risk for bleeding, which is dangerous after surgery.

These are examples of common NSAIDS:

- *Aspirin: Ecotrin, Bayer Aspirin, Aspir-trin, and Acutrin*
- *Ibuprofen: Advil, Motrin, Nuprin, Samson, IB Pro*, and Midol
- Dayquil, Ibudone, Dimetapp, and Vicoprofen are each names of mixtures of medications that contain ibuprofen.
- Naproxen: Aleve, Naprosyn, Anaprox, Treximet, and Vimovo also have naproxen in them.
- Salsalate: disalicylic acid and salicylisalic acid

It is easy to tell whether your pain medication is an NSAID or contains one. It probably says on the label. If you are not sure, just ask your doctor or call a pharmacist to find out. These are some of the familiar NSAIDs and some of their brand names.

Sources: [4, 5, 6, 7]

You probably will not be taking steroid medications to control pain, even though they are pretty strong. Common names include cortisone, prednisolone, hydrocortisone, and betamethasone. Steroids slow down healing so recovery from surgery can actually take longer.[8]

Getting Your Kitchen Ready for Post-Surgery Recovery

Plan to be on a clear liquid diet for a couple days following the RYGB. In the beginning, you will want to have ice chips or crushed ice to suck on since it is easier than gulping water and aggravating your newly rearranged gastrointestinal system. You can buy ice chips at a convenience store or supermarket if your fridge does not make them.

Table 16 illustrates standard guidelines for a clear liquid diet.[9] Make sure to have enough options and large enough quantities in your home so that you do not risk running out after surgery. You are not going to be able to drive yourself to the grocery store for a wheel or lift heavy items, such as a 24-pack of ready-to-drink iced tea.

Allowed	Not Allowed
✓ Water	✗ Any solid or semi-solid food
✓ Broth	✗ Nectar
✓ Popsicles	✗ Canned fruit
✓ Gelatin	✗ Milk
✓ Tea	✗ Protein shakes
✓ Coffee	✗ Meal replacement beverages
✓ Sports drinks	✗ Juice with pulp
✓ Pulp-free fruit juices	✗ Cream (e.g., in coffee)

Table 16: Standard guidelines for a clear liquid diet

Ways to Make Post-Op Recovery Easier

You will feel tired, sore, and possibly sick when you get home from the hospital. Your first priority is to recover from surgery. These are a few things you might want to take care of before the RYGB to make your life easier later:

- Do the laundry
- Clean the house
- Go grocery shopping for your own liquid diet and for your family's food

Getting to and from the Hospital

You may be used to driving yourself around, but getting to and from the hospital for the gastric bypass is another story. You will probably need to arrange for a ride.

Transportation to and from the Hospital

A few patients go home the day after laparoscopic RYGB.[10] If you are among them, do not try to drive yourself home even if you think that you feel okay. You may still be groggy from anesthesia and pain medications, exhausted from the surgery, and in pain. It is safer and easier to get a ride.

When you schedule your surgery, your surgeon will be able to estimate what time you will be ready to go home assuming that you do not have complications. Most patients stay an average of three days.[11] Keep in mind that the following unpredictable factors can delay your hospital discharge time:

- Changing from a laparoscopic to open procedure
- Complications from surgery that require more care in the hospital
- Taking longer than average for the anesthesia to wear off

Preparing ahead of Time

The day before you expect to leave the hospital, contact your driver to tell him or her what time you think you will be ready to go home the next day. Make a plan for meeting each other. A likely place is at the hospital discharge center. Another option is to call your ride when you are ready to come home or when you begin check out of the hospital.

Be sure to have these items with you when you check into the hospital for your surgery:

- Your ride's name and phone number
- A back-up contact or the number of a taxi company in case your first choice is not able to come and get you
- A soft cushion to protect your sore abdomen from the seatbelt and bumpy ride home

Transportation and Medical Tourism

If you are getting bariatric surgery as part of a medical tourism package, a ride to and from the clinic or hospital should be part of the package. The hospital might have dedicated shuttles to take you around. If not, be sure to have a few different taxi numbers on you so that you can get back to the hotel and rest without worrying about how to get there. Call the numbers before your surgery to be certain that the companies have English-speaking representatives and are still in business.

Packing for the Hospital

Packing your bags ahead of time reduces stress and prevents you from forgetting things. Your surgeon's office may be able to provide you with a standard packing list. It is likely to include the following items.

What to Pack...

Paperwork and Contact Information

- Papers from the surgeon's office
- Your insurance company's name, phone number, fax number, any contact names you have, and a copy of your pre-approval letter for reimbursement

- Personal contacts. Write down names and phone numbers of people for the hospital to contact in case of an emergency or for you to call if you need to or simply want to talk. Write each person's relationship to you.
- A way to pay for what you need. You may have unexpected minor expenses, such as a bottle of water or extra cushion for your stomach from a convenience store on the way home.

Medications and Supplements

- *Prescription medications:* Take enough for your expected hospital stay plus enough for a couple extra days just in case you stay in the hospital longer than you expected. Be sure to have the medications in a powder or liquid form so you can still take them after the surgery even though you cannot swallow whole pills.
- *Instructions for your prescription medications:* For each, write down the time you take it, the dose, and whether you take it with food. These instructions can be helpful because you might be a little groggy after your surgery or a nurse might be administering your medications. Do not forget to write down any special instructions that your family physician or surgeon gave you for taking your medications around your time of surgery.
- *Pain medications:* These may be prescription or over-the-counter. Pack the medications that your surgeon recommends.
- *Dietary supplements:* As long as your surgeon has cleared each one, pack your dietary supplements in powder or liquid form, as well as instructions for taking them.

Comfortable Clothing

- Loose-fitting clothes, with special attention to a loose-fitting waist. An elastic waistband will feel much more comfortable on your sore stomach than a tight-fitting belt or zippered waistband after your surgery. Ask the hospital how many changes of clothes to bring; most likely, you will just wear one set to the hospital and wear a hospital gown for most of your time in the hospital.
- Enough changes of underwear and socks—plus a couple extras—for the amount of time your surgeon estimates you will be in the hospital
- A warm sweater just in case you get cold
- Wear a pair of comfortable sneakers to the hospital.
- Pack a pair of non-slip or rubber-soled slippers.

Personal Items

- Toothbrush and toothpaste
- Hairbrush or comb
- An extra hairband or scrunchie if you have long hair and need it tied back

- Hand lotion and chapstick to prevent dryness
- Hand sanitizer in case you want to wash your hands but are too tired to get up after surgery
- Shampoo and conditioner
- Soap or shower gel

Entertainment

- *Reading material:* magazines, books, a Kindle, or newspapers
- *Games:* crossword puzzle or Sudoku books
- *Music:* a CD player and CDs or an iPod
- *Video:* a laptop with a DVD player and a couple of DVDs to watch
- *Extra batteries and/or your battery charger(s):* for your music player, laptop, cell phone, and Kindle
- *Your cell phone:* Charge it up before you go to the hospital.
- *Pencil, pens, and paper*
- *The BariatricPal.com app for smartphone or Kindle!* You can connect to the community and stay in touch while you are at the hospital! Be sure to download it for free before going to the hospital.

Miscellaneous

- Continuous positive airway pressure, or CPAP, machine if you have sleep apnea. If you normally sleep with a CPAP machine, ask your surgeon whether you should take it to the hospital with you. The facility might be able to supply you with one so you do not have to lug your own.
- Reading glasses
- Your teddy bear, lucky horseshoe, or whatever else gets you through life's challenges

A small rolling suitcase is ideal because it is big enough to fit the essentials and you do not have to lift it off of the ground. You will not be able to do heavy lifting after surgery.

Leave a Few Things at Home!

Leave the non-essentials at home, so you do not have to worry about losing them at the hospital. Do not bring these items.

Luxury Items

- Dress clothes and shoes. You will be in a hospital gown, and dress clothes and shoes will be uncomfortable anyway.
- Makeup and other nonessential toiletries, such as eyebrow tweezers
- A full range of shower and bath items. Save the luxurious bath for when you are home in the comfort of your own bathtub.

Valuable Items

- Jewelry: All it does is draw attention to you and invite theft. Leave it at home.
- Too much cash: Just bring enough for an emergency taxi ride and a few dollars extra for unexpected expenses. Too much cash, especially when travelling, is asking for trouble.

Above All, Relax!

Do not worry too much about forgetting things. The hospital will take care of the absolute essentials and will probably be happy to make up for anything you forget, such as a magazine or hand sanitizer. The focus now is for your surgery to go as well as possible.

Additional Packing Considerations for Medical Tourism

Medical tourism is not as complicated as you may think. That is especially true if you have opted for an all-inclusive package deal or if your surgeon's clinic is used to working with foreigners. They will guide you through the preparation so you can be sure that you have taken care of everything before getting on that plane. Most of your packing will be the same for Mexico or Venezuela, but there are extra items to consider. Your surgeon may supply you with a specialized list for tourists.

Extra Daily Essentials

- *Extra clothing:* Do not count on doing a laundry while you are gone. You almost certainly will not have one available to you at a low cost in your hotel. You definitely do not want to have to find and use a Laundromat while you are trying to recover from the gastric bypass surgery! Keep in mind that you do not need a lot of extra clothes, because you will be in a hospital gown.
- *Extra underwear:* Yes, it is embarrassing, and no, it is not likely…but diarrhea is a definite possibility after getting RYGB. Do not worry about cleaning dirty underwear; instead, just pack a few extra pairs. They are light and small, so they are easy to pack.
- *Toiletries:* Double-check to make sure you have what you need. You can buy things like toothpaste and shampoo anywhere in the world, but sometimes it is nicer to have the brands from home that you are used to.

Special Items for Travelers

- *A pocket dictionary:* This lets you get your point across quickly. You can use the occasional Spanish word instead of waiting for a Spanish-speaking healthcare professional to go and find an English-speaking colleague to translate.
- *A phone card:* Cell phone fees can be astronomical when calling home from another country. Ask your surgeon what most patients do when they want to call the U.S. You might end up using your hospital or hotel landline telephone with a calling card for only a few cents per minute. Be sure to ask your hotel or hospital if there is a surcharge for using their phones—some places add a dollar or more per minute.

- *Passport:* Check, double-check, and triple-check your passport. Make sure that it is current and that it is good through at least six months after your planned return date.

- *List of contact:.* Include your regular list of family members and friends, as well as the name, address, and phone number of your hotel; your primary care physician; your regular pharmacy; and the name, phone number, and fax number of the surgeon who will be taking charge of your aftercare.

- *Plane tickets, if necessary:* Check for your outgoing and return plane tickets if you have paper tickets. If you have e-tickets, also called paperless tickets, you will just need a photo ID and major credit card to check in at the airport.

- *Money:* Major credit cards, debit cards, and bankcards are accepted almost nearly everywhere in the world. Carrying less cash means less worry about losing it or getting it stolen. Weeks or months before you leave, call your credit card company or bank to make sure your card will be accepted at most places in your destination city. Take more than one card, if you have them, in case for some reason one does not work. A small amount of extra cash can always come in handy, and most places will accept dollars instead of the local currency of Mexican pesos. Using dollars instead of pesos, however, may be more expensive.

Getting Help

Be prepared for anything. Always be aware of available resources when you are traveling in a foreign country, especially if you are traveling alone and planning to have a minor surgery. These are some things to consider:

- Know what to do and where to go if you lose your passport. Contact the nearest U.S. Embassy. U.S. Embassy locations in Mexico include popular bariatric surgery destinations, such as Monterrey and Tijuana.[12,13]

- Write down the contact information of your hospital and hotel and keep it with you at all times. Have the name of the hospital and hotel, the name of your surgeon, and the address and telephone numbers of the hospital and hotel.

- Carry the company's contact information if you are getting the RYGB as part of a medical tourism package.

- Write down the phone number of your credit card company or bank so that if you lose your card or it does not work, you can cancel it and get a replacement quickly.

The Last Few Hours Are Finally Here!

You are packed and ready for surgery! What exactly do you do on the day before surgery? What will happen when you get to the hospital? This section will prepare you for these final few hours before the RYGB.

Last-Minute Checks

Take a final glance at your checklist to make sure you have packed everything and that you followed all of your surgeon's pre-surgery instructions. If you do not already know, call the hospital to find out where your ride should drop you off and where to check into the hospital. These extra tasks can help distract you from surgery.

Pre-Surgery Diet and Medications

Food that is in your stomach when you go under general anesthesia can enter your lungs and cause a dangerous situation. To avoid this, patients should fast for at least six hours before surgery. The fast also reduces nausea and vomiting that are common when you wake up from surgery.[14] Your surgeon is likely to recommend an overnight fast with no food or drinks besides water after 10:00 p.m.

Overnight Fast

The overnight fast is a common procedure before surgery.[15] It not only makes the anesthesia safer but also makes surgery easier by preventing food in your stomach from interfering with your surgeon's view of your stomach. You can only have water and not other beverages, such as the following:

- Diet drinks
- Tea or coffee
- Anything with caffeine

Medications

Each medication may have a different set of pre-surgery instructions, so read through them to make sure you are following your physician's or surgeon's instructions correctly for each medication. If you are not sure, call your surgeon or the pharmacy. Blood thinners, such as warfarin (with the popular brand name of Coumadin) and Plavix, can increase bleeding during and after surgery. Your doctor will probably have you skip your dose on the day of surgery. If you are on insulin to control your blood sugar levels, you will probably take a smaller dose than usual. That is because you will not be eating carbohydrates during the day, so your blood sugar levels will not spike as much as they usually do.

Do Not Forget Your "Before" Pictures!

They are not absolutely necessary, but this is your last chance to catch yourself as a pre-surgery patient who is ready to leave obesity in the past! Your "before" pictures are the ones you get to contrast with your "after" pictures. You can pull them out of your wallet or even paste them on your refrigerator to motivate you when times get tough. They remind you that whatever you are going through is worth it so that you never have to take another "before" picture again.

Checking into the Hospital

Hospital staff will take charge of your care as soon as you check into the hospital. When it is nearly time for surgery, you will meet with your surgeon, the anesthesiologist, and possibly other members of the surgical team, such as nurses, who will be there during the procedure. The surgeon or a nurse will double-check everything for the last time. You will need to confirm that have not eaten since the day before, that you have followed the liquid diet as instructed and that you have taken your medications as instructed. To help prevent surgery mistakes, you should also be asked to confirm that you are there for the gastric bypass.

> **Tip**
>
> Chapter 3, "All About the Roux-En-Y Gastric Bypass (RYGB)," identifies the members of your surgical team and describes the surgery.

Then someone will wheel you to the holding area outside of the operating room in a wheelchair. You will have an IV placed into you so that the anesthesiologist can deliver anesthesia during your surgery. You will also be hooked up to a heart rate monitor and an oxygen monitor. These devices let the anesthesiologist see how you are doing during surgery and how much anesthesia to give you.

You will be wheeled to the operating table and helped to lie on your back in a comfortable position with your head on pillows. The anesthesiologist will place a mask over your nose and mouth to breathe through. The mask delivers oxygen. The first part of the anesthesiology process is the induction process to calm you down. It might happen through an injection or through an endotracheal tube, a pipe that goes from the mask and down your throat, to breathe through. You will breathe in a gas that relaxes you and numbs pain. Next, you will be put to sleep with an anesthetic through your IV tube. While you are asleep, the anesthesiologist will also deliver a muscle relaxing drug so that your muscles do not twitch as a reflex during surgery.

The next time you wake up, your gastric bypass will be complete, and you will be ready to lose weight for life!

✍ Summary

☛ Now you know everything about preparing for the surgery. You know how to prepare your home, what to pack, and what else to bring if you are going abroad. You know what to eat the night before surgery, how you are getting to the hospital, and what will happen once you get there. You are ready for the Roux-en-Y gastric bypass!

☛ Next we continue from when you wake up from surgery. Chapter 11 will help you recover as quickly and smoothly as possible. There will be bumps along the way, but a bit of preparation can smooth your journey.

Time to Take Action: Last-Minute Checklist

A checklist is always helpful when you're packing for an overnight stay. Here's what you might want to take to the hospital. Just check them off when they're in your suitcase or purse.

_____ Any paperwork from your insurance company or the hospital

_____ Passport if going to Mexico

_____ All of your prescription medications

_____ Change of underwear and socks

_____ Non-slip slippers or light sneakers

_____ Toothbrush and toothpaste

_____ Hairbrush or comb

_____ Lotion or hand cream

_____ Chapstick or lip balm

_____ Hand sanitizer

_____ Book, magazines, MP3 player, or any other entertainment

_____ Cell phone (fully charged)

Contact Information (name and telephone number):

_____ Your primary care physician

_____ Your ride home from the hospital

_____ Your insurance company

_____ The number and address of the nearest U.S. consulate
(if you are going to another country for your RYGB)

Your own items:

_____ Lucky rabbit's foot

_____

_____

_____

1   Schumann R, Jones SB, Cooper B, Kelley SD, Bosch MV, Ortiz VE, Connor KA, Kaufman MD, Harvey AM, Carr DB. Update on best practice recommendations for anesthetic perioperative care and pain management in weight loss surgery, 2004-2007. Obesity (Silver Spring). 2009;17(5):889-894.

2   Acetaminophen. Medline Plus, National Institutes of Health. Web Site. http://www.nlm.nih.gov/medlineplus/druginfo/meds/a681004.html. Updated 2012, 15 January. Accessed October 4, 2012.

3   Dugdale DC, Zieve D. Pain medications - narcotics. MedlinePlus, National Institutes of Health. Web site. http://www.nlm.nih.gov/medlineplus/ency/article/007489.htm. Updated 2011, May 22. Accessed October 4, 2012.

4   Aspirin. Acetaminophen. Medline Plus, National Institutes of Health. Web Site. http://www.nlm.nih.gov/medlineplus/druginfo/meds/a682878.html. Updated 2011, 16 March. Accessed October 4, 2012.

5   Ibuprofen. Medline Plus, National Institutes of Health. Web Site. http://www.nlm.nih.gov/medlineplus/druginfo/meds/a682159.html. 2010, 1 October. Accessed October 4, 2012.

6   Salsalate. Medline Plus, National Institutes of Health. Web Site. http://www.nlm.nih.gov/medlineplus/druginfo/meds/a682880.html. Updated 2010, 1 September. Accessed October 4, 2012.

7   Naproxen. Medline Plus, National Institutes of Health. Web Site. http://www.nlm.nih.gov/medlineplus/druginfo/meds/a681029.html. Updated 2012, 15 June. Accessed October 4, 2012.

8   Corticosteroid (oral route, parenteral route). (2012). *Mayo Clinic*. Retrieved from http://www.mayoclinic.com/health/drug-information/DR602333/METHOD=print

9   Dugdale DC, Zieve D. Diet – clear liquid. Medline Plus, National Institutes of Health. Web site. http://www.nlm.nih.gov/medlineplus/ency/patientinstructions/000205.htm. 2010, November 21. Accessed October 4, 2012.

10 Elliott JA, Patel VM, Kirresh A, Ashrafian H, Le Roux CW, Olbers T…Zacharakis E. Fast-track laparoscopic bariatric surgery: a systematic review. Updates Surg, 2013.

11 Kelly JJ, Shikora S, Jones DB, Hutter M, Robinson MK, Romanelli J, Buckley F, Lederman A, Blackburn GL, Lautz D. Best practice updates for surgical care in weight loss surgery. Obesity, 2009;17(5):863-870.

12 Venezuela: Country Specific Information. U.S. Department of State. Web site. http://www.travel.state.gov/travel/cis_pa_tw/cis/cis_1059.html. Accessed October 6, 2012.

13 Mexico: Country Specific Information. U.S. Department of State. Web site. http://travel.state.gov/travel/cis_pa_tw/cis/cis_970.html. Accessed September 17, 2012.

14 Mayo Clinic Staff. General anesthesia. Mayo Clinic. Web site. http://www.mayoclinic.com/health/anesthesia/MY00100/METHOD=print. 2010, June 26. Accessed October 6, 2012.

15 Dugdale DC, Zieve D. Diet – clear liquid. Medline Plus, National Institutes of Health. Web site. http://www.nlm.nih.gov/medlineplus/ency/patientinstructions/000205.htm. 2010, November 21. Accessed October 4, 2012.

11

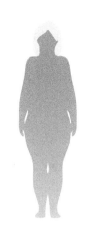

Your Time at the Hospital After Surgery

Congratulations! You are now a gastric bypass patient! Despite your careful research and preparation for surgery, this moment feels like the true start to your weight loss journey and new lifestyle. With all the planning and effort you put in to get here, you deserve to treat yourself right to get the full advantages of having the RYGB.

This is a very important period in your weight loss journey because what you do now affects your short-term recovery and long-term success with the gastric bypass. This chapter describes what to expect as you recover from surgery and how to prevent or reduce complications. The chapter covers:

- Your stay in the hospital
- The first few days at home
- Returning to normal activities and to work

By the end of this chapter, you will be a pro with your new digestive system! You will be well on your way back to your normal life and ready to focus on losing weight for good.

Your Time at the Hospital after Surgery

The Roux-en-Y gastric bypass takes about two to four hours.[1] The procedure tends to be shorter if your surgeon is experienced; it is longer if you have an open gastric bypass instead of a laparoscopic one or if there are complications. One or two hours after the procedure is over, you will gradually wake up under the watch of hospital nurses. Next, you will likely go to your hospital room, where one or more nurses will care for you until you leave the hospital.

Fully Regaining Your Consciousness as the Anesthesia Wears Off

The anesthesia will slowly wear off, and you will start to regain consciousness one or two hours after the RYGB. You probably will not remember much of the next few hours, because you will still be groggy from surgery. Bustling nurses will take care of you, so you do not need to worry about anything.

The PACU

Most surgery patients wake up in a special room called the post-anesthesia care unit, or PACU. The PACU is a room that is equipped with a bunch of high-tech equipment to monitor vital signs such as blood pressure and heart rate. Some patients may be hooked up to IVs giving them medications, fluids, or nutrients.[2] You will probably have an IV in your arm to provide fluids and prevent dehydration because by the time you wake up from surgery, you will not have had anything to drink for several hours. You might also have a tube in your throat to help you breathe.[3]

A nurse or team of nurses will monitor you closely as you fully regain consciousness. They will look at the machines you are hooked up to and check that everything is okay, and they might make some adjustments in your IV. Every couple of minutes or so, they will ask you how you feel, and they can add pain medications or medications to reduce nausea if you are overwhelmed. They might ask you silly personal questions such as your name or address just to make sure that you are thinking clearly. The nurses might pay so much attention to you that they can even get annoying as you go from being mostly asleep to fully alert. That is a good sign though: If you are awake enough to feel pestered, you are recovering pretty well!

The Humorous Side of the PACU

You might not remember much about your conversations with the nurses in the PACU. If you are like many patients, you will ask why the nurses are in the PACU and what operation they had. You will think you are listening to and understanding the nurses' answers, but you will ask the same questions again within minutes! Once you are alert enough to stop repeating your questions and recognize that some of the other patients are repeating their own questions just like you were, you might find the behavior pretty funny—and start to admire the patience of the nurses as they continue to cheerfully answer the same questions repeatedly.

You Might Start to Feel Post-Surgery Pain

After surgery, anesthesia, muscle relaxants, and pain medications begin to wear off. As you become more alert and less medicated, the pain will intensify in your stomach area where the surgeon made the incisions to insert the laparoscopic tools or to access your stomach. You might feel pain right in your abdomen where the surgeon cut and stitched your stomach and small intestine. Shoulder pain is common after a laparoscopic procedure because of the extra gas that might still be in your abdominal cavity. The pain will increase as your pain medications are wearing off. The nurse may give you medications to manage the pain.

Leaving the PACU

You will stay in the PACU until the nurse is sure that your heart rate, breathing, and blood pressure are stable. If you have obstructive sleep apnea, you will be in the PACU for about three extra hours until you are completely over the effects of anesthesia to make sure that you do not fall asleep and stop breathing without your CPAP machine.[4] Then you will go to your hospital room.

Staying Hydrated Right after Surgery

Dehydration is a real threat after surgery if you and your nurses are not careful. The IV in the PACU provides enough fluid to prevent dehydration, but you need to start drinking fluids when your IV is removed. You might not want to because you will be feeling nauseous or in pain, but nurses will continue to encourage you to drink.

Ice chips, or chopped or shaved ice, are a good choice for your first post-surgery food:

- It is pure water, so it helps prevent dehydration.
- It is solid, so you cannot eat it too quickly. Wait until it melts in your mouth before swallowing.
- It helps you progress to taking small sips of regular water.

You cannot avoid all discomfort after Roux-en-Y gastric bypass, but you can make your transition to a liquid diet easier by following a few tips:

- Take small sips and drink slowly. Small pieces of ice are perfect for forcing you to do both of these. Take very small spoonfuls or even a piece at a time. Stick with tiny sips when you progress to water.

- Make sure the ice melts and warms in your mouth before you swallow to avoid aggravating the sites of surgery.

- Avoid very hot or cold liquids because they can be painful on your surgery wounds.

- Sit up to make it easier for foods to go down. A motion called peristalsis is pretty effective at pushing foods and beverages downward in your gastrointestinal tract.[5] That is why kids can swallow without choking while they are standing on their heads. However, some weight loss surgery patients experience heartburn or reflux,[6] and you can reduce your risk by eating and drinking in an upright position.

- Avoid carbonated beverages. This isn't just because of the calories in full-sugar sodas. You should even avoid diet beverages such as diet soft drinks and sparkling waters. The bubbles not only make you feel bloated and possibly nauseous, but it can also stretch your stomach pouch and cause problems later.

- Keep sipping. It is hard to drink a lot at this time, so focus on sipping your fluids continuously to make sure you get enough.

Following these guidelines is good practice for the future. Eating slowly and avoiding carbonated beverages will reduce stomach stretching so that weight loss is easier. Also, eating only in an upright position helps prevent esophageal reflux, heartburn, and unpleasant feelings of being overly full. Eating only when seated at the table in an upright position is also a great habit to get into because it prevents you from mindless eating and drinking while you are preparing food or relaxing on the couch.

Healthy Recovery in the Hospital

If you do not have serious complications, you will be in the hospital or clinic for about two to seven days. The average stay is five days.[7] You might be eager to get home, but staying in the hospital lets you make rapid progress. Take advantage of the opportunity! These are some benefits of staying in the hospital:

- *Trained medical professionals are on hand if anything goes wrong.* Most likely, nothing serious will go wrong. Instead, you will only use the medical professionals' expertise as they reassure you that you are fine. You may feel nauseous or be vomiting or even a little dizzy from the anesthesia, and you will almost certainly have some pain in your stomach or shoulder. During these first several hours, you are not sure which symptoms are serious and which are simply uncomfortable. When you are in the hospital, you can describe each symptom to a nurse to find out whether it is worth worrying about and what its cause is.

- *You do not have to worry about going to the bathroom when you are exhausted and in pain after surgery.* Initially, you might use a catheter to urinate if you are having trouble or cannot stand up to get to the bathroom. When you are ready to go into a bathroom, having a trained medical professional to help you is safer than going by yourself and easier—and less embarrassing—than asking your spouse or someone else to help you. Bariatric nurses are able to support obese patients by using special equipment and teamwork as necessary. Hospital bathrooms are equipped with features like handrails to grab onto and high-seated toilets so that you do not have to bend your knees as far to sit on the toilet.

- *You do not have to worry about putting on a brave face for your kids.* Most parents do not want their children to see them when they are not at their best. You are going to be weak and tired after surgery. Staying in the hospital away from your children prevents them from having to see you in a weakened state at home. Also, it prevents you from feeling pressure to play with them or help out around the house.

- It builds your confidence. You might be a nervous wreck, or at least a little unsure of yourself, right after your surgery. After all, it is a life-changing experience and a dramatic change in your body. Depending on nurses at this time lets you relax and focus on recovery. You can ask all of your little questions and get sound advice from your nurse without having to worry about feeling stupid or making a mistake that will delay recovery. By the time you are discharged, you will be better able to recognize your signs and symptoms and know what to do about them.

- *It builds your family's confidence.* Your own emotions affect your family's reactions. If you are anxious and concerned, they will be too. If you are confident and reassuring from the moment you walk in the door at home, your family will feel much more comfortable. You can set the example so that they do not feel uneasy around you.

- *It helps your family to help you.* Pay attention to how the nurses take care of you in the hospital. That will give you some ideas of what to ask your family members to do for you. They are probably eager to help you out but do not want to hurt you and do not know what to do until you tell them their roles in your recovery.

Your Stay in the Hospital

Your only job in the hospital is to recover. Follow your surgeons' and nurses' instructions so that you can be confident that you are laying the best possible foundation for your future with the gastric bypass. Before surgery, you might be worried that staying in the hospital for so long will be boring, but the days will probably pass faster than you think. You will be tired from surgery, and you will have a few other things to concentrate on:

- *One or more appointments with your surgeon:* Your surgeon will need to check your progress and permit you to be released from the hospital when it is time.

- *One or more appointments with your nutritionist or dietitian:* We will talk about appointments with the dietitian later in the chapter.

- *Visits from your family and/or friends:* The hospital will probably have regular visiting hours when your family can come see you in your room or you can visit with them in a hospital lounge or another public place.
- *Carefully planned meals:* You will be on a liquid diet, and your nurse should automatically bring you your meals and snacks. You should also have water near you at all times, including at night, so you can stay hydrated.

Unplanned Time

Surgery is exhausted. The down time in the hospital will help you recover. Surgery is tough on your body not only because of the actual surgical procedure and cuts but also because of the barrage of anesthesia and medications from your surgery. Your down time is when you can take naps, read books, do crossword puzzles, watch DVDs, log on to BariatricPal.com, and do all the other activities you packed for yourself. As you feel stronger, you might start to take short walks in your room and the hospital halls during your free time.

Staying Active

Staying active can help you feel better and may even speed up recovery. Staying active can be as simple as standing up every few minutes during the day, walking around your hospital room, or going down the corridor. Slow walking is a great activity for increasing your blood flow and helping your surgery wounds to heal.

Pain Medications

The first day and night may be very painful because the anesthesia will wear off and the pain from surgery will be in full force. You will continue to have pain for several days or weeks, but the worst of it should be over within days. Nurses will continue to provide pain medications as you need them. Your surgeon may prescribe certain pain medications, such as opioids or narcotics. These include codeine, vicodine, and oxycodone.[8]

Another common pain medication after bariatric surgery is ketorolac.[9] Like ibuprofen and aspirin, ketorolac is a non-steroidal anti-inflammatory drug (NSAID) used to treat pain.[10] Compared to normal NSAIDS such as ibuprofen and aspirin, ketorolac is only available by prescription. Using ketorolac can help you decrease the amount of narcotic painkillers that you need, but you shouldn't take it for more than a few days as your doctor recommends. Side effects of ketorolac may be similar to those that you are fighting after surgery, including diarrhea, nausea, and fatigue.

Leaving the Hospital and Going Home

You will be in the hospital for about two to seven days. As you progress, your surgeon will probably give you a closer estimate of when you can expect to go home. Then you can make plans or confirm your plans for getting home.

Getting Discharged from the Hospital

You need an official discharge before leaving the hospital. You will be eligible for discharge after your surgeon examines you and gives you the go-ahead. At a major hospital, the discharge station may be a large desk at the front of the bariatric surgery ward. In a smaller clinic, you might be discharged at the front reception desk.

The process does not take long. You will go through the usual medical checkout procedures, such as paying your co-pay or the full or partial amount of services depending on your financing plan. The receptionist should confirm your next appointment with the surgeon and may also verify your next dietitian appointment if your dietitian's office is in the same medical facility. You may need to sign some paperwork or fill out some forms. If you are still having trouble walking far or being on your feet for a long time, a nurse might wheel you to the curb outside to wait for your ride in a wheelchair.

Some surgeons prevent patients from driving themselves home for their own safety. The receptionist at discharge may require you to identify the person who is ready to drive you. That person might even need to come into the discharge area so that the receptionist can see him or her in person.

What to Ask Before You Leave the Hospital

Most of the steps of the discharge process are pretty clear, so you do not have to worry about remembering them. There are a couple of important things to be sure you know before you leave the hospital:

- *Find out the best phone number to use if you have questions when you are at home.* This is probably different than the general hospital number that you might use to make appointments or call for general questions. You might get a direct number to your surgeon or surgeon's staff so that you do not have to spend time on hold or going through telephone menus. You may be calling this number a lot over the next several days!

- *Get an off-hours number.* This does not necessarily need to be an emergency number, but it could be. Before you leave the hospital, make sure you know which number to call at any time of the day or night and on weekends.

- *Be sure you understand your post-surgery instructions.* Your surgeon should have provided you with written instructions and gone over them with you. They should guide you through the entire recovery process, including your gradual return to regular physical activity, your dietary progression from liquids to solid foods, any changes in how to take your regular prescription medications, and specific instructions for using pain medications.

- *Make sure you have your diet guidelines.* Instructions for what to drink and eat during the next several weeks should be written clearly. Ask about anything that is unclear or confusing.

On the Ride Home

Keep resting as much as possible. To use that pillow that you put in the car or packed for yourself before surgery, place it under your seatbelt and over your abdomen to reduce stomach pain. The pillow reduces jarring and irritation from the seatbelt, especially when the car bounces or turns.

Anxiety is normal when you leave the hospital and you are no longer under constant medical supervision, but try to stay calm. Your surgeon would not have let you go home if he or she did not think you were ready. And you are not completely on your own. Your hospital and surgeon are just a phone call or drive away.

Your First Few Days at Home

Getting home can be empowering. You are now able to take charge of your own fate. You will start, over these days and weeks, to feel capable of doing anything you set your mind to—including losing the weight you want by following your post-surgery instructions. You will undoubtedly make mistakes along the way, but you can overcome setbacks by staying positive and focusing on your goals.

Some Pain Is Normal

Your surgery wounds will hurt. The pain should be less intense than in the hospital by the time you get home, but you will probably still feel pain in the surgical incisions on your abdomen as well as deeper in your stomach and intestines where the surgeon made cuts and stitches. The pain may feel like muscle soreness or a sharper pain.

These are some additional possible sources of discomfort:

- Your shoulder or neck may continue to ache for as long as there is extra gas in your abdominal cavity. That is the gas that was pumped in during the laparoscopic procedure if that is what you had.

- Nausea is possible because of the pain as well as the pain medications. You need to call your doctor if the nausea becomes so bad that you cannot drink and you start to become dehydrated. That can happen within several hours.

Pain Medications & Alternative Pain Management Strategies

Your pain medications will be similar to those in the hospital. You can continue taking prescription narcotics if your surgeon recommends them and/or the prescription non-steroidal anti-inflammatory drug called ketorolac. At this time, your surgeon might suggest using less of the prescription medications and more over-the-counter options, which are typically milder and less risky. Examples include ibuprofen, aspirin, and acetaminophen, also known as Tylenol. Your surgeon will probably suggest taking pain medications only as needed and to

> **Tip**
>
> The earlier portion of this chapter, dedicated to your hospital stay, discusses the different types of common painkillers and which are most likely to be prescribed for treating your pain after the surgery. **Chapter 6, "Considering Roux-En-Y Gastric Bypass? ...What You Need to Know,"** discusses the possible side effects and complications after surgery.

take as few as possible to manage the pain. Limiting your painkillers to only when you really need them is healthier:

- It reduces the amount of chemicals in your body
- It builds mental toughness
- Some kinds of painkillers can be addictive
- Some pain medications can delay healing from surgery or increase your risk of having an ulcer
- Pain medications can interfere with your regular medications, which may already be affected by your surgery and changes in diet

Unfortunately, minimizing your use of pain medications requires you to endure some pain. These strategies can help you cope with the pain. Practicing these strategies can help you get better at managing pain without drugs. As you find yourself growing stronger, do not forget to tell yourself how proud you are of yourself for handling this tough situation.

- *Distract yourself by focusing on something else*: This takes your mind off of the pain. You can turn to an old hobby or use your post-surgery recovery time as an opportunity to start a new hobby, such as blogging or sewing.
- *Talk yourself through it:* Reassure yourself either out loud or in your head that you are fine. Take inventory of your pain—try to identify exactly what hurts, how bad it is, and what is causing the pain. Then think about how bad it *could* be and how strong you are for not letting it bother you. The pain might not seem so bad once you have stared it in the face.
- *Go social:* Phone a friend, write some emails, or visit BariatricPal.com. Members there will sympathize. They will keep you company and will not ask you to hide the pain. Time can fly by when you are absorbed in your telephone or online conversations, and the pain can become more bearable before you have to give in to the urge to take medication.
- *Get moving:* Activity can distract you and calm you. It also increases circulation, so you might feel less pain. Any activity that you do can be helpful. That might mean that you stand up and sit down a few times, using the edge of a table for support, or it might mean that you walk around the house for a few minutes. Doing arm circles and swinging your legs back and forth can be enough to reduce pain without needing to stand up if that is too much for you.
- *Use a heating pad and/or ice pack:* Place the heating pad on the area of pain, whether it is your stomach, shoulder, or neck. If you want, alternate with ice packs. Heat increases blood flow and is soothing. Ice is a natural painkiller and anti-inflammatory. Follow the instruction on the heating pad and ice packs so you do not get burned or risk frostbite. Only use them for the recommended length of time stated on the label, usually 10 to 20 minutes, and wrap them in a towel instead of applying them directly to your skin.
- *Delay taking pain medications:* If you have your doctor's approval to skip doses, try to

postpone your next dose by a few minutes at a time and see if you can stretch that out for longer. These are some examples:

- Can you hold out until the next commercial break? What about until the end of the television program you are watching?
- Can you walk to the end of the driveway and back before taking pain medication?
- *Reduce your dose.* That will help you get some pain relief while still reducing the amount of chemicals in your body.

Distracting yourself is a valuable skill for the rest of your weight loss journey. Sometimes you will feel hungry before it is time for a meal or snack. Your new mental discipline can help you accomplish other tasks instead of giving in to your hunger and going straight to the refrigerator.

> **Tip**
>
> Chapter 18, "The Benefits of a Strong Support System," talks about creating a list of people to call when you feel as though you are about to slip off of the diet.

When to Consult Your Surgeon

In addition to pain, you may experience other side effects from the Roux-en-Y gastric bypass. Most do not require medical attention, but consult your doctor if you have any doubts.

- Around 6 to 10 percent of RYGB patients require readmission to the hospital within 30 days of surgery.[11]
- Around 14% of RYGB patient develop a complication within 30 days of surgery. [12]

Dumping Syndrome

Dumping syndrome is a side effect of the RYGB that is more likely if you eat high-fat or high-sugar foods. Chapter 5, Risks of RYGB, describes dumping syndrome more fully. Symptoms may include nausea, vomiting, cramping, and diarrhea. Although it is unpleasant, dumping does not usually require medical attention. Call your doctor if you need help figuring out how to modify your diet so that it does not cause trouble or if your dumping syndrome is so bad that you cannot keep food down. Twelve percent, or one in eight, patients have severe dumping.[13]

Fever and Redness

A temperature of 101 or more degrees can be a sign of an infection. About 1 to six percent of bypass patients get infections after surgery.[14] Infections can start at the incisions from surgery, and they may also appear red and become more painful.[15] An untreated infection can spread to the rest of your body. Sepsis, or the spread of an infection to your blood, can develop if conditions were not sterile during surgery or if you do not treat your original infection quickly; between 1 and two percent of RYGB patients get sepsis.[16] Another possible cause of fever is a blood clot, which can be fatal. A pulmonary embolism blocks blood flow to your lungs, while a deep vein thrombosis blocks blood flow to your legs. A fever does not always require medical treatment, but you should consult your surgeon to check.

Shortness of Breath or Chest Pain

Shortness of breath can be a sign of a few different conditions that require attention:

- Pneumonia occurs in about 1% of gastric bypass patients[17] and is caused by an infection. Symptoms may include chest pain and coughing.

- Blood clots may be another cause of shortness of breath. Blood clots are well-known complications of surgery, and other symptoms include painful, red, or swollen legs. A pulmonary embolism is a blood clot that affects your lungs,[18] and deep vein thrombosis, or a blood clot in your thigh or lower leg, is another post-surgery concern.[19]

- Shortness of breath is a potential sign of a pulmonary embolism. Swollen legs can happen if a blood clot is blocking the blood flow to them. If you have swollen legs, you might need to go to the hospital and get an ultrasound so that your surgeon can see if there is a blood clot.

Nausea

Nausea is a common effect of anesthesia. If you are nauseous while in the hospital, the nurses may give you anti-nausea medications. Painkillers can cause nausea too. You need to call your surgeon if your nausea gets so bad that you cannot stomach fluids. You can get dehydrated and require hospitalization if you go for more than a few hours without drinking fluids.

Vomiting

Vomiting can have a variety of causes, and some of them are serious. Furthermore, the force of repeated vomiting can lead to dehiscence, or splitting of your surgery wounds. It is safest to call your surgeon if you vomit more than once and do not know the cause. These are some possible causes of vomiting after the RYGB:

- *As a side effect of taking narcotic painkillers on an empty stomach:* Your surgeon may be able to suggest a better pain medication schedule for you.

- *As a sign of an anastomotic leak:* Leaks and fistula occur in up to five percent of bypass patients,[20] and they can be fatal if not treated. Other symptoms of leaks include fever, stomach pain, frequent urination, and a rapid heart rate.

> **Tip**
>
> See Chapter 5, "Roux-En-Y Gastric Bypass: Risks and Considerations," for an-depth discussion of the potential side effects and complications from the gastric bypass surgery. The chapter goes into symptoms of potentially serious or mild complications and which patients are most likely to experience them. Chapters 13 and 14 discuss your post-surgery diet and how to safely eat after RYGB.

- *Eating too much:* You can vomit if you eat more than your stomach pouch can comfortably hold. This is not a big concern when you are on the liquid diet during the first week or two after surgery. It is more likely to become a problem when you start eating real foods. You can prevent overeating by limiting yourself to the amount of food on your diet plan and by eating only until you are full.

Sharp Stomach Pain

Sharp stomach pain that comes on suddenly or becomes worse can be a signal that something is wrong and you need to call your surgeon. Some post-surgery pain is normal as your surgery wounds heal, but the pain should gradually decrease. A sudden increase in pain or a noticeable change in the type of pain you feel can be a sign of these problems and may need medical attention:

- Gastritis[21]
- Anastomotic leak
- Splitting of surgery wound

Most of your symptoms will not be due to a medical emergency; your surgeon will be able take care of your problem fairly easily. The tried and true guidelines never go out of style though; if you think you have a medical emergency, call 9-1-1. If you think you need emergency care, go to the nearest emergency room. It is always better to be safe than to risk a complication.

Keep Letting Your Wounds Heal

If you had laparoscopic RYGB, your skin will have four to six small scars where your surgeon made surgical cuts.[22] Your surgery wounds will be slightly larger if you had an open procedure. Your job at home is to allow your wounds to continue to heal just as they were in the hospital. Your hospital discharge guidelines might include instructions for your cuts. Wounds should be kept clean and dry to prevent infections and to allow the sides of the cuts to close properly. At first, you may need to sponge off to wash yourself instead of taking a shower to keep your wounds dry.

Your surgeon's other instructions for care are also important. You might have to change the dressings, or bandages, regularly, and there might be an antibiotic cream or ointment to put over the cuts to prevent infections. If you have stitches, your surgeon might need to take them out for you, although some kinds of surgical stitches are made out of materials that will eventually dissolve by themselves so that you do not need to get the stitches removed.

Your surgery scars will eventually disappear or become nearly invisible, and they probably will not bother you. If they do, there are some treatment options that you can consider later on when you are closer to your goal weight and your body stops changing so much.

Relaxation and Recovery

The best thing to do when you get home from the hospital is relax so that you can recover as quickly and as well as possible. This will make your weight loss journey easier. Here are a few suggestions to reduce strain on your body:

- Do not do hard chores if they are not absolutely necessary. Do not vacuum, rearrange furniture, or scrub floors.

- Do not lift heavy objects. The effort can lead to dehiscence, or splitting of your wound.

- If you have children, be sure to review some ground rules. At this time, your children should not be jumping on you or demanding to be picked up.

- Loving spouses and caring family members and friends may also need gentle reminders not to hug you.

Taking a Break from Stress

Surgery takes an emotional toll, and mental rest is as important as physical rest. The surgery itself was tiring, and the stress of planning for surgery and the relief of having it over can be exhausting! The pre-surgery nerves and post-surgery sense of relief are normal.

Taking the mental break that you need may require a conscious effort not to get worked up about things that are not that important. This may be a good time to begin a new habit of setting aside time each day for yourself. Now you might devote this time to deep breathing and relaxation. Your personal time might soon evolve into your daily exercise time, starting with stretching and eventually developing into what will become your regular routine.

> ### Tip
>
> Chapter 16, "Physical Activity to Control Weight Loss," discusses starting a safe exercise routine. It also gives some suggestions on fitting in your daily exercise and learning to love it.

Support Is Important Too

Take advantage of your friends and family and let them help you. Almost all of us have close friends or family members who are not only willing but anxious to help by doing anything they can to make recovery easier. These are some of the simple but significant ways that your supporters can aid you:

- Check on you, in person or over the phone, at regular intervals during the day if you are home alone

- Drop off your children at school and pick them up after school, as well as take them to any afterschool activities that they have

- Babysit for a few hours to give you a little bit more quiet time

- Lift something heavy for you, such as a full laundry basket or some bags of groceries

- Run a few errands since you should not drive a car for a couple days after surgery until the anesthesia and pain medications are completely out of your system
- Ask you how you are feeling and really listen to the answer

Asking friends and family members for help may seem a little awkward to you. That is especially true if you are used to doing everything on your own or if you have a regular pattern in which everyone knows their own roles so you do not really directly ask each other for help. They might not know exactly what to do to be helpful and might feel like it is not their place to offer because they worry that you will be insulted. It is up to you to take the first step and ask for help. Both you and your supporters will be so glad you did. Once you start the conversation, the ice will be broken. You can let them know specific things they can do to help, and they will feel more comfortable asking what they can do.

Returning To Normal Activities and Work

When you first get home from the hospital, you will be tired and you will not feel like doing much. That is for the best because resting is what you need. You will become more active as you get your energy back. Within a few weeks, you can be back in full swing with work and life—but do not increase your activity levels too quickly.

Keep Moving but Do Not Strain

A small amount of light activity is good for you even when you are tired. It speeds up your blood flow so that more oxygen and nutrients are delivered to your surgery location, and your wounds might heal faster. You can keep doing the same things at home that you were doing in the hospital: standing up and sitting down repeatedly, walking around, or even walking up and down the driveway.

Do Not Lift Heavy Objects

Avoiding lifting or straining to move heavy objects is a good idea after any surgery. You do not want to strain so much that you put pressure on your abdomen and risk gastric staple line dehiscence. Everyone has a different idea of what is "heavy," but a good initial goal might be to limit yourself to lifting less than 8 pounds, which is the weight of a gallon of milk. After that, you can increase your limit by no more than about one pound per day. If you are not sure whether something is heavy, just err on the safe side and do not lift it.

Since you might not even realize how much weight you lift in your daily life, here is a list of everyday objects that are too heavy for right after surgery:

- Suitcases and bags of groceries
- Heavy (full) pots and pans, such as when you are making soup or a pot roast
- Furniture
- Vacuum cleaners
- Strollers
- Children (even if they say "please" when they ask you to carry them!)

Keep Moving as You Progress to Normal Activities

Any kind of light activity around that you can comfortably do without straining helps you heal faster, feel better, and progress more easily to your regular activities. Standing up frequently instead of sitting still is a great way to start. You can even set a timer to remind you to stand up every 15 or 30 minutes.

Other very light activities include walking around the house or down the driveway; easy chores, such as folding clothes; and stretching. When you feel comfortable, walk slowly, play golf, and play with your children without lifting them up. Water activities, such as water aerobics and swimming, are great choices because they are low-impact, so they do not strain your joints. Be sure to get your surgeon's okay before getting into the pool because you do not want to get your incisions wet before they heal.

In general, the more active you were before your surgery, the faster you can increase your activity levels after the surgery. You are also going to be able to do more activities sooner if your surgery was laparoscopic and you have not had any serious complications or severe side effects from the surgery. Usually, patients with a lower pre-surgery BMI can get back to regular activities faster.

When you think about the return to normal activities, keep in mind that any timeline that you see for adding in new activities is just an estimate. You might return to certain activities faster than other weight loss surgery patients, and you might take a little longer to progress to other activities. That is okay. The important part here is to listen to your body. Take your time adding in new activities and increasing the amount you do because you do not want to risk hurting yourself or delaying your recovery from surgery. Immediately stop any activity that causes pain. If the pain does not stop when you stop the activity, call your doctor or surgeon for advice.

Going Back to Work

If you work, going back to work is a big milestone. It is one thing to recover from surgery and get used to your new body and lifestyle in the comfort and privacy of your own home. It is quite another thing to go take on responsibilities at work while dealing with your new gastrointestinal system in public.

You can probably return to work within a few weeks of surgery if you did not have complications. You need to wait awhile longer if you are having post-surgery complications or if your job requires you to be very active or lift a lot of weight. Do not rush your return to work no matter how eager you are to get back there. You are still recovering from surgery and do not want to put yourself at risk for any setbacks that can occur if you get too ambitious. Also, if you feel sick at work, be strong enough to let yourself come home and recover more fully.

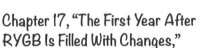

Tip

Chapter 17, "The First Year After RYGB Is Filled With Changes," has advice about returning to work and knowing what to expect from your colleagues. You will learn about handling medical problems at work, figuring out who your true work friends are, and how you can deal with the sensitive topic of eating. We will talk about some of the different options for how much and exactly what you want to tell various people about your bariatric surgery.

Summary

☛ This chapter took you from the operating room in the hospital to getting back to work and other regular activities. Now you know what to expect when you wake up from surgery, how your hospital stay will go, and what you can do at home to make your recovery from surgery as fast and smooth as possible.

☛ These days and weeks are important in laying the foundation for your future success as a gastric bypass patient. Patience during recovery can help you get through this time with the best possible results. Your wounds will heal faster if you do not try to rush anything; you will be at lower risk for developing complications, and your future weight loss should be easier.

Time to Take Action: Prepare for the Post-Surgery Challenges!

Shortly after getting RYGB surgery, post-surgery pain and strong hunger may be two of the biggest challenges that you will face. This form can help you prepare for these challenges so that you can overcome them more easily.

What do you expect the pain to feel like? How do you expect the hunger to feel?

List at least five things you can tell yourself when the going gets tough

- e.g., It'll be worth it because …
- I've worked so hard for it that I can't stop now…
- It'll get better soon

1. _____
2. _____
3. _____
4. _____
5. _____

List at least three activities you can do to distract yourself from the pain or hunger.

- e.g., call my best friend Martha
- Do the crossword puzzle in the newspaper.

1. _____
2. _____
3. _____
4. _____
5. _____

1   Zieve D, Rogers A. Gastric bypass surgery. Medline Plus. Web site. http://www.nlm.nih.gov/medlineplus/ency/article/007199.htm. Updated 2012, June 4. Accessed February 12, 2013.

2   Bhimji S, Zieve D. General Anesthesia. MedlinePlus, National Institutes of Health. Web site. http://www.nlm.nih.gov/medlineplus/ency/article/007410.htm. Updated 2011, January 26. Accessed October 24, 2012.

3   Schumann R, Jones SB, Cooper B, Kelley SD, Bosch MV, Ortiz VE, Connor KA, Kaufman MD, Harvey AM, Carr DB. Update on best practice recommendations for anesthetic perioperative care and pain management in weight loss surgery, 2004-2007. Obesity (Silver Spring). 2009;17(5):889-894.

4   Schumann R, Jones SB, Cooper B, Kelley SD, Bosch MV, Ortiz VE, Connor KA, Kaufman MD, Harvey AM, Carr DB. Update on best practice recommendations for anesthetic perioperative care and pain management in weight loss surgery, 2004-2007. Obesity (Silver Spring). 2009;17(5):889-894.

5   Dugdale DC, Zieve D. Peristalsis. Medline Plus, National Institutes of Health. Web site. http://www.nlm.nih.gov/medlineplus/ency/article/002282.htm. Updated 2011, November 17. Accessed October 24, 2012.

6   Madalosso CA, Gurski RR, Callegari-Jacques SM, Navarini D, Thiesen V, Fornari F. The impact of gastric bypass on gastroesophageal reflux disease in patients with morbid obesity: a prospective study based on the Montreal Consensus. Ann Surg, 2010;251(2):244-8.

7   Shinogle JA, Owings MF, Kozak LJ. Gastric bypass as a treatment for obesity: trends, characteristics and complications. Obesity Research, 2005;13(12):2202-2209.

8   Dugdale DC, Zieve D. Pain medications - narcotics. Medline Plus, National Institutes of Health. Web site. http://www.nlm.nih.gov/medlineplus/ency/article/007489.htm. Updated 2011, May 22. Accessed October 25, 2012.

9   Schumann R, Jones SB, Cooper B, Kelley SD, Bosch MV, Ortiz VE, Connor KA, Kaufman MD, Harvey AM, Carr DB. Update on best practice recommendations for anesthetic perioperative care and pain management in weight loss surgery, 2004-2007. Obesity (Silver Spring). 2009;17(5):889-894.

10 Keterolac.. Medline Plus, National Institutes of Health. Web site. http://www.nlm.nih.gov/medlineplus/druginfo/meds/a693001.html. Revised 2010, October 1. Accessed October 25, 2012.

11 Hutter MM, Schimer BD, Jones DB, Ko CY, Cohen ME, Merkow RP, Nguyen NT. First report from the American College of Surgeons – Bariatric Surgery Center Network laparoscopic sleeve gastrectomy has morbidity and effectiveness positioned between the band and the bypass. Ann Surg. 2012;254(3):410-422.

12 Hutter MM, Schimer BD, Jones DB, Ko CY, Cohen ME, Merkow RP, Nguyen NT. First report from the American College of Surgeons – Bariatric Surgery Center Network laparoscopic sleeve gastrectomy has morbidity and effectiveness positioned between the band and the bypass. Ann Surg. 2012;254(3):410-422.

13 Laurenius A, Olbers T, Näslund I, Karlsson J. Dumping syndrome following gastric bypass: validation of the Dumping Symptom Rating Scale. Obes Surg. 2013.

14 Huang C-K. Single-incision laparoscopic bariatric surgery. J Minim Access Surg. 2011;7(1):99-103.

15 Pech N, Meyer F, Lippert H, Manger T, Stroh C. Complications, reoperations and nutrient deficiencies two years after sleeve surgery. J Obesity. 2012.

16 Hutter MM, Schimer BD, Jones DB, Ko CY, Cohen ME, Merkow RP, Nguyen NT. First report from the American College of Surgeons – Bariatric Surgery Center Network laparoscopic sleeve gastrectomy has morbidity and effectiveness positioned between the band and the bypass. Ann Surg. 2012;254(3):410-422.

17 Hutter MM, Schimer BD, Jones DB, Ko CY, Cohen ME, Merkow RP, Nguyen NT. First report from the American College of Surgeons – Bariatric Surgery Center Network laparoscopic sleeve gastrectomy has morbidity and effectiveness positioned between the band and the bypass. Ann Surg. 2012;254(3):410-422.

18 Pulmonary embolism. National Heart, Lung and Blood Institute. Web site. http://www.nhlbi.nih.gov/health/health-topics/topics/pe/printall-index.html. 2011, July 1. Accessed October 26, 2012.

19 Dugdale DC, Zieve D. Deep venous thrombosis. National Heart, Lung and Blood Institute. Web site. http://www.nlm.nih.gov/medlineplus/ency/article/000156.htm. Updated 2012, February 19. Accessed February 15, 2013.

20 Griffith PS, Birch DW, Sharma AM, Karmali S. Managing complications associated with laparoscopic Roux-en-Y gastric bypass for morbid obesity. Can J Surg. 2012 Oct;55(5):329-36.

21 Dugdale DC, Longstreth GF, Zieve D. Gastritis. Web site. http://www.nlm.nih.gov/medlineplus/ency/article/001150.htm. Updated 2011, January 31. Accessed October 28, 2012.

22 Zieve D, Rogers A. Gastric bypass surgery. Medline Plus. Web site. http://www.nlm.nih.gov/medlineplus/ency/article/007199.htm. Updated 2012, June 4. Accessed February 12, 2013

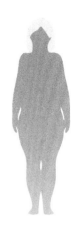

12

Aftercare: Your Post-Surgery Care Program

The last chapter discussed your very early post-surgery recovery phases in the hospital and provided advice on speeding up your recovery at home. This chapter talks about continuing your recovery with proper medical care. Your postoperative care program, or aftercare program, is a long-term program to keep you healthy and improve your weight loss with the RYGB. Your formal care program typically lasts for months or years after surgery and should be considered for life.

This chapter talks about:

- Post-surgery appointments with your surgeon
- Likely medical tests
- Other healthcare appointments post-surgery
- Support groups and other sources of support
- Staying positive and persistent during this time

By the end of the chapter, you will know what to expect during your post-surgery care. You will also know why each part is important so you stay motivated to keep getting the care you need. Working with your medical team members and following their guidance are important now because your actions now affect your future health and weight loss with the gastric bypass.

Aftercare: Your Post-Surgery Care Program

The quality of your post-surgery care program can be an important influence in your weight loss success and health after gastric bypass. As explained in Chapter 7, "*Planning For the Gastric Bypass*," the aftercare program is an important consideration when choosing your surgeon and medical team. Benefits of a comprehensive care program include:

- Lower risk of complications
- Better weight loss
- Lower risk of psychological problems
- More nutrition education opportunities

Your post-surgery care program is designed to improve your health and increase weight loss. It is likely to include these components:

- Follow-up appointments with the surgeon
- Regular medical tests to monitor your nutrient status and health conditions
- Appointments with a dietitian or nutritionist for nutrition counseling and meal planning
- Meeting with a clinical psychologist or psychiatrist, either in a group or a one-on-one setting, for your mental health
- Going to regular support group meetings

Your surgeon will probably encourage or require you to attend medical appointments for the several months following your surgery. Ideally, postoperative medical care will last for life. You will always be following a careful diet, working to avoid complications from the gastric bypass, getting medical tests and attending support group meetings.

Post-Op Care: Surgeon Appointments and Medical Tests

Your surgeon will probably examine you at least once or twice in the hospital to make that your gastric bypass shows no signs of leaking. Your surgeon also needs to examine you before approving your discharge from the hospital. Before you go home, your surgeon should give you your post-surgery instructions and answer any questions.

Surgeon Appointments throughout Your Weight Loss Journey

You will continue to see your surgeon after you get discharged from the hospital. You may have a couple of appointments with your surgeon during your first few weeks after leaving the hospital. These appointments will probably be scheduled before you leave the hospital after surgery. Appointments will become less frequent until they are monthly and eventually annually.

Typical Schedule of Surgeon Appointments

The American Society for Metabolic and Bariatric Surgery, or ASMBS, recommends the following appointments for bariatric surgery patients:[1]

- 1 to 6 times during the first six months
- 1 to 2 times during the next six months
- 1 to 2 times during the first year
- Annually for the rest of your life

You will need more appointments if you have nutritional deficiencies, if you do not lose weight as fast as expected, or if you develop complications.

Post-Op Care for Medical Tourism RYGB Patients

If you got the Roux-en-Y gastric bypass in Mexico or anywhere else that is too far to commute to for your aftercare program, your care should continue with a physician closer to home. Before surgery, your surgeon should have helped you plan for your post-surgery care. If not, you can still look around for a surgeon who will care for you. Try asking your own surgeon for recommendations or look around just as you would if you were searching for a surgeon for the original RYGB procedure.

What Happens in Your Regular Appointments?

Just like when you visit your primary care doctor, you will get weighed when the nurse checks you in. Now that you are on your weight loss journey, your weigh-in at the surgeon's office has a special meaning! Your surgeon should give you a chance to ask about any concerns or symptoms. If you are having trouble, your surgeon may recommend medical tests, such as a radiological scan using a blue dye to diagnose an anastomotic leak.[2] Your surgeon may routinely order blood tests to check your cholesterol levels, blood sugar levels, and nutritional status. You and your surgeon should discuss any abnormal results.

Medical Tests to Expect in Your Post-Surgery Care Program

Even if you have no alarming symptoms, your continuing care should include regular screening tests. If your surgeon works in a large clinic or hospital with its own laboratory, you can probably get your tests done on the same days that you see your surgeon for post-surgery follow-up appointments. These are some of the tests you can look forward to.

Nutritional Assessments

The gastric bypass puts you at risk for nutritional deficiencies because of a limited food intake and nutrient malabsorption. We will go over the specific vitamins and minerals in more detail later, but these are some of the more likely nutritional tests you will get on a routine basis:[3]

- Iron
- Vitamin B12
- Vitamin D
- Folate
- Albumin (to measure protein)

Blood Tests for Chronic Health Conditions

Although nobody likes getting pricked with a needle to get blood drawn, these blood tests are gratifying! Your improving values as you lose weight help justify your hard work to follow the gastric bypass diet. Many of your obesity-related chronic conditions will improve as you lose weight, and your blood tests will show it. If you had diabetes or pre-diabetes before the surgery, your blood sugar levels will probably come way down—you may even be able to get off blood sugar medications. The same is true for indicators of heart disease, such as total cholesterol, LDL cholesterol, and triglyceride levels.[4] These are also likely to drop as you lose weight. You may even be able to get off of your medications for cholesterol and triglycerides.

> **Tip**
>
> Chapter 13, "Post-Surgery Diet: From Liquid Diet to Solid Foods," Chapter 14, "RYGB Diet 101," Chapter 15, "The RYGB Diet & Nutrition," discuss nutrients and nutrient deficiencies in more detail. You will learn which nutrients you need to pay special attention to, which foods they are in, why you might not be getting enough, and how to prevent deficiencies.

Blood Pressure

This is another important measure that is probably going to get near the healthy range as you lose weight and start to exercise. Obesity raises your blood pressure, and losing weight to lower your blood pressure is healthy for your heart and kidneys. Your physician may eventually recommend that you stop your blood pressure-lowering medications.

Bone Density Scan

This one is not frequent, because of its cost, but it is a great test to see how healthy your bones are. When you lose weight fast, your bones can become less dense. As they get weaker, they are more likely to fracture. Nearly 40 million Americans have osteoporosis, or weak bones, and many do not realize it until they break a hip after what should have been a minor fall.[5] Older women at highest risk for osteoporosis can get bone density scans every two years, but your doctor might also recommend one if your weight loss is very fast or you are not getting enough calcium and vitamin D.

Dietitian Appointments

A comprehensive aftercare program includes regular follow-up appointments with a dietitian, with appointments starting one to two weeks after surgery, when you are still on a liquid or pureed food diet. Appointments become less frequent over time, and you might meet the dietitian at one, two, three, six, and nine months after surgery before switching to an annual schedule.[6]

The RYGB diet is challenging, and your dietitian can be the proverbial rock during your weight loss journey. He or she can help you plan meals, set reasonable goals, and overcome dietary problems that you encounter.

Choosing Foods and Planning Menus

The RYGB diet allows some foods and limits or even forbids many others. Your dietitian will let you know which foods and liquids are okay and which are not allowed during each stage of the RYGB diet as you progress from liquids to solid foods and continue losing weight. Some foods are allowed, but you might develop intolerances to them. Your dietitian can help you figure out alternative foods to maintain good nutrition.

Food Lists to Menu Planning

You are changing your whole pattern of eating, and menu planning with the dietitian can prevent you from feeling overwhelmed. Even when you know which foods are okay from your food list, you need to know additional information to plan menus for entire days and have your meal plan as nutritious as possible.

- *How much* of each food to eat
- *When* to have meals, snacks, and fluids
- *What* to eat within a day
- *How to meet* your nutrient requirements through diet and supplements

You and your dietitian can work on planning daily and weekly nutritious, low-calorie meals and menus. At first, you will probably rely on the dietitian to do most of the work.

As you get more experience, you will get better at planning your own meals.

Ideas and Recipes to Prevent Boredom

Eating foods from lists can be very boring…until your dietitian shares new recipes for you to try. Dietitians are trained to be able to suggest interesting ways to use foods using simple recipes so you do not have to be a chef. Your dietitian can also give you ideas on what to contribute to a potluck dinner and what to choose when you are at a restaurant with friends.

Part of your appointment time with the dietitian will include goal setting. Some of the goals that you set will have to do with weight loss, but others will be unrelated to the numbers you see on the scale. They will be things such as stopping your meal when you are full or remembering to take your supplement every day. Dietitians can also help you troubleshoot if you are not hitting your weight loss goals or if you are having digestive problems that can be related to your RYGB diet. Your dietitian can assess your diet and point out a few problems with it that you might not have even realized. Minor changes can make a big difference in your weight loss results.

Post-Operative Nutritional Assessment

In addition to working with you on your diet and weight loss, the dietitian may help ensure that your nutritional status is good. There are some standard ways to do this.

Weight and Body Fat

The dietitian should assess your nutritional status at each post-surgery appointment. Monitoring your weight, BMI, and percent excess body weight lets the dietitian know that you are losing weight as hoped and that you are eating the right amount of calories at each stage of weight loss. If you are not losing weight as fast as you expected, the dietitian can work with you to figure out how you can change your diet to hit your goals.

Checking Your Blood Tests

The dietitian should also review any of your nutrient-related blood tests. If you have deficiencies of protein or any vitamin or mineral, the dietitian can suggest foods and supplements to try to keep your nutrient levels normal.

Assessing Your Diet

At each appointment, your dietitian will probably assess your diet by asking what you typically eat. When you have your diet assessed, the dietitian may notice that your intake of certain nutrients is low. For example, if you are not eating fortified grains or many vegetables or beans, you might have a low intake of folate or folic acid. In that case, the dietitian may recommend that your doctor order a folate test to check your status.

The dietitian might not even need tests to make some recommendations. For example, a fish oil supplement can be a healthy choice if you do not eat seafood.

Dietary assessment can be helpful in other ways:[7]

- Identify causes of dumping syndrome, nausea, or vomiting

- Figuring out times when you can drink more fluids
- Recognizing the need to increase your dietary variety

Additional Roles

Your dietitian or nutritionist might also work with you on the following issues:[8]

- Choosing foods that promote healthy weight loss because they are nutritious, low in calories, and filling. Examples include egg whites, chicken breast, seafood, fat-free dairy products, vegetables, whole grains, and fruits.

- Avoiding foods and beverages that interfere with weight loss because they are high in calories and not very filling. Examples include refined carbohydrates, such as sugary foods and white bread, fried foods, other high-fat foods, and sugary beverages.

- Reviewing your medications to make sure you are taking what you should

- Psychological issues, such as emotional eating, getting social support, and improving your body image

Your frequency will depend on factors like your insurance, your surgeon's recommendations, your own preferences, and your dietitian's regular procedure. You will meet more often if you are having trouble following your meal plan, and you might meet less often if you are really nailing your eating, losing weight at the rate you want, and feeling confident about where you are headed.

Email and smartphone apps make contacting your dietitian easy. You can even send your food record electronically to ask for advice.

It Is Okay If You Do Not Have a Dietitian

Because of money or logistics, not everyone has the opportunity to meet with a dietitian often, especially if you are self-pay or your insurance has stricter limits on your dietitian appointments. That is okay. Take advantage of any professional nutritional help you can get from a qualified nutritionist or dietitian, and be aware of the many other resources available to help you with your diet:

> **Tip**
>
> Chapter 7, "Planning For the Gastric Bypass," Chapter 8, "Roux-En-Y Gastric Bypass Costs, Insurance, and More," Chapter 9, "Pre-Surgery Tips," give you more information on what a dietitian does and what you can expect during appointments. Chapters 13 and 14 have information on the post-surgery diet right after surgery and on the RYGB diet that you will be following as part of your long-term lifestyle change for weight loss and management.

- Your surgeon or clinic probably has standard instructions for bariatric patients. You might receive lists of allowed foods and their serving sizes at each stage of recovery from surgery and your long-term gastric bypass diet. You should also receive lists of foods to avoid, limit, or try cautiously. Clinic staff should be able and willing to answer your questions, no matter how detailed.

- This book is a relatively detailed guide to the post-surgery and long-term RYGB diet.

This book introduces the following topics:

- Which foods you can and cannot have at each stage
- How to make a meal plan
- Choosing healthy foods
- Eating proper serving sizes
- Staying aware of nutrient deficiencies
- Figuring out what to do when you have a reaction to a certain food

- BariatricPal.com is a social networking platform with hundreds of thousands of members who are bariatric surgery patients, including tens of thousands of members specifically interested in RYGB. You can benefit from their experiences. Because of personal experience, postoperative gastric bypass patients are ideal for answering very detailed questions, such as about specific types or amounts of food or certain symptoms or health conditions. Surgeons may not be able to answer these questions with such a personal perspective. Another benefit of this online community is that people are online at all times of the day and night, so you are likely to be able to message or chat with community members whenever you need them.

- Other online sources are likely to provide what you need in terms of food lists and basic information. As discussed in Chapter 7, "*Planning for the Gastric Bypass*," you will soon learn which sites seem trustworthy and which do not.

Meeting with a Mental Health Professional

Not all surgeons require regular post-surgery appointments, but you should have regular contact with a mental health professional in, group or one-on-one settings. You should also have the option of making appointments if you want them.

Post-operative Psychological Challenges

Emotional and mental challenges are normal responses to the dramatic life changes after your gastric bypass. The RYGB is life-changing even without complications and with desired weight loss. The process is long, hard, and a mental strain. Even your visible results can be emotionally challenging—as delighted as you might be to get the body you want, looking, feeling, and being treated like a whole new person can be stressful. Your relationships can change when some people inevitably start to treat you differently than they used to when you were obese. They can be uncomfortable around you or make you feel abnormal for being a bariatric surgery patient.

How a Psychologist Can Help

A mental health professional that sees you regularly in support group meetings or private appointments can get to know you well enough to recognize warning signs of mental struggles when they appear. To promote your mental health, continue to see a psychologist or at least know where to find one for years after the RYGB surgery.

Strategies for Positive Thinking

The power of positive thinking is cliché, corny, and true. Negative thinking can put you in a self-defeating rut. On the contrary, positive thinking can keep you motivated and give you strength to succeed in your diet program. A mental health professional can teach you tricks for turning lemons into lemonade just by changing the way you react to a situation—without changing the actual circumstance. Some people are naturally positive; others need more practice. A psychologist can suggest ways to improve your positive thinking strategies.

Knowing Yourself a Little Better

Psychologists know how the mind works and how powerful it is. Some of us are naturally good at knowing ourselves, and some of us are not. Improving your self-awareness and learning to respond appropriately to doubts or fears will make you stronger. For example, you might notice that your most powerful cravings for sweets come in the evening after dinner. Your psychologist might think through the situation with you and have you dig deep within yourself. You might, in fact, realize that you are not really craving sugar; instead, maybe you are in the habit of having dessert because you associate it with well-being from your childhood. A psychologist might suggest an alternative, such as reading a bedtime story to your daughter, which keeps you feeling safe but does not hurt your diet.

Detecting Signs of Depression

Extreme obesity can lead to depression. If you had mild depression before surgery, you may have fewer symptoms after surgery when you are losing weight.[9] However, there is a small risk of depression after the RYGB surgery. These factors can contribute to depression:

- *Realizing that your obesity was hiding an underlying issue*: Now that you are losing weight, it is harder to hide behind your obesity, and you have to confront the issue.
- *Many life changes*: You look different, feel different, have a different body, have different relationships with people, and have different physical abilities. All these changes can be overwhelming.

A psychologist can monitor you for depression and get you treated in its early stages. Treatments might include one-on-one therapy with the psych, extra group support sessions for weight loss surgery patients, or both.

Setting Goals and Troubleshooting

Goal-setting helps you stay focused. A psychologist can help you with setting more general goals than the ones you set for your weight loss or with the dietitian. You can learn strategies for setting realistic long-term and short-term goals. You can plan how you will achieve them and how you can evaluate your progress along the way.

Overcoming Troubles with Your Weight Loss

A mental health professional can help you address emotional or psychological problems that may be interfering with your weight loss. In fact, the American Society of Metabolic and Bariatric Surgery, or ASMBS, recommends psychological attention as part of your care plan if you are struggling with weight loss after bariatric surgery.[10] Psychological factors, such as not understanding how RYGB works or not being able to stick to the right diet, can prevent satisfactory weight loss. A psychologist can help.

Even without directly talking about your diet, your psychologist can be pivotal in your long-term weight loss success. Take advantage of the mental health professional services that you are entitled to from your insurance or through working with your surgeon, and you will probably notice that you also approach other aspects of your life with a healthier and more productive attitude.

Support Groups

Support groups are almost indispensable to effective postoperative care. They are so important to your success that before agreeing to perform bariatric surgery, your surgeon may ask you to sign a contract stating that you will attend group sessions for months or years after surgery. You might start with weekly or biweekly meetings; eventually, as you get closer to your goal weight and lifetime maintenance, you may have the option of going monthly. Weight loss surgery patients are encouraged to attend bariatric surgery group support meetings for life.

How Support Groups Can Help

Why are support groups so effective at turning you into a success story? Meetings are educational and motivational, so you can learn what you need to know and have the motivation to do what you need to do to lose weight. These are a few ways that support groups can help:

- *Provide social support*: Your weight loss journey can feel lonely even if your family and friends are very supportive. They do not feel the exact same things that you do.

- *Give you confidence*: You will meet some gastric bypass patients who are in exactly the same situation that you hope to eventually be in: maintaining goal weight for life. Knowing that they were once morbidly obese and were able to lose weight with the same operation as you can give you confidence that you, too, can achieve your goal weight.

- *Keep your spirits up:* Group meetings are opportunities to relax and just be yourself. Seeing others who are experiencing the same things as you and are managing to embrace it positively can motivate you to be just as upbeat.

- *Expose you to new ideas:* Many meetings will likely include guest presentations. You might hear from plastic surgeons, long-time bariatric patients, or dietitians. You might discover chances to volunteer as a weight loss surgery patient advocate.

- *Long-term success:* Strategies that you learn from the many health professionals and patients at meetings can be useful for years.

Mindfulness and RYGB

Participating in support group meetings can improve your mindfulness, which is the ability to "be in the moment," or be aware of your feelings and surroundings. It lets you think more clearly so you can connect your current thoughts and actions to consequences in the future. These are some examples of how mindfulness can benefit you:

- Choosing high-protein, fat-free egg whites instead of bacon and eggs for breakfast because you know that your current craving will pass and you will be better off later if you choose the egg white

- Choosing to exercise instead of watch TV because you recognize that you will feel better after you work out and you will lose weight faster, even though watching TV is more comfortable at this moment

Support Groups and Sticking to Your Diet

Only a fraction of bariatric surgery patients stick to their diets exactly as instructed. The rest may eat foods that are not recommended, drink beverages while eating solid foods, have larger portions, or eat fewer meals and snacks than recommended. Poor eating behaviors can interfere with your short-term and long-term weight loss and increase your risk for complications, such as vomiting and dehydration.

Attending support group meetings can help you maintain your good nutrition habits or improve your bad habits in a variety of ways:

- The other group members and the group leader can suggest strategies to make following your diet easier. They might share recipes to make your nutritious diet more interesting or suggest; healthier options for satisfying cravings and ways to remember to eat frequently and measure your portions.

- You can learn which foods are more and less likely to cause problems at various stages of your weight loss journey.

- Going to regular meetings can keep you motivated because you will know that you will be seeing the other group members each week or month. That will give you a sense of accountability during the week or month as you are working hard to make the right choices and stay on track.

- Group meetings can help you track time. You might even start setting goals based on your next meeting. For example, you could set the goal of getting in an extra cup of water each day in the week before your next meeting.

Sources:[11,12]

Support Group Meeting Locations and Leaders

Many surgeons, especially the ones that work in larger clinics and hospitals or that specialize in bariatric surgery, and organize their own support groups. Meetings will probably be held in the hospital building. Surgeons that do not run their own groups may direct you to a nearby facility to attend meetings with other local bariatric surgery patients.

Structure of Group Meetings

A typical meeting might last for one to two hours and have a consistent format. Group leaders may change from meeting to meeting. Regular leaders may include:

- Your surgeon or another local surgeon whose patients are in your group

- A clinical psychologist or another mental health professional or counselor

- A nurse or other bariatric healthcare professional

- A peer counselor or bypass or other bariatric patient who has been successful after his or her own surgery and is interested in helping other patients see the same results. Guest lecturers are also likely.

> **Tip**
>
> Chapter 17, "The First Year After RYGB Is Filled With Changes," discusses possible cosmetic surgeries for RYGB patients that have lost a lot of weight.

Typical Meeting Agenda

Often the meetings start with a round of introductions. You might be asked to say your name and some basic information, such as where you are in the RYGB process: just thinking, choosing a surgeon, approaching surgery, or postoperative and losing weight already.

After the introductions, the main part of the meeting might include a presentation by the meeting leader or an invited guest. For example, in one weight loss surgery meeting that I attended, the guest lecturer was a surgeon whose specialty was removal of excess skin for formerly obese patients that had lost a lot of weight. In his presentation, he described the process of removing extra skin from the underarms and talked about who would be good candidates for the procedure.

After the main presentation, the floor will probably be opened up for questions about the presentation and then for general questions about anything related to the bypass. Do not be afraid to ask all of your worrying or embarrassing questions. Nobody else was born knowing the answers, and every other weight loss surgery patient has experienced their own embarrassing side effects in public. They have had the same experiences with diarrhea, vomiting, and getting too full very quickly—or if they have not had surgery yet, they are worried about these things. They want to know just as badly as you do about how to prevent it—and a lot of the other patients will have excellent tried-and-true advice for you.

You might meet your new best friends at RYGB support group meetings. Just as in any other group, you will like some people and more than others. You share your experiences of years of obesity and a commitment to becoming healthy using bariatric surgery. That is some deep stuff, and it can be the basis for some amazing friendships.

Cognitive Behavioral Therapy

Some group sessions might be based on principles of cognitive behavioral therapy, or CBT.[13] This is especially likely if you have a psychologist leading your meetings. You might also use CBT techniques in individual sessions with your psychologist. CBT has been used in treating psychosocial disorders, such as depression and addictions, as well as for managing chronic diseases. CBT can be applied to bariatric surgery patients in these ways:

- Increasing adherence to your diet
- Preventing vitamin and mineral deficiencies
- Sticking to the recommended amounts of exercise
- Improving your monitoring and management of diabetes and high blood pressure
- Improving your body image, self-esteem, and relationships with others

CBT focuses on the ability to control your thoughts and actions. It provides a variety of methods to increase the likelihood that you will perform the healthy actions you want. These might include learning more about the benefits of eating a varied diet, asking your family and friends to praise you for measuring your food, setting a timer so you remember to eat each meal or snack, and keeping only nutritious foods in the house.

Alternatives to Attending Support Group Meetings In-Person

In-person support groups are nice because you have the opportunity to meet people and get involved. Unfortunately, they are not always practical or possible for you. They may be too far from home or incompatible with your schedule.

Videoconferences and Conference Calls

Videoconferences and conference calls are increasingly common options to live meetings, and you do not have to drive to them. You can attend from your own home. You just need some basic equipment such as computer speakers and a microphone. Using your own webcam lets people in the meeting room or at their computers see you too. You will need some sort of software, which is usually available for a free download, and instructions for installing the software will be easy to find and follow from the hosting company's website.

The group meeting's organizers can tell you how to "attend" the meeting. You might be able to access the meeting from the group's website, or you might need to log in to a conference-hosting service and/or make a telephone call. Many everyday companies offer remote meeting hosting.

Other Options

You can still get the social support you need even if live meetings do not fit into your schedule. Recorded videos of live meetings are available from a few sources. You can watch webcasts and webinars at any time, such as while your children are in bed or while you are walking on the treadmill. Often you can even participate by sending in your questions before or after the actual event. Discussion forums provide additional support group options. You can participate in online conversations on your own time or schedule group live chat sessions with other forum members.

Staying Positive Post-Surgery!

The first few weeks after surgery can be tough. You might have stomach pain from your healing wounds, gastrointestinal symptoms, nausea, hunger, and anxiety about your future lifestyle. You might be tired of seeing your surgeon and dietitian so often and of getting so many medical tests. Measuring your food, selecting appropriate foods, taking your multivitamins, and getting enough water can all be burdensome.

The worst part might be that your weight might not even come off as fast as you had expected, because your focus during this time is on recovery, not weight loss. You might start wondering whether the RYGB was worth it.

Give Yourself a Pep Talk Instead of Giving Up!

These concerns are normal and reasonable, but do not let them get you down. It is normal to get a bit down after any event that big, no matter how phenomenal the results are. Even gold-medal Olympians can feel a bit lost after the Games—they just dedicated at least four years of their lives to their dreams and suddenly feel let down after they finally win the Olympic gold. Like Olympians, you can get through this emotional low time and continue to work hard so that everything will eventually fall into place and be worth it.

Always Look Ahead

Do not even start wondering whether you *should* have gotten the RYGB or not. You got it, and that is what you have to work with. Your job now is to do the best you can with what you have.

Remind Yourself of the Important Things

To get through this hard time, remind yourself:

- *You are not alone.* Nearly all bariatric surgery patients go through the exact same challenges and come out on top if they keep following the right diet.

- *Things will get better.* This period of trials and tribulations will eventually end. Challenges will always be present, but this will probably be the most difficult time.

> **Tip**
>
> During this time, your support system is crucial. **Chapter 17, "The First Year After RYGB Is Filled With Changes,"** talks about different sources of support, both in your life and online, to turn to when you are starting to doubt yourself or you need a little extra encouragement or motivation.

- *This is a lifelong journey.* The goal is not to lose weight as quickly as possible. It is to lose weight and maintain your weight loss for life. After a few years, you will realize that it will not matter exactly how fast you lose weight. It will not matter whether it takes you one year, three years, or five years to hit your goal weight. What *will* be important from this time is that you stuck to your program, made healthy choices to avoid health complications, and developed the skills you need to control your weight for life.

Keep It in Perspective

These weeks may seem endless as you are going through them; later they will seem like a flash. For now, keep reminding yourself why you got surgery, what your weight loss will mean to you and your family, and how proud you will be of yourself when you finally get into the swing of things as an experienced RYGB patient.

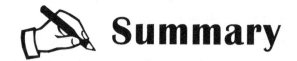

Summary

☛ This chapter described a standard postoperative care program to increase success with the RYGB. You should have regular appointments with your surgeon to be sure that you are healing well and preventing complications. You can expect to have certain medical tests regularly too. The dietitian and psychologist can provide valuable support and information, so take advantage of these experts when you can! Support group meetings can serve a variety of roles from informative, to supporting, to motivational.

☛ These can be challenging times, so we ended the chapter with a little pep talk that can come in handy if you are feeling a little down on yourself. Many weight loss surgery patients find that things get *a lot* better if you can just stick it out now.

☛ This chapter covered pretty much everything you need to know about your aftercare program—except for your diet. That is important enough to deserve a chapter on its own because a good post-surgery diet will speed your recovery from surgery and lay the foundation for steady weight loss and good eating habits in the future. In the next chapter, you will learn all about your diet for the first several weeks after RYGB surgery.

Your Turn: Keep Your Post-Surgery Appointments Straight!

You are going to have a lot of appointments after your surgery. This form can help you keep them straight so you know when they are, where they are, and how to prepare. We recommend using this template for each of your appointments so that you always stay on top of your medical care.

Date of appointment:

Time of appointment:

Appointment with (Name) _____ , (position or title) _____

Location of appointment (may need hospital name and specific building and room number)

Preparation required (e.g., fasting, bringing medical history or results from recent blood tests, diet log to show a dietitian, list of questions to ask):

Other notes (e.g., do you need a ride?)

RYGB Patient Story: Kristy

Kristy from Oklahoma has a family that many people only dream of having. Married for 22 years, she has a 20-year-old daughter and sons who are 16 and 13. She works at USPS. This woman tells us how she took responsibility for her weight and used the RYGB as a tool to lose nearly 200 pounds from a pre-surgery weight of 340 pounds down to 149 pounds and a healthy BMI of 23.3.

On Taking Charge of Her Weight

I struggled with weight for years. My family moved around a lot when I was growing up, and I blamed weight gain on that. Next, after having each baby, I blamed the extra weight on "baby weight." Then I started working nights and I blamed my weight on that. It was just a constant blame game. Everything caused me to be fat but me!

The turning point for me was losing my Dad. I felt like my whole world was falling apart. I realized that the only thing I could control was getting as healthy as possible for my family so that I could be around for many years to enjoy them. Since I had yo-yo dieted my whole life, I knew I needed a tool that would help me lose the weight permanently. I did a ton of research, lurked a lot on the BariatricPal.com forum, and in October of 2011, started the process of getting my gastric bypass. The process seemed long, but it gave me time to educate myself some more and for the doctors to make sure I was healthy enough for the surgery. I had surgery in February of 2012.

On the Highlights and Challenges after Surgery

Surgery has made so many differences…here are some highlights:

- *Now that I can shut the door in regular public bathroom stalls, I don't have to use the handicapped stall when I use a public restroom.*

- *I'm not out of breath all of the time.*

- *I'm not the "fat" mom.*

- *My kids tell me that I'm skinny!*

- *When I fall into my husband's arms, they wrap all the way around me!*

The biggest benefit is that I love myself! I have a general sense of overall happiness, but I'm still getting used to the changes. I still tend to want to wear big clothes to hide my body even though I look smaller when I wear clothes that fit. I have to wrap my mind around the fact that even after losing 107 pounds, I still have 68 more pounds to go to my original goal weight of 165 pounds. How did I let myself get so big?

On Social Support and Her Advice

I love that I can get online anytime and see something that educates me and/or motivates me. BariatricPal.com is just like a family! The best tips that I have are to eat your protein, exercise, and drink your water. Overall, be patient with the weight loss. I still feel leery about offering tips or advice for weight loss, but mainly I just want everyone to know that I have gotten my confidence back and I am truly happy!

1   Mechanick JI, Kushner RF, Sugerman HJ, Gonzalez-Campoy M, Collazo-Clavell ML, ... Dixon J. American Association of Clinical Endocrinologists, The Obesity Society and American Society for Metabolic and Bariatric Surgery medical guidelines for clinical practice for the perioperative nutritional, metabolic and nonsurgical support of the bariatric surgery patient. Obesity. 2009;17:S1-S70.

2   Griffith PS, Birch DW, Sharma AM, Karmali S. Managing complications associated with laparoscopic Roux-en-Y gastric bypass for morbid obesity. Can J Surg. 2012 Oct;55(5):329-36.

3   Ziegler O, Sirveaux MA, Brunaud L, Reibel N, Quillot D. Medical follow-up after bariatric surgery: nutritional and drug issues. General recommendations for the prevention and treatment of nutritional deficiencies. Diabetes Metab. 2009;35(6 Pt 2):544-547.

4   Mechanick JI, Kushner RF, Sugerman HJ, Gonzalez-Campoy M, Collazo-Clavell ML, ... Dixon J. American Association of Clinical Endocrinologists, The Obesity Society and American Society for Metabolic and Bariatric Surgery medical guidelines for clinical practice for the perioperative nutritional, metabolic and nonsurgical support of the bariatric surgery patient. Obesity. 2009;17:S1-S70.

5   NIH Senior Health: Built with You in Mind. (n.d.). Osteoporosis: what is osteoporosis? National Institutes of Health. http://nihseniorhealth.gov/osteoporosis/whatisosteoporosis/01.html. Accessed October 29, 2012.

6   Aills L, Blankenship J, Buffington C, Furtado M, Parrott J. ASMBS Allied Health nutritional guidelines for the surgical weight loss patient. Surg Obes Relat Dis. 2008;4(5Suppl):S73-S108

7   Aills L, Blankenship J, Buffington C, Furtado M, Parrott J. ASMBS Allied Health nutritional guidelines for the surgical weight loss patient. Surg Obes Relat Dis. 2008;4(5Suppl):S73-S108.

8   Aills L, Blankenship J, Buffington C, Furtado M, Parrott J. ASMBS Allied Health nutritional guidelines for the surgical weight loss patient. Surg Obes Relat Dis. 2008;4(5Suppl):S73-S108.

9   Mechanick JI, Kushner RF, Sugerman HJ, Gonzalez-Campoy M, Collazo-Clavell ML, ... Dixon J. American Association of Clinical Endocrinologists, The Obesity Society and American Society for Metabolic and Bariatric Surgery medical guidelines for clinical practice for the perioperative nutritional, metabolic and nonsurgical support of the bariatric surgery patient. Obesity. 2009;17:S1-S70.

10 Mechanick JI, Kushner RF, Sugerman HJ, Gonzalez-Campoy M, Collazo-Clavell ML, ... Dixon J. American Association of Clinical Endocrinologists, The Obesity Society and American Society for Metabolic and Bariatric Surgery medical guidelines for clinical practice for the perioperative nutritional, metabolic and nonsurgical support of the bariatric surgery patient. Obesity. 2009;17:S1-S70.

11 Elkins G, Whitfield P, Marcus J, Symmonds R, Rodriguez J, Cook T. Noncompliance with behavioral recommendations following bariatric surgery. Obes Surg, 2005;15:546-51.

12 McVay MA, Friedman KE. The benefits of cognitive behavioral groups for bariatric surgery patients. Bariatric Times. 2012;9(9):22-28.

13 McVay MA, Friedman KE. The benefits of cognitive behavioral groups for bariatric surgery patients. Bariatric Times. 2012;9(9):22-28.

13

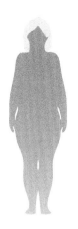

Post-Surgery Diet: From Liquid Diet to Solid Foods

Food is central to your weight loss. You are eager to start the diet that will get you the weight loss results you want, but you cannot start it immediately after surgery. Instead, you will have to patiently go through the post-surgery diet before focusing entirely on rapid weight loss.

Recovery needs to be your focus for several weeks after RYGB. For now, minimizing side effects and preventing complications are higher priorities than losing weight. The post-surgery diet helps you do this by gradually progressing from a liquid-only diet to a solid diet. These are the stages of your diet progression after bariatric surgery:[1]

- Liquid diet
- Pureed diet
- Soft foods diet
- Regular RYGB diet

This chapter covers the first three phases. The next chapter will cover the solid foods phase. That phase is what you will follow as your regular RYGB diet for the long term as you continue to lose weight.

This chapter covers the following topics:

- Why the post-surgery diet is absolutely critical for your health and weight loss
- What you can and cannot eat during each phase of the diet
- When to go on to the next stage
- What to do if you have a reaction to a specific food
- Food lists and sample meal plans for each phase

So are you ready to start eating for health and recovery? Here is how!

A Bit about the Post-Surgery Diet

You have already progressed in your gastric bypass journey, but you are still not ready to focus strictly on losing weight. If you can be patient for the next few weeks and concentrate on recovering and setting a good base for the future, you will be setting a better foundation for your future weight loss and health.

Why You Need to Follow the Post-Surgery Diet

Following the post-surgery diet as closely as you can is absolutely necessary. "Cheaters never prosper" is completely true in this case. The effects of cheating can be far more serious than simply stalling your weight loss temporarily and can include:

- Interfering with weight loss for the long term. Stretching your stomach pouch by overeating will reduce the restriction that you feel, so you will tend to eat more. That makes the gastric bypass much less effective
- Gastrointestinal symptoms, such as diarrhea, bloating, cramping, and constipation

- Nutrient deficiencies or food intolerances
- Serious complications, such as leaks or infections

These are additional reasons to follow the post-surgery RYGB carefully:

- It lets you get used to eating smaller portions at meals and snacks instead of large meals.
- It builds on the skills that you were working on before surgery to plan meals and monitor your intake.
- It helps you develop new necessary skills, such as chewing your food slowly, eating only until you are full, and avoiding beverages at meals.

A Few Challenges to Expect

You should have plenty of motivation to follow the post-RYGB diet, but you will face some challenges. Knowing what to expect can help you prepare for and overcome them.

- *Slow weight loss*: You might lose a lot of weight right after surgery, but you might not. The focus now is on healing properly by eating the right foods or liquids and preventing nutritional deficiencies. You only have this one chance to heal properly, so take advantage of it.
- *Slow progress:* Each stage will take at least a week and likely more to get through.[2] You will only add in a few new kinds of food at a time. Sometimes a new food can cause discomfort and delay your progression. Be patient and listen to your body, and remember that weight control is not a race. It is about losing weight and maintaining your weight loss, whether hitting goal weight takes 5, 10, or 20 years.
- *Change*: You will be unable to eat many foods that you used to enjoy, and you will have to get used to different eating patterns, such as small meals and snacks.
- *Hunger, especially when you are on a liquid diet*: The gastric bypass makes your stomach smaller so it fills up quickly, but the strategy does not work so well when you are on a liquid diet because liquids empty quickly from your stomach. Another reason why you may be hungry is that it takes about 20 to 60 minutes for your hunger and satiety hormones to respond to food and tell your brain that you are full.[3] This means that you should practice eating slowly and stopping before you are completely full. Many obese patients may have been ignoring their fullness signals for years.
- *Crabbiness:* You are hurting. You are hungry. You are stressed. You are barely losing weight. A voice inside of you tells you that you might as well give up, but do not! You can get through this.
- *Mistakes:* Nobody is perfect, and neither are you. You will inevitably eat something that is not on the diet, measure a portion wrong, or forget to take your multivitamin. The difference between successful weight loss and ongoing struggles is whether you get back on track.

- *The unexpected:* You might start to enjoy the tastes of healthy foods as you reduce sugar and fat in your diet. Junk food might not taste so good any more. You might notice that, for the first time in a long time, you are full! Hours or a day might pass without fixating on food. That is when you can be confident that the RYGB will work for you.

Remind yourself that it is all about the end goal! Each tiny success will increase your confidence and your ability to stay on track. As long as you follow the diet rules, you *will* lose weight.

Kitchen Equipment to Get You Started

You do not need much, but a bit of kitchen equipment will help with your post-surgery diet. Having the right tools and utensils makes it easier to stick to your meal plan. These items are almost indispensible:

- *Measuring cups and measuring spoons:* "Eyeballing" it will no longer work. Get into the habit of measuring each portion of everything you put into your mouth. If your meal plan calls for a quarter-cup of cream of wheat made with one tablespoon of milk, measure out a quarter-cup of cream of wheat and a tablespoon of milk. Even experienced chefs can underestimate portions and slow weight loss by accidentally taking in way too many calories.

- *Kitchen scale:* A kitchen scale is invaluable for measuring foods that do not fit neatly into cups and spoons. Examples include meat and fish. Scales are also useful for measuring foods, such as dry cereal, that can settle during packaging, so their actual weight and volume is not exactly the same as what is listed on the package. For solid food, weight is always more accurate than volume (cups and spoons). Analog kitchen scales have dials that point to the weight of the food when you put it on the scale. Digital, or electronic, kitchen scales are more precise; they display the weight in ounces or grams on a screen for you. They can run on batteries or be electric.

- *Blender:* A full-size blender can handle pretty much anything you throw into it, and you may find yourself using it several times a day during the pureed foods phase. A hand blender can be a good option for the semi-solid foods phase. It is easier to clean than a full-sized blender. Be aware that it may leave a few small chunks in your food.

- *Strainer:* Straining food lets you get rid of any chunks. Different grades of strainers have bigger or smaller holes to meet your needs. Strainers with smaller holes are better for early stages of your bypass diet.

- *Storage bags and containers:* Storage bags and containers can store single servings of food. They

> **Tip**
>
> **Checking Your Kitchen Equipment before Surgery**
>
> Chapter 10, "Final Preparation for RYGB," recommends taking some time before surgery to get your entire home and kitchen ready. This includes gathering the kitchen items that you will need after surgery. The more preparation you do before surgery, the easier your recovery will be.

help you plan ahead. You can use them to carry food with you when you know you will not be able to measure your portions when it is time to eat later. They are also useful for letting you make an entire, multiple-serving recipe. Before you serve yourself your single portion, pack up the rest of your recipe into single-serving portions in individual plastic storage containers or little bags to put in the fridge or freezer. Then you will always have the right amount of food on hand.

What Do I Look for When Purchasing Measuring Cups and Spoons?

You might be a lifelong baker or chef, but you might be someone who thinks gourmet cooking means defrosting a bag of frozen vegetables to serve with Chinese takeout. If that describes you, buying kitchen utensils might be daunting or even undesirable—it might make you fear that the next step will be to make complicated recipes. But do not worry. You can easily get the measuring utensils that you need to lose weight—not tie you to the kitchen!

This is some basic information to help you get what you need:

- A standard full set of measuring cups includes a ¼-cup, a ☐-cup, a ½-cup, and a 1-cup measure. They will probably come together in a single package.

- A full set of measuring spoons has a ¼, ☐, ½, and 1 teaspoon measure plus a 1-tablespoon spoon. They will probably come together as a single product. Most measuring spoons that come in sets have holes on the other end of their handles. A single ring goes through each spoon so that the spoons are all attached and you will not lose them.

- A glass measuring cup is useful for measuring liquids and sometimes solid foods. It usually has a capacity of 2 cups, and each ¼ cup is marked from the bottom (0) to the 2-cup fill line near the top. The cup might also have metric markings up to 500 milliliters. Since the glass is clear, you can see from the side exactly how much fluid or food is inside the glass. Compared to other kinds of glass, heat-resistant will not crack when it is hot, so you can put hot liquids in it or microwave it. Pyrex is the most familiar brand name for heat-resistant kitchen glassware.

Except for your glass measuring cup, it does not matter what your measuring cups and spoons are made from. Metal, such as stainless steel, is most common; some people prefer plastic because they like the way it feels and it does not get hot. Metal utensils with plastic handles are easy to grasp and to clean.

If you are a newbie in the kitchen, inexpensive sets are ideal choices. You can upgrade them later if you want.

Do you need help converting measurements? **Chapter 14, "RYGB Diet 101,"** has a handy chart for you!

You may already have these items on hand. If not, you can get them at any kitchen supplies store or mass merchandiser and most grocery and drug stores. Many dollar stores have measuring cups and spoons that are perfectly adequate.

Phase 1 – Liquid Diet

You cannot eat solid food right after surgery. Instead, you will be on a liquid diet.[4] Most, but not all, surgeons recommend a clear liquid diet for one to two days after surgery. The full liquid diet, which is less restrictive, begins after the clear liquid diet or right after surgery. It lasts until about 10 to 14 days after surgery if you have no complications and you are ready to progress, but you can be on it for longer.[5] Strict adherence to the diet can help you in the following ways:

- It provides essential nutrients.[6] The short-lived clear liquid diet is not nutritionally adequate, but a full liquid diet can provide enough calories and protein to be safe for weeks.[7]

- It allows your stomach and small intestine to heal after surgery. Solid foods can prevent your seam lines from sealing up properly, causing a leak and the need for another surgery. Infection is another risk of aggravating your surgery wounds with solid food.

- It reduces nausea.

- A liquid diet reduces your risk of discomfort, such as reflux, or regurgitation, heartburn, and gastrointestinal symptoms.

- It prevents dehydration.

Choices on a Clear Liquid Diet

The clear liquid diet is described in Chapter 10, "Final Preparation for RYGB." You cannot have any solid foods. *Table 17* is a reminder of the liquids that you can and cannot have on a standard clear liquid diet.[8] If your surgeon has slightly different lists, follow those.

Allowed	Not Allowed
✓ Water	✗ Any solid or semi-solid food
✓ Broth	✗ Nectar
✓ Popsicles	✗ Canned fruit
✓ Gelatin	✗ Milk
✓ Tea	✗ Protein shakes
✓ Coffee	✗ Meal replacement beverages
✓ Sports drinks	✗ Juice with pulp
✓ Pulp-free fruit juices	✗ Citrus juice and tomato juice (too acidic)
	✗ Cream (e.g., in coffee)

Table 17: Liquids You Can and Cannot Have

Choices on a Full Liquid Diet

The full liquid diet continues to promote recovery.[9] This diet can be nutritious enough for several weeks if needed, so do not feel pressured to rush through it. Be sure that you can tolerate each new fluid before moving on. Here is a run-down of some common options on the liquid diet.

Water

Water is calorie-free, it naturally helps reduce your appetite, and it is convenient. Staying hydrated promotes recovery, gives you energy, and helps you lose weight, so do not limit your water intake. Here are some tips to increase your consumption:

- Always have some water available!
- Keep bottles in the car and in your office, and store extras.
- Keep a filled water bottle or pitcher of water and a glass on your desk so you remember to drink throughout the day.
- Jazz up your water if you do not like it plain. Try adding a sprig of fresh mint (you can buy a bunch at the grocery store) or use a slice of lime or lemon to freshen it up—just make sure you do not eat the mint leaf or get any lemon seeds in your water while you are on a liquid diet!
- Try ice water—some people find it more refreshing when it is ice cold.

Diluted Juice

Apple, grape, and other juices and nectars are allowed on the full liquid diet, but dilute them by making 50/50 solutions with water. So, instead of having four ounces of juice, have two ounces of juice mixed with two ounces of water. This reduces the calories and helps prevent dumping syndrome. Fruit juices provide potassium and vitamin C. Choose 100 percent juices instead of juice drinks with added sugars because sugar does not provide essential vitamins and minerals. Avoid acidic juices, such as grapefruit, tomato, and orange.

Broth or Bouillon

Clear soup, such as chicken, beef, and vegetable broth, does not have many nutrients, but it can provide some variety in the liquid diet when most of the rest of your liquids are sweet. These are some options for this diet phase:

- Flavored cubes that you dissolve in boiling water
- Flavored powder that you dissolve in boiling water
- Ready-to-heat broth or bouillon in cans or cartons
- Thin cream soups without any chunks, e.g., cream of tomato soup
- You may be able to have pureed, watered-down soups, but be certain they do not have any pieces of food in them. Ask your surgeon or dietitian because different health care providers have different recommendations.

Reduced-Fat Milk or Soy Milk

Skim or non-fat milk, 1% low-fat milk, and calcium-fortified soy milk provide protein and calcium. Protein is necessary for your wounds from surgery to heal, and it helps suppress hunger. Calcium is necessary for bone health. Chapter 15 talks more about calcium and other nutrients. Whole milk and flavored milk and soy milk products, such as chocolate, vanilla, or strawberry, are higher in sugar and calories than regular milk and unflavored soy milk. Lactose-free, soy, and almond milk are good choices if you have lactose intolerance after RYGB.

Sugar-Free, Diet, or Light Beverages

These are usually calorie-free or very low in calories, with about 5 or 10 per cup. Check the nutrition label to make sure, though, because some "light" or "reduced-calorie" beverages might have 50 or more calories per cup. These are some good options:

- Crystal Light
- Sugar-free Kool-Aid
- Diet Snapple (without caffeine)
- Powdered sugar-free flavored water mixes. These are handy because you can carry them in a pocket or purse and add them to water no matter where you are.

Avoid caffeinated beverages, such as coffee and energy drinks, and carbonated options, such as diet sodas. Caffeine can increase your stomach acid secretion and risk for ulcers. Carbonated beverages can make you feel overly full and, worse, permanently stretch your stomach pouch so it is not as restrictive.

Gelatin and Popsicles

These treats can make you feel as though you are cheating on your diet, but you are not. Ice cream is not allowed though.

- Sugar-free ice pops and gelatin are very low in calories.
- Powdered gelatin is easy to make yourself, but it needs to chill for a few hours before you can eat it.
- Ready-to-eat gelatin in single-serving cups is easy to carry with you. It can be in the baking aisle, with powdered gelatin, or in the refrigerator section.
- You can make frozen juice pops by freezing 100% juice in paper cups with a popsicle stick in each one.

Protein Shakes

Getting enough protein each day can be challenging after surgery, but it is necessary for minimizing your loss of lean muscle tissue mass and for speeding wound healing after surgery. Protein shakes can help while you are on the liquid diet since they are not rough on your stomach. Another benefit of many types of protein shakes is that they are fortified with vitamins and minerals that can be tough to get from your liquid diet after surgery. Sugar-free or low-carbohydrate shakes can be lower in calories and are less likely to lead to blood sugar spikes. Ask your surgeon or dietitian which brands are recommended and where you can purchase them.

Protein Supplements

Protein supplements, such as powders and powdered egg whites, can help you get to your recommended minimum of 65 to 75 grams of protein each day. You can dissolve them in water, juice, or milk so they are easy to work into the liquid diet. Choose sugar-free varieties if you are opting for flavored protein powder.

Table 18 is a summary table of what you can and cannot have on a full liquid diet.[10] Ask your surgeon or nutritionist to verify your choices.

Allowed	Unlikely – Ask Surgeon	Not Allowed
✓ Everything on the clear liquid diet	? Cream of wheat	✗ Bread, pasta, rice
✓ Butter, margarine, oil, cream	? Applesauce	✗ Nuts, beans, seeds
✓ Protein shakes	? Pureed potatoes	✗ Meats, poultry, fish
✓ Low-fat milk or soymilk	? Watery oatmeal	✗ Cheese
✓ Protein shakes and meal replacements		✗ Fruit
✓ Protein powders (protein supplements)[11]		✗ Vegetables
✓ Sugar, honey and syrups		✗ Ice cream and frozen yogurt

Table 18: Summary of what you can and cannot have on a full liquid diet

What Is the Difference between Natural Sugars and Added Sugars, and How Do They Fit into My Diet?

"Natural sugars" are found naturally in many foods, while "added sugars" are added during food processing or preparation. They make foods taste sweeter. Added sugars are what you probably think of first when you think of sugar. They include the following:

- White sugar (table sugar)
- Brown sugar, cane sugar
- Honey
- Molasses
- Corn syrup and high-fructose corn syrup
- Maltodextrin and dextrose
- Invert sugar

These are some common natural sugars:

- Lactose, or "milk sugar," is in milk and other dairy products.
- Fructose, or "fruit sugar," gives a sweet taste to fruit. It is also in vegetables. Fructose counts as an added sugar when manufacturers add it (or high-fructose corn syrup) to sweeten other foods, such as soft drinks, ice cream, and candies.
- Glucose is in many foods, including breads, cereals, and other grains; fruit; vegetables; and dairy products.

Are Added Sugars or Natural Sugars Better for Weight and Health?

All kinds of sugars, whether they are natural or added, are carbohydrates. They have four calories per gram, and they are not very filling. Chemically and nutritionally, *added sugars and natural sugars have the same effect on your body.*

But...

Added sugars can harm your diet more than natural sugars:

- Added sugars are often in high-calorie foods that do not fit into the RYGB diet. Examples include baked goods, sugary beverages, sugar-sweetened cereals, and flavored yogurts.
- Natural sugars are in many healthy foods, including fat-free yogurt, whole grains, fruits, beans, and vegetables.

What You Can Do

Limiting foods with added sugars is an effective strategy to help you lose weight and eat a more nutritious diet. It can also help you prevent dumping syndrome, which is discussed in more detail in Chapter 5, Risks of Gastric Bypass Surgery.

These tips can help you limit your sugar intake:

- Read the list of ingredients on food labels. Limit foods that list one or more types of added sugars near the beginning of the ingredients list.
- Choose no sugar added and sugar-free options
- Check the nutrition facts panels on food packages and choose foods with under 5 grams of sugar per serving.

Source: [12]

Liquids to Avoid

Not all liquids are allowed after the gastric bypass surgery because they can delay healing and increase your risk for long-term complications. You should also avoid any liquid that you are not tolerating, even if it is officially on your "allowed" list.

Acidic Juices: You know how painful the acid from citrus fruits can be if you have ever bitten into an orange when you had a cut in your mouth. It hurts! Acidic juices, such as tangerine, orange, and grapefruit juice, can cause the same pain to your surgery wounds. Tomato juice, vegetable juice, and tomato soup are also high in acid and should be avoided if they bother you.

Carbonated Beverages:[13] Your choices are already limited, and a refreshing diet soft drink or bottle of flavored or unflavored bubbly water may be tempting. But carbonation can make you feel full and nauseous pretty fast. Worse, the bubbles can lead to stretching of the stomach pouch, which will reduce the restrictive effects of the surgery or increase your risk of having a leak.

Caffeinated Beverages: Caffeine is a diuretic, which means it makes your body lose water. Normally it is not a big problem and does not even affect your hydration levels. After RYGB, though, drinking enough fluids to stay hydrated is difficult. Other reasons to avoid caffeine are that it can causes ulcers or heartburn and it can irritate the stomach and delay healing. These are common sources of caffeine:

- Hot and iced coffee and coffee drinks, such as mochas and lattes
- Some hot and iced tea, including some types of diet Snapple
- Energy drinks and many sports drinks
- Hot chocolate made with cocoa powder for baking
- Hot chocolate from packets usually only has a small amount of caffeine.

Calories and the Liquid Diet: Weight loss is all about eating fewer calories than you burn. You may be surprised to learn that calories can add up pretty quickly on the liquid diet, even though you are not eating solid food. Drinking a lot of high-calorie liquids can prevent weight loss. These are a few high-calorie fluids to limit or avoid because of their calories, even though they are technically permitted on a liquid diet.

Cream or Cheese Soup: Unlike broth and bouillon, soups with cream or cheese bases can have over 200 calories per cup. That is 400 calories in a two-cup can, which is a standard size. Cream of mushroom soup, cream of chicken or tomato soup, clam chowder, and broccoli cheese soup are high in calories. Broth and bouillon can take just as long to eat and be just as satisfying while only having 10 to 20 calories per serving.

Diet Shakes: Diet shakes, nutritional supplement shakes, liquid meals, and protein shakes such as Ensure and Boost can have 200 to 400 calories per serving. They are allowed on your liquid diet and are high in essential nutrients, but discuss them with your dietitian to see exactly how they fit into your meal plan. Some diet shakes are high in sugar and are not that high in protein, fiber, or essential vitamins and minerals. These will just add calories without making you feel full.

Hot Beverages with Cream and Sugar: Black coffee and plain tea are nearly calorie-free, but coffee and tea with cream and sugar are higher in empty calories; that is, calories without extra nutrients. Cream and creamers contain unhealthy saturated or trans fats. Each 8-oz. cup of sweetened coffee with cream or creamer can have 80 to 200 or more calories; the same is true for tea with milk and sugar or honey.

Fruit Drinks and Other Sugar-Sweetened Beverages: Fruit drinks have about 120 calories per cup, which is the same amount of calories as 100% fruit juices. But fruit *drinks* are almost pure added sugars, and they do not have the natural nutrients that are found in fruit *juices*. They also have artificial flavors and colors. They are basically the same as fruit punch. Instead, choose 100% fruit juice for its nutritional benefits or sugar-free beverages for their taste.

Whole Milk: It has all the protein and calcium of fat-free milk, but each cup of whole milk has 150 calories. A cup of fat-free milk has 80 calories. Whole milk is high in unhealthy fats.

Keeping Calories in Check during Phase 1 of the RYGB Diet

Healing, not calorie-counting, is the top priority during Phase 1, Liquids. However, high-calorie choices now can seriously stall your weight loss. Plus, you might want to start choosing low-calorie options now so that it is already a habit when you get to later phases of the RYGB diet.

These sample meal plans (*Table 19*) with calorie counts can help you see how much your choices affect calorie counts on the liquid diet.

Meal or Snack	High-Calorie Sample Day	Lower-Calorie Sample Day
Breakfast	High-protein, full-sugar meal replacement shake (300 calories) ½ cup regular gelatin sprinkled with 10 grams unflavored protein powder (80 calories)	4 ounces apple juice diluted with 4 ounces of water and mixed with 15 grams unflavored protein powder (110 calories) ½ cup sugar-free gelatin sprinkled with 10 grams unflavored protein powder (50 calories)
Snack 1	8-ounce Special K protein shake (190 calories)	8-ounce sugar-free protein shake (130 calories)
Lunch	12-oz. low-fat milk with 15 grams chocolate-flavored protein powder (260 calories)	12 ounces skim milk with 15 grams sugar-free chocolate-flavored protein powder (170 calories)
Snack 2	½ cup sugar-free ice pop 8 ounces low-fat milk (150 calories)	½ cup sugar-free ice pop 4 ounces fruit juice diluted with 4 ounces water (80 calories)
Dinner	8 ounces (1 cup) cream of chicken soup (without chunks) made with whole milk and 10 grams protein powder (200 calories)	8 ounces (1 cup) chicken broth with 10 grams protein powder (60 calories)
Snack 3	8 ounces low-fat milk and 10 grams flavored sweetened protein powder (200 calories)	8 ounces skim milk and 10 grams sugar-free protein powder (130 calories)
Total Calories	1380 calories	730 calories

Table 19: Sample meal plans during phase 1 of the RYGB diet

"Solid Liquids" Are Not Liquids

Some foods seem like liquids, especially if you really, really want them to be. But they are not. A liquid has to pour freely as you are eating it. Unless your surgeon or dietitian specifically tells you that you can have some of these "solid liquids," they are not allowed on a liquid diet. Do not sneak them in and interfere with your future success with the RYGB.

- *Ice cream:* Ice cream melts into a liquid, but it is a food, not a liquid. Avoiding ice cream right now is better for your health anyway. It can have 300 to 600 calories per cup and more cholesterol-raising saturated fat and blood sugar-spiking sugar than you should get in a day.

- *Yogurt:* It is high in protein, calcium, and probiotics (healthy bacteria that live in your gut and may boost your immune system. You can eat it later but not now on the liquid diet. You eat it with a spoon.

- *Pudding:* Pudding is one of those "recovery" foods that we think of when someone is healing and needs a simple comfort food. But it is not a liquid, so save it for the next phase of your RYGB diet. Hot chocolate is a better way to get your chocolate fix during the liquid phase, and vanilla and banana-flavored protein shakes can be substitute fixes for your craving for comforting tastes.

Hydration after Gastric Bypass

Water makes up more than half of the body weight of the average middle-aged adult.[14] Staying hydrated may have been easy and natural before surgery, but dehydration is a real threat after surgery.[15] It can occur within hours if you do not drink enough water or get your fluids from other sources.

Why do you need water?

- It is necessary for maintaining a normal body temperature, for every metabolic reaction in your body, and for digesting, absorbing, and using nutrients[16]

- It prevents dehydration signs and symptoms, such as dark yellow or a small amount of urine, less sweating than usual, headaches, nausea, confusion, and dizziness

- It can prevent mid-afternoon headaches

- It helps control weight because it naturally reduces hunger and is calorie-free

Adequate water is even more important when you are recovering from surgery because it allows your wounds to heal. You need a minimum of 1.5 liters, or six 8-ounce cups, of fluids per day. That includes the amount of fluid you have at meals plus water and other liquids that you drink throughout the day.

After you get past the liquid diet and pureed foods diet after surgery, you will not be having water and other beverages with your meals or just before or after meal times. Avoiding beverages at meals helps prevent overeating and the risk of stretching your stomach pouch, and it slows the passage of food through your stomach so that you feel full for longer after your meal. You can meet your fluid requirements by drinking liquids throughout the day in between meals. Aim for one to two cups between meals and snacks to hit your 1.5-liter (6-cup) goal.

Nutritional Supplements: Vitamins and Minerals

Because of your low food intake and the nutrient malabsorption after gastric bypass surgery, dietary supplements are necessary to prevent nutrient deficiencies. You should begin taking them before surgery or in the liquid diet stage. Your surgeon or dietitian can tell you which supplements to take, their quantities, when to take them, and anything else to check for on the label when you are buying each supplement.

Most Common Vitamin and Minerals of Concern

Post-surgery, you are at higher risk for deficiencies of certain vitamins and minerals because of the foods they are in and how your body absorbs them. These are some of the vitamins and minerals of greatest concern for RYGB patients:[17]

- *Calcium:* Calcium is necessary for maintaining your bone mineral density so that your bones stay strong as you get older. A restricted diet can cause osteoporosis and bone fractures (broken bones) later on.

- *Vitamin D:* You need vitamin D so that your body uses calcium properly. Your skin can make vitamin D when you are out in the sun, but many of us are not out in the sun for long enough to make enough vitamin D, so we need to get it from our diet or supplements.

- *Vitamin B-12:* This vitamin works with folic acid to keep your heart healthy and prevent anemia.

- *Iron:* This mineral is necessary for preventing anemia, which can make you tired and susceptible to infections. It occurs in about half of female RYGB patients that are menstruating because of significant losses of iron each month during menstruation.

- *Vitamin A:* This vitamin can become deficient on a very low-fat diet because you need to eat fat for your body to be able to absorb it. Your diet will be low in fat after the gastric bypass, putting you at risk for deficiency.

- *Thiamin (vitamin B1):* This is a vitamin that you need for metabolism. Severe deficiency is very rare, but it is possible if you have periods of vomiting. Slightly low status is likely in gastric bypass patients.[18]

- *Vitamin K:* Like vitamin A, vitamin K can only be absorbed when you have fat in the diet. Deficiency is rare for most people, but after bypass, you may need supplements.

- *Zinc:* This mineral is necessary for a strong immune response and for proper metabolism. It is in a lot of high-protein foods, but you can become deficient because of your low food intake on the RYGB diet and because absorption depends on your dietary fat intake.[19]

Multivitamin and Mineral Supplement

Having most of your vitamins and minerals in a single formula can save you a lot of trouble. A standard daily supplement usually has about 50 to 100 percent of the daily value of most vitamins and minerals, such as the B vitamins; vitamins A, C, D, E and K; and many minerals, such as zinc, calcium, copper, iron (for women), and chromium. You may need additional supplements, such as a calcium or iron supplement.

Form of Supplementation

On your liquid postoperative diet, you cannot take vitamins and minerals in regular pill form. You can get your vitamins and minerals using liquid or powdered multivitamin and mineral supplements instead of large pills or capsules. Another option is to use a pill grinder to grind up your regular hard pills so you can sprinkle the powder on your food.

Vitamin and mineral supplements continue far beyond the liquid diet phase. You will probably be on them for life because of your limited diet and nutrient malabsorption.

Sample Menus for Phase 1 – Liquid Diet

Table 20 is a sample daily menu for your post-surgery clear liquid diet, which lasts for only one to two days and will finish while you are in the hospital. The diet involves sipping on as many clear fluids as you can handle.

Sample Meal Pattern[20]

Meal or Snack	Sample Day on the Clear Liquid Diet
Breakfast	½ cup sugar-free gelatin
	2 ounces of apple juice diluted with 2 ounces of water
Snack 1	½ cup sugar-free gelatin
Lunch	8 ounces (1 cup) beef-flavored broth
	½ cup apple juice
Snack 2	½ cup decaffeinated diet iced tea
Dinner	½ cup vegetable-flavored broth
	½ cup of gelatin
	2 ounces of grape juice diluted with 2 ounces of water
Snack 3	1 sugar-free popsicle
	½ cup of apple juice

Table 20: Sample daily menu for your post-surgery clear liquid diet

Table 21 is a sample menu for a day on the full liquid diet, which will last for about two weeks. On the full liquid diet, your focus should also be on getting enough protein.[21] Be sure to drink plenty of water throughout the day to prevent dehydration.

Meal or Snack	Sample Day for the Full Liquid Diet
Breakfast	4 ounces apple juice diluted with 4 ounces of water and mixed with 20 grams unflavored protein powder ½ cup sugar-free gelatin sprinkled with 10 grams unflavored protein powder
Snack 1	8-ounce sugar-free protein shake
Lunch	12 oz. low-fat milk with 10 grams sugar-free chocolate-flavored protein powder
Snack 2	½ cup sugar-free ice pop 4 ounces fruit juice diluted with 4 ounces water
Dinner	8 ounces (1 cup) cream of chicken soup without chunks and with 10 g protein powder
Snack 3	8 ounces low-fat milk and 10 grams protein powder

Table 21: Sample menu for a day on the full liquid diet

Phase 2 – Pureed Diet

Transition to the pureed diet phase is a big step because it means that your recovery is going well and you are not having any serious complications with the gastric bypass. Getting through the liquids phase successfully should also prove to you that you *can* stick to the RYGB diet.

In the pureed foods phase, you get to add real foods back into your diet! You will have to select your foods very carefully, but your diet will be far more interesting and satisfying than the liquid diet. The purposes of this phase are to continue to allow your body to recover from surgery, to meet your nutrient needs, and to lose a little more weight. This phase will last from about two to four weeks after surgery.

Tips for Success in Phase 2

You are more experienced and stronger than you were in phase 1, but you are not yet fully recovered from surgery. You are still getting used to the gastric bypass, and you have a long way to go in your weight loss journey. For these reasons, following Phase 2 properly is just as important as it was to follow the liquid diet properly. These guidelines may help.

Be Patient

The liquid diet is boring and not very satisfying, so getting excited about getting to Stage 2 is natural. Do not go overboard with your new options though. Instead, add in only one new food at a time and do not eat it again for another few days if you think it causes you trouble. Be prepared to go back to your liquid diet for a day or two if you have symptoms like a sore throat or nausea. Also be ready to stop eating when you feel full, even if it is only after one bite. You are still at risk for nausea or stretching your stomach pouch if you eat the wrong foods or eat too much.

Pureed Foods – Not Chunky!

Some foods, such as pudding, are naturally smooth. Others, such as applesauce, may have small chunks. Puree and strain it before eating these kinds of foods to prevent any little chunks from irritating your surgery stitches. Your blender or hand blender and strainer will come in handy during this phase.

Approaching Meals and Snacks

Right after surgery, the size of your stomach pouch is only about 15[22] to 39[23] milliliters, or about ½ to 1 ½ fluid ounces. That is not much. Your original stomach was more than 1,000 milliliters, or 4 cups (32 fluid ounces). As you add in non-fluid foods during phase 2, you may notice a new sensation — fullness.

Fullness is a good and normal feeling that should come after a meal. You may need to relearn how to recognize fullness, since you may be used to ignoring it. You may also experience early satiety — an intense feeling of fullness that comes on before you finish the food that you had planned. You will not be able to comfortably eat more. At that point, the meal or snack will be over even if you have only eaten a bite or if you have food left over.

You cannot predict when early satiety will happen, so be prepared for it:

- Eat your protein first so that you are still likely to meet your protein requirements.
- Eat your vegetables and fruits next because they provide important nutrients and health benefits.
- Do not fight it. You cannot control it, so do not let it upset you. Just pack up or throw away your food.

Foods on a Pureed Foods Diet

Phase 2 includes all of the liquids from Phase 1 plus a few foods. Everything needs to be pureed or of a pureed texture. These are some examples of foods for a pureed diet.[24],[25] Remember, everything needs to be perfectly smooth. You can try putting it through a strainer if you are not sure whether it qualifies as "pureed."

Cottage Cheese: Cottage cheese may become one of your staples. Fat-free and 1% low-fat cottage cheese are high in protein and calcium and low in calories and carbohydrates. Puree small-curd cottage cheese to make it perfectly smooth.

Yogurt: Yogurt is another high-protein, high-calcium choice. It also provides probiotics, which are healthy bacteria that can boost your immune system and regulate digestion. Fat-free yogurt is lowest in calories and the least likely to cause an upset stomach. You can also limit your calories, carbohydrates, and sugar by choosing plain yogurt. If you prefer flavored yogurt, choose one with no added sugars. Instead, it should be sweetened with a calorie-free sugar substitute, such as aspartame, sucralose (brand name Splenda), or stevia instead of added sugars such as corn syrup or sugar. Be sure to choose yogurt without chunks of fruit chunks in it.

Tofu: Tofu is another good source of protein, and fortified tofu has calcium. Only silken tofu is allowed on your pureed foods diet. Veggie burgers and other meat substitutes, such as tofu meatballs and sausages, are not okay for right now.

Ricotta Cheese: It is a great dairy choice on the post-surgery RYGB diet because it is high in calcium but almost free from lactose. That means that it is low-sugar and less likely to cause symptoms of lactose intolerance or dumping syndrome than yogurt. Choose low-fat or fat-free ricotta to limit the calories.

Peanut Butter: Creamy peanut butter has less protein than cottage cheese and yogurt, but it has some, plus other beneficial nutrients, such as heart-healthy fats, vitamin E, fiber, and magnesium. Its thickness and sticky texture can be welcome when you are limited to pureed foods, which are often watery. Chunky peanut butter is not okay for this phase of the RYGB diet. Be sure to take only tiny bites and chew each one for a long time so that it mixes well with your saliva and is not as sticky when you swallow it.

Tips for the Pureed Foods Diet

To puree a chopped food, such as diced cooked potato or chopped ripe melon, place it in a blender or food processor. Add enough liquid to cover the blades, cover or close the blender or processor, and turn it on. If you are using a hand blender, place the food in a bowl, add a small amount of liquid, and blend. Be sure to submerge the blade of the hand blender — keep the blade below the level of food to avoid making a mess!

Foods during this stage should be no thicker than applesauce or watery mashed potatoes. If your food is thicker than that, stir in liquid until the consistency is right.

Little tricks can make the pureed food stage tastier and easier to stick to. As long as you stick to the allowed ingredients, you can try pureeing foods using ingredients aside from pure water. These are some examples:

- Add cinnamon and cloves, ginger, or pumpkin pie spice to mashed bananas and canned pumpkin.
- Puree potatoes in broth or with fat-free milk and nutmeg.
- Add herbs and spices, such as black pepper and thyme, to pureed potatoes and sweet potatoes.
- Blend plain Greek yogurt with applesauce, cinnamon, and calorie-free sweetener.

Pudding: Chocolate, banana, and vanilla pudding can be treats during this phase of recovery. Ready-made puddings are often in single-serve containers. If the entire 4-ounce (one-half cup) container is too big for your tiny stomach pouch, be prepared to store the rest for another meal. Stick with sugar-free pudding to limit calories and prevent dumping syndrome.

Mashed Bananas: Make sure to remove the strings when you peel your banana and to puree it thoroughly so that it does not still have chunks when you eat it. Bananas are high in carbohydrates. They are naturally sweet and are sources of dietary fiber, potassium, magnesium, and vitamin C

Cooked Fruits: Some kinds of cooked fruits are allowed on a pureed foods diet, but be sure to check with your nutritionist or surgeon before eating them. Smooth applesauce and pureed and peeled, cooked, or canned peaches, apples, and pears are good choices if you puree them well. If you are making your own from fresh, peel them first. Stay away from stringy or fibrous fruits, such as canned mandarin oranges, and avoid fruits with small seeds, like raspberries. Avoid fruit jams, which are high in sugar and low in nutrients and likely to cause dumping syndrome.

Pureed Potatoes, Sweet Potatoes, and Squash: Peeled, cooked, pureed potatoes and sweet potatoes are likely allowed on your pureed foods diet. If they are still too thick after you puree them, try adding some water and pureeing them a little more. Stringy yams should be avoided. Frozen and canned, cooked winter squash and pumpkin are other high-potassium, nutritious choices on your pureed foods diet. Be sure to choose plain canned pumpkin and not canned pumpkin pie filling with sugar and spices.

Soft Hot Cereal: Fortified cream of wheat and farina are nutritious choices for this phase, but you might need to stay away from oatmeal, even though it is healthy, because of its chunks. Let the cereal cool down before you eat it because your stomach wounds may still be sensitive to very hot and very cold temperatures.

Soup: You can add more soups in addition to the broth and bouillon that you had on the liquid diet. Be absolutely certain that they have no chunks. It is safer to strain your recipe or the can of soup before eating it to get it smooth enough. Cream soups are high in calories and fat, so choose reduced-fat versions. They will not be part of your regular diet when you get to the semi-solid food stage and beyond.

Your dietitian or surgeon might have slightly different recommendations for what you can and cannot have in Phase 2. Some gastric bypass patients, for example, can have pureed canned tuna within two to four weeks after surgery. Your dietitian may also recommend a specific order to introduce food in so you start with the ones that are least likely to cause problems.

> **Tip**
>
> **Learning from Others' Experiences**
>
> If you want to compare your own experiences to those of other RYGB patients, you might want to log onto BariatricPal.com. Experienced members there can share memories of their own Phase 2 recovery diets. They can tell you about which foods worked for them and which did not. Just keep in mind that everyone's journey is slightly different.

Your healthcare team and your body should be your guides. Some foods might not agree with you even though they are on the approved list. On the other hand, you might find that you are able to progress faster than average with other foods. Some people are very sensitive to spicy foods, and you might need to avoid things like chili powder and curries until you are certain that your surgical wounds have healed completely.

Allowed	Not Allowed[26]
✓ Phase 1 liquids	✗ Raw and cooked vegetables
✓ Pureed, reduced-fat cottage cheese	✗ Meat
✓ Fat-free yogurt without chunks	✗ Bread and cold cereal
✓ Hard or soft silken tofu	✗ Most grains, such as rice and pasta
✓ Pureed cream and thin soups	✗ Nuts and seeds; peanut and nut butter
✓ Pureed watery potatoes and sweet potatoes	✗ Raw fruit
✓ Mashed bananas	✗ Fruit with seeds or peel
✓ Some cooked, peeled fruits	✗ Fruit jam
✓ Beans	✗ High-calorie, unhealthy choices, e.g., ice cream and butter
✓ Unsweetened applesauce	

Table 22: Foods Allowed/Not Allowed in Phase2

Stage 2 Includes Some High-Calorie Foods That You Will Not Be Eating Later

At this point, you are still eating some high-calorie foods and beverages, such as cream soups and protein shakes. These liquid calories are okay now because you are still focusing on getting the nutrients you need to promote healing from surgery, but soon they will not be allowed. When you get to the soft foods stage and your long-term solid foods diet, you will depend on highly nutritious solid foods for your nutrients and calorie-free or low-calorie beverages to stay hydrated.

Developing Good Eating Habits for Life with the Roux-en-Y Gastric Bypass

Phase 2, the pureed foods diet, is a good opportunity to start practicing the eating patterns that you will be following in the future. You are not yet eating the full range of solid foods that you will be eating in a couple of months, but you should be following the same general guidelines as you will for your weight loss journey. These are some of the behaviors that will help you lose weight and prevent side effects.

Eating Slowly

This is important in your success because it lets you feel full before you have eaten as much food. Start in Phase 2 by taking small bites from a shallow spoon and setting the spoon down in between each bite. Savor each bite and chew it thoroughly before swallowing — as you should do anyway on a pureed diet to be sure that you are not swallowing any chunks! Then, pause for a few seconds before filling up your spoon and lifting it to your mouth for the next bite. Remembering to do this will take a lot of effort at first, but it will soon become habit. Another benefit of eating slowly is that you will concentrate more on eating and be able to enjoy your food more!

Eating Protein First

This is important for making sure you meet your requirements each day, even if you have early satiety as described above. Eating your protein food first at a meal has additional benefits. First, protein is a filling nutrient. It helps you stay full for a little longer after you eat so that you do not get hungry for the next meal as soon.[27] Plus, it helps to stabilize your body's blood sugar levels so you have more energy and do not have wild swings.

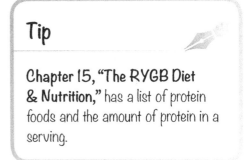

Tip

Chapter 15, "The RYGB Diet & Nutrition," has a list of protein foods and the amount of protein in a serving.

- Choose high-protein foods first when you are selecting foods for a meal or snack.

- Eat your protein food first at each meal.

- Make your protein intake a priority by focusing on it early in the day.

Focusing on Fullness

You ate a lot more than you needed to during those years of fighting obesity. This might have been because you ignored your biological hunger and fullness signals and instead ate for other reasons, such as pleasure, comfort, or habit. Now you are going to only eat what you *need* to based on hunger. It will take you a while to learn to recognize the signals that you are full. Your small stomach pouch fills quickly, but it can take 20 or more minutes for your brain to recognize that you are full. At first, the signals can be very faint. To give yourself time to get full and retrain your brain to recognize fullness, you might have to pause your eating before you feel full.

Making Healthy Food Choices

It is not your main focus yet, but you can start thinking about making healthy food choices. It is not a big deal; it is as simple as making little decisions such as these:

- Choosing cottage cheese instead of mashed potatoes because you feel that you need the protein more than the carbohydrates

- Choosing pureed carrots instead of cream of wheat because you want the vitamin A

- Choosing yogurt instead of a protein shake because you know it will keep you full for longer

Measuring Your Portions

Portion control is essential for losing weight and keeping it off. Measuring your portion sizes is the only sure way of making sure you are in control of how much you are eating. Continue to use your measuring cups and spoons and kitchen scale stay in control.

Staying Hydrated

Consuming enough fluids remains a challenge for many bariatric patients.[28] Staying hydrated is even harder in Phase 2 than Phase 1 because, in Phase 2, you do not drink fluids with your meals or snacks. Instead, you should only have beverages at least 30 minutes before or after eating.[29] Stay focused on making it a priority to drink plenty of water each day, with a goal of one to two cups between meals. The deeper you can get this habit engrained in your mind, the easier it will be to maintain the pattern when you move on to solid foods and are depending on the small stomach pouch to fill up quickly and stay full for longer so you can suppress hunger and lose weight.

Sample Menus for Phase 2 – Pureed Foods Diet

Table 23 displays two sample menus for your pureed foods diet. Each has five small meals or snacks and is designed to be high in protein to meet your needs.[30] You can switch servings of similar foods as long as you watch your portion sizes and choose high-protein options first. Do not forget to drink plenty of water between meals.

Meal or Snack	Day 1 Sample	Day 2 Sample
Breakfast	2 tablespoons cream of wheat made with fat-free milk 1 scoop protein powder in two ounces of fruit juice diluted with 2 ounces of water 2 tablespoons cottage cheese	½ cup cottage cheese ½ medium mashed banana
Snack 1	1 tablespoon protein powder in ½ cup fat-free milk	½ cup cooked pureed carrots
Lunch	8 ounces of vegetable soup 2 ounces fat-free ricotta cheese	8 ounces of beef broth with 20 grams of unflavored protein powder ½ cup cream of wheat
Dinner	¼ cup mashed potatoes made with fat-free milk and 2 tsp. olive oil	¼ cup mashed sweet potatoes ¼ cup light silken tofu
Snack 2	1 tablespoon peanut butter ½ cup applesauce	½ cup sugar-free vanilla pudding with 10 grams protein powder

Table 23: Sample Menus for Phase 2 – Pureed Foods Diet

Phase 3 – Soft Foods Diet

Your wounds are nearly healed within three or four weeks of gastric bypass surgery. You may be ready to progress to Phase 3, the soft foods (semi-solid foods), phase if you are not experiencing surgery complications and you are able to tolerate all of the foods in the pureed foods diet. You can choose from a much wider variety of foods in Phase 3. The phase may last until five to eight weeks after surgery.

Tips for Success in Phase 3

Stay Patient: You are much stronger now, but you do not want to risk any setbacks at this point. Adding foods too quickly or eating foods that are not allowed can lead to a leak or dumping syndrome. As you did in Phase 2, only add in one new food at a time, and be prepared to go back to the pureed or even liquid diet for a few days if you cannot tolerate a new food.

Be Ready for Change: Phase 3, the soft foods diet, is a transition period. It bridges the post-surgery recovery period and the time when you are back to your full range of normal activities. It is a time to shift from recovery mode to weight loss mode. You will start to focus on nutrients in addition to protein. By the end of Phase 3, your diet will be very similar to your long-term diet.

Keep Watching Your Portions: Continue to measure the serving size of each food and beverage at every meal and snack. That helps keep your calories in check so you lose weight as expected. It also helps prevent from eating too much and developing nausea or stretching your stomach pouch.[31] A larger stomach makes the surgery less effective by reducing the amount of restriction that you feel.

Foods on a Soft Foods Diet: The increased range of allowed foods can make your diet healthier and more interesting than before. This phase is more variable than the previous stages, and some of the specific food recommendations and prohibitions from your surgeon and dietitian may be different from the ones on this list. Follow their advice. These are some foods that you can probably add in this phase.

Canned Tuna and Other Chunk Proteins: Canned tuna and other chunk proteins, such as canned chicken and imitation crabmeat, are very convenient. They are high in protein, low in fat, and already cooked. Most choices are boneless, but some, such as canned salmon, have bones and can irritate your stomach pouch.

Ground Meat: Cooked extra-lean ground beef, turkey, and chicken are high in protein and iron and good choices for a semi-solid diet. To make sure that the meat is ground finely enough, puree it yourself before cooking it, and strain it after cooking. Choose only high-quality meats to avoid gristle.

Eggs: Eggs are high in protein and ideal for a soft foods diet because they do not have anything crunchy or fibrous in them. Soft-boiled and scrambled eggs are especially good choices. Egg whites contain all of the egg's protein, and they are fat-free and cholesterol-free. Yolks in moderation can be part of a healthy diet too.

Cooked Vegetables: Vegetables are healthy enough to be your top priority after protein. Canned vegetables are the safest choices when you are first introducing them into your postoperative diet because they are thoroughly cooked and very soft. You can also use peeled fresh and frozen vegetables as long as you cook them well and avoid seeds. Canned green beans; frozen green peas; and peeled, chopped, and boiled carrots are great choices to start with.

Cooked Grains: Well-cooked white pasta and white rice are okay for most people on a soft diet, and fortified ones are rich in B vitamins and iron. To be safe, you can blend them with water after cooking them to make them thinner and smoother. Bread and cold cereal are not yet okay on this diet.

Fresh Fruit: Ripe, soft peeled pears and nectarines and melon may be tolerated on a soft foods diet. Avoid dried fruit because it is tough. It is also high-calorie. Just like citrus juices, citrus fruits such as oranges and tangerines can be irritating because of their acid. Hold off on them until later in your weight loss journey.

Beans, Peas, and Lentils: Beans and lentils are high-protein and soft enough for a semi-solid diet, but they often cause gassiness. If your surgeon or dietitian recommends them, start with only a tiny portion, such as a tablespoon, and wait for at least a day to see if you tolerate them well. You can also try diluting them with water or broth and pureeing them. If you cannot tolerate whole beans, you might be able to get away with hummus or dip made with garbanzo beans or chickpeas. If you are able to tolerate beans, low-sodium canned beans and lentils and fat-free refried beans are good options. If you choose dried beans or lentils, be sure to soak them overnight and cook them very thoroughly.

Low-Fat Cheese: It is high in protein and a good source of calcium. You can use it to add flavor to foods by melting it on meat, adding it to your scrambled eggs, or sprinkling shredded cheese on soup. Reduced-fat and fat-free cream cheeses are okay but not as nutritious as low-fat cheddar, mozzarella, and other aged cheeses.

Foods from Phases 1 and 2 While in Phase 3

By the time you are in Phase 3, the soft foods stage, you can easily physically tolerate all of the liquids from Phase1 and the pureed foods from Phase 2. But that does not mean that all of those options are part of your semi-solid foods diet. Phase 3 is about promoting weight loss as you transition to making healthy selections.

Stop Drinking Your Calories

Fluids were your only sources of calories during the Phase 1 liquid diet, and your food choices were so limited during Phase 2 that you probably depended on protein shakes and other beverages with calories to meet your nutrient requirements. Phase 3, the semi-solid foods stage, reduces these choices. High-calorie beverages decrease the effectiveness of the gastric bypass because they do not make you feel full. This is especially true for sugar-sweetened beverages, such as coffee drinks, sports and energy drinks, and fruit drinks. Fat-free and 1% low-fat milk can remain in your diet because it is so healthy, but you will still need to monitor your portion sizes. Water, tea, coffee, and non-carbonated diet drinks are good choices because they are low-calorie or calorie free.

Make Nutritious Choices

All of the foods from Phase 2 are allowed during Phase 3, but some are better choices than others during Phase 3. Nutritious, high-protein foods, such as fat-free yogurt and cottage cheese, should be regular parts of your diet. On the other hand, cream soups are choices to limit or avoid because they are not high in the nutrients you need. Protein shakes can help you reach your protein goals, but when possible, opt for solid protein sources, such as egg whites, because they are more filling.

Sample Menus for Phase 3 – Semi-Solid or Soft Foods Diet

A typical Phase 3 diet includes four or five small meals each day, with water or other non-caloric liquids in between them. Your surgeon and dietitian may suggest having only three meals per day or having three meals with three snacks. Follow their advice. The Phase 3 meal pattern is similar to the meal pattern you will be following on the full solids diet, or Phase 4. Remember to separate your liquids and solids by at least 30 minutes to avoid dumping syndrome, increase fullness, and prevent your stomach pouch from stretching. If the meals are too big for you, stop eating. You do not have to finish your planned food.

Meal or Snack	Day 1 Sample	Day 2 Sample
Breakfast	½ cup cottage cheese 3 tablespoons farina made with 1 percent low-fat milk and sprinkled with protein powder 1 tablespoon smooth peanut butter	3 tablespoons banana mashed with 1 tablespoon protein powder ½ cup plain fat-free yogurt sprinkled with cinnamon and a sweetener packet ¼ cup protein shake
Snack 1	1 cup fat-free plain yogurt	1 cup (8 ounces) sugar-free protein shake
Lunch	2 ounces canned tuna ½ cup applesauce ¼ cup pureed sweet potatoes	1 ounce canned chicken breast 4 tablespoons canned green beans 3 tablespoons fat-free cottage cheese
Dinner	2 ounces lean ground turkey ¼ cup pureed peas ½ cup silken tofu	2 ounces cooked white fish with no bones ½ cup vegetable soup with 2 tablespoons protein powder 3 tablespoons well-cooked pureed pasta 1 tablespoon peanut butter
Snack 2	½ cup sugar-free chocolate pudding 1 soft-boiled egg	2 ounces fat-free ricotta cheese 1 tablespoon peanut butter ½ cup cooked cream of wheat

Table 24: Sample Menus for Phase 3 – Semi-Solid or Soft Foods Diet

Table 24 displays two sample menus for the Phase 3 diet. They provide the recommended 70 to 80 grams of protein and 1.5 liters of water. You can swap foods from these suggested menus as long as you swap similar foods, such as green beans for carrots, and keep the emphasis on protein foods. Your surgeon and dietitian might have additional sample menus or suggest specific foods to include or exclude; listen to their advice!

Handy Food Lists

This chapter has a great deal of important information. It is a good source to refer to as you progress through your postoperative diet. You can also look at the following food charts listing the foods you can have in each of the first three stages. You might find them helpful on your refrigerator or as grocery lists.

Phase 1: Liquid Diet Foods for One to Two Weeks after Surgery

- Water
- Caffeine-free tea or coffee
- Diet juice drinks, e.g., Crystal Light or sugar-free Kool-Aid
- Fruit juices, nectars, or ciders (avoid citrus juices)
- Gelatin
- Popsicles, especially sugar-free
- Protein shakes (full liquid only)
- Protein powder
- Non-fat (skim) or 1 percent low-fat milk (full liquid only)
- Calcium-fortified soy milk (full liquid only)
- Broth or bouillon

Phase 2: Pureed Foods until Three or Four Weeks after Surgery

- Phase 1 plus…
- Fat-free cottage cheese
- Cream soups
- Creamy peanut butter
- Pudding
- Yogurt without fruit chunks
- Canned fruit
- Applesauce
- Mashed bananas
- Silken tofu (the soft kind)
- Creamed soup

- Pureed potatoes with water
- Cream of wheat and farina

Phase 3: Semi-Solid or Soft Foods until about Six to Eight Weeks after Surgery

- Phases 1 and 2 plus…
- Canned tuna or chicken
- Extra-lean ground beef, chicken, or turkey
- Eggs, egg whites, or fat-free, cholesterol-free egg substitute
- Rice
- Pasta
- Fresh fruit
- Cooked vegetables (not broccoli, asparagus, or celery)
- Low-fat or fat-free cheese
- Imitation crab meat or fresh crab meat
- Fish—be very careful of bones

✍ Summary

☛ This chapter took you through your post-surgery recovery diet from surgery to four to eight weeks after surgery. You should be proud of yourself for making it from the clear liquid diet all the way through the soft foods diet. It means you have been diligent about sticking to the plan. You are doing everything possible to achieve successful weight loss with the RYGB.

☛ The next chapter covers the gastric bypass diet that you will be following for years as you lose weight and keep it off. You will learn what you can eat and start to understand how to put together your own healthy meal plans. You will keep practicing your new eating skills as you try to lose weight and get healthy.

Time to Take Action: Getting Some Practice in Monitoring Your Diet and Yourself

The gastric bypass diet is all about you and your long-term lifestyle changes. The period of post-surgery recovery is ideal for thinking about your food intake and how you feel while you eat. The more you practice, the more natural it will become. For this worksheet (*Table 25*), choose a single day and fill out the answers to the questions below for each meal and snack.

Meal or Snack	What did you eat?	How hungry were you before the meal or snack? How hungry and satisfied were you afterwards?	Record other notes here. Did you have any trouble with sticking or obstruction? Did you enjoy the food? Did you chew it well?
Breakfast	Half-cup of cottage cheese, quarter-cup applesauce	Starving before. Still hungry afterwards, but hunger died down later.	No troubles. Had cooked apple yesterday and felt nauseous, but today's applesauce was fine.
Snack 1 (if applicable)			
Lunch			
Snack 2 (if applicable)			
Dinner			
Snack 3 (if applicable)			

Table 25: Monitoring Your Diet and Yourself

1   Aills L, Blankenship J, Buffington C, Furtado M, Parrott J. ASMBS Allied Health nutritional guidelines for the surgical weight loss patient. Surg Obes Relat Dis. 2008;4(5Suppl):S73-S108.

2   Aills L, Blankenship J, Buffington C, Furtado M, Parrott J. ASMBS Allied Health nutritional guidelines for the surgical weight loss patient. Surg Obes Relat Dis. 2008;4(5Suppl):S73-S108.

3   Smeets AJ, Westerterp Plantenga MS. The acute effects of a lunch containing capsaicin on energy and substrate utilization, hormones and satiety. 2009;48(4):229-34.

4   Snyder-Marlow G, Tayle D, Lenhard MJ. Nutrition care for patients undergoing laparoscopic sleeve gastrectomy for weight loss. J Am Diet Ass. 2010;110(4):600-607

5   Aills L, Blankenship J, Buffington C, Furtado M, Parrott J. ASMBS Allied Health nutritional guidelines for the surgical weight loss patient. Surg Obes Relat Dis. 2008;4(5Suppl):S73-S108.

6   Snyder-Marlow G, Tayle D, Lenhard MJ. Nutrition care for patients undergoing laparoscopic sleeve gastrectomy for weight loss. J Am Diet Ass. 2010;110(4):600-607

7   Dugdale DC. Diet – full liquid. Medline Plus, National Institutes of Health. Web site. http://www.nlm.nih.gov/medlineplus/ency/patientinstructions/000206.htm. Updated 2010, November 21. Accessed October 9, 2012.

8   Dugdale DC. Diet – clear liquid. Medline Plus, National Institutes of Health. Web site. http://www.nlm.nih.gov/medlineplus/ency/patientinstructions/000205.htm. Updated 2010, November 21. Accessed October 9, 2012.

9   Aills L, Blankenship J, Buffington C, Furtado M, Parrott J. ASMBS Allied Health nutritional guidelines for the surgical weight loss patient. Surg Obes Relat Dis. 2008;4(5Suppl):S73-S108.

10 Dugdale DC. Diet – full liquid. Medline Plus, National Institutes of Health. Web site. http://www.nlm.nih.gov/medlineplus/ency/patientinstructions/000206.htm. Updated 2010, November 21. Accessed October 9, 2012.

11 Snyder-Marlow G, Tayle D, Lenhard MJ. Nutrition care for patients undergoing laparoscopic sleeve gastrectomy for weight loss. J Am Diet Ass. 2010;110(4):600-607

12 Gropper, S.S., & Smith, J.L. (2008). *Advanced Nutrition and Human Metabolism* (5th ed.). Wadsworth Publishing: Belmont, California.

13 Aills L, Blankenship J, Buffington C, Furtado M, Parrott J. ASMBS Allied Health nutritional guidelines for the surgical weight loss patient. Surg Obes Relat Dis. 2008;4(5Suppl):S73-S108

14 Panel on Dietary Reference Intakes for Electrolytes and Water, Standing Committee on the Scientific Evaluation of Dietary Reference Intakes. Dietary reference intakes for water, potassium, sodium, chloride and sulfate. National Academies Press. Web site. http://www.nap.edu/catalog.php?record_id=10925. 2005. Accessed October 10, 2012.

15 Aills L, Blankenship J, Buffington C, Furtado M, Parrott J. ASMBS Allied Health nutritional guidelines for the surgical weight loss patient. Surg Obes Relat Dis. 2008;4(5Suppl):S73-S108

16 Myklebust, M., & Wunder, J. Healing foods pyramid: water. University of Michigan Health System. Retrieved from http://www.med.umich.edu/umim/food-pyramid/water.htm. Updated 2010. Accessed October 10, 2012.

17 Aills L, Blankenship J, Buffington C, Furtado M, Parrott J. ASMBS Allied Health nutritional guidelines for the surgical weight loss patient. Surg Obes Relat Dis. 2008;4(5Suppl):S73-S108.

18 Xanthakos SA. Nutritional deficiencies in obesity and after bariatric surgery. Pediatr Clin North Am, 2009;56(5):1105-1121.

19 Ziegler O, Sirveaux MA, Brunaud L, Reibel N, Quillot D. Medical follow-up after bariatric surgery: nutritional and drug issues. General recommendations for the prevention and treatment of nutritional deficiencies. Diabetes Metab. 2009;35(6 Pt 2):544-547.

20 Snyder-Marlow G, Tayle D, Lenhard MJ. Nutrition care for patients undergoing laparoscopic sleeve gastrectomy for weight loss. J Am Diet Ass. 2010;110(4):600-607

21 Snyder-Marlow G, Tayle D, Lenhard MJ. Nutrition care for patients undergoing laparoscopic sleeve gastrectomy for weight loss. J Am Diet Ass. 2010;110(4):600-607

22 Buchwald H. ASBS 2004 consensus conference statement: bariatric surgery for morbid obesity: health implications for patients, health professionals and third-party payers. Surgery for obesity and related diseases, 2005;371-381

23 Aills L, Blankenship J, Buffington C, Furtado M, Parrott J. ASMBS Allied Health nutritional guidelines for the surgical weight loss patient. Surg Obes Relat Dis. 2008;4(5Suppl):S73-S108.

24 Snyder-Marlow G, Tayle D, Lenhard MJ. Nutrition care for patients undergoing laparoscopic sleeve gastrectomy for weight loss. J Am Diet Ass. 2010;110(4):600-607

25 Aills L, Blankenship J, Buffington C, Furtado M, Parrott J. ASMBS Allied Health nutritional guidelines for the surgical weight loss patient. Surg Obes Relat Dis. 2008;4(5Suppl):S73-S108.

26 Snyder-Marlow G, Tayle D, Lenhard MJ. Nutrition care for patients undergoing laparoscopic sleeve gastrectomy for weight loss. J Am Diet Ass. 2010;110(4):600-607

27 Protein: moving closer to center stage. (2012). The Harvard School of Public Health Nutrition Source. Web site. http://www.hsph.harvard.edu/nutritionsource/protein/. Accessed October 11, 2012.

28 Aills L, Blankenship J, Buffington C, Furtado M, Parrott J. ASMBS Allied Health nutritional guidelines for the surgical weight loss patient. Surg Obes Relat Dis. 2008;4(5Suppl):S73-S108.

29 Mechanick MD, Kushner RF…Dixon J. American Association of Clinical Endocrinologists, The Obesity Society, and American Society for Metabolic & Bariatric Surgery medical guidelines for clinical practice for the perioperative nutritional, metabolic, and nonsurgical support of the bariatric surgery patient. Obesity, 2009;17(S1):S3-72.

30 Snyder-Marlow G, Tayle D, Lenhard MJ. Nutrition care for patients undergoing laparoscopic sleeve gastrectomy for weight loss. J Am Diet Ass. 2010;110(4):600-607

31 Snyder-Marlow G, Tayle D, Lenhard MJ. Nutrition care for patients undergoing laparoscopic sleeve gastrectomy for weight loss. J Am Diet Ass. 2010;110(4):600-607

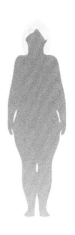

14

RYGB Diet 101

The last chapter talked about laying the foundation for successful weight loss after the gastric bypass surgery. The chapter progressed from your liquid diet through the pureed food diet to the soft foods diet. You are ready for the solid foods stage when you are comfortable with the foods in Phase 3, the soft foods diet. You can finally focus on rapid weight loss and nutritious choices!

This chapter covers Phase 4, the solid foods diet. Phase 4 is the long-term food plan that can take you to your goal weight and beyond. In fact, you will follow this meal pattern for as long as you want to control your weight and maximize your nutrient intake. On Phase 4, you continue to add new foods slowly and gradually.

This is what you will find in this chapter:

- Foods that you can and should have
- Foods to be try carefully, limit, or avoid
- Tips for success
- Meal patterns and sample menus for the RYGB diet

Overview of Phase 4 – The Solid Foods Diet

The solid foods diet is more accurately called a lifestyle instead of a phase. As long as you have no setbacks, you will be following this diet for the long term. Occasionally you may have trouble with solid foods and temporarily need to go back to a soft or pureed foods diet until you feel better, but those times should be rare and short. In general, the solid foods diet is your daily diet for life. These are the goals:

- Lose weight and then maintain your goal weight
- Prevent gastric bypass complications
- Prevent nutritional deficiencies
- Eat a healthy overall diet

Your Focus Shifts to Weight Loss and Health

After cautiously focusing on healing during the first three post-op diet phases, you can finally focus on weight loss! You will lose weight fastest by sticking to the recommended portion sizes and food choices.

Full-Speed Weight Loss Ahead!

Most bariatric surgery patients can lose about one to two pounds per week by following the diet's food choices, meal patterns, and portion sizes. You will regularly see and feel changes in your body when you lose weight at this rate. You will be healthier, and more likely to stick to the diet, when you select nutritious foods. We will talk about making nutritious choices later on.

It Takes about 1 to 2 Years or More to Hit Your Goal Weight

You already know that the Roux-en-Y gastric bypass is not a quick fix for obesity. It is a lifelong approach to managing your weight. It can take one, two, or even more years to hit your goal weight. That may seem like a long time, but it is hardly anything compared with the years and years that you struggled with obesity. And you will feel better, look better, and be healthier long before you hit your final goal weight.

How long might it take for you to lose the weight? This worksheet (*Table 26*) can help you estimate the time.

Step	Write Your Numbers in This Column	Sample 1	Sample 2	Sample 3
1. Write your pre-surgery weight.		362 pounds	279 pounds	295 pounds
2. Write your goal weight.		174 pounds	134 pounds	164 pounds
3. Subtract your goal weight from your pre-surgery weight (Line 1 – 2).		188 pounds	145 pounds	131 pounds
4. Write your expected rate of weight loss.		1 pound per week	2 pounds per week	1.5 pounds per week
5. Divide the amount of weight you want to lose by your rate of weight loss (Line 3 divided by line 4) to get the number of weeks it will take to get to your goal.		188 weeks (about 3.5 years)	67 weeks (about 15 months)	86 weeks (about 21 months)

Table 26: Estimate Time to Lose Weight

These are the examples used in *Table 26*:

- *Sample 1:* You are 5'10", and your starting weight is 362 pounds (BMI of 52); you are about 188 pounds over a goal weight of 174 pounds (BMI of 25). If you lose 1 pound per week, it will take about 3.5 years to hit your goal weight.
- *Sample 2:* If you are 5'4" and your pre-surgery weight is 279 pounds (BMI of 48), you are about 134 pounds over a goal of 145 pounds (BMI of 25). If you lose 2 pounds per week, it will take about 67 weeks, or 15 months, to lose your excess weight.
- *Sample 3:* If you are 5'8" and your starting weight is 295 pounds (BMI of 44), you are 131 pounds over a goal of 164 pounds (BMI of 25). If you lose 1.5 pounds per week, it will take about 20 months to hit your goal.

All gastric bypass patients have their own best rates of weight loss, so do not try to compare yourself to others. As long as you are eating healthily and following your surgeon's and dietitian's advice, you can be confident that you are doing the right thing.

Reducing Complications while Losing Weight

You will always be at risk for developing complications. Examples of complications that can develop long after surgery are dumping syndrome, with symptoms such as nausea, vomiting, shakiness, and diarrhea; leaks; staple line disruptions; and gastroesophageal reflux disease.[1] You can lower your risk of these effects by following these tips—which you will continue to see in this chapter because they are important both for your safety and for your weight loss.

- Separate solids and liquids by at least 30 minutes
- Have only the recommended portions of food
- Stop eating when you are full—remember, your stomach pouch is smaller than it used to be, and you do not want to stretch it
- Only try one new food at a time, and wait for a day or two to make sure you are tolerating it well
- Chew slowly and thoroughly to prevent anything sharp from irritating surgery stitch lines
- Avoid high-sugar, high-fat foods to avoid dumping syndrome

Shifting to Healthier Eating Habits

Gastric bypass is a chance to start over. You remove all solid foods from your diet and add them in slowly over several months. This long process can help you retrain your taste buds and develop new healthy habits, such as automatically reaching for the nutritious choice instead of the junk.

The other major shift, besides in your taste buds, is in how much you eat. Gone are the days of overloading a huge plate, wolfing it down, and going back for more. Now you will measure out your food, chew each small bite slowly, enjoy your meal, and leave the table—without reaching into the fridge for a post-meal snack!

Foods on the Solid Diet

During Phase 4, you add foods one by one until you are eventually able to eat nearly all healthy foods. Many gastric bypass patients find one or more foods that do not agree with them. Do not worry if you find that you cannot tolerate certain foods. Just avoid the trouble foods and choose healthy alternatives to keep your diet interesting and nutritious.

Food Lists for the Solid Diet

These are lists of some common foods that will probably become pretty regular in your diet. Pay attention to the serving sizes—remember to measure carefully!—because they are probably a lot smaller than you are used to. They are also smaller than "standard" serving sizes that you might see on food packages. Do not forget that you can always stop eating before you finish your food if you feel full and you do not have to eat the entire serving. Your stomach pouch is only a fraction of the size of your original stomach, and you do not want to stretch it or feel sick from eating too much.

Protein Foods – The Base of Your Diet

These are high in protein, low in carbohydrates and fat, and high in other essential nutrients. They are the cornerstones of your diet because they will help you reach your daily protein needs of about 65 to 80 grams. Eat protein foods first at meals.

These foods are almost pure protein. Each of these servings has about 7 grams of protein:

- 1 ounce of lean meat, such as lean steak, tenderloin, or pork
- 1 ounce of skinless chicken or turkey breast
- 1 ounce of extra lean ground beef, chicken, or turkey
- 1 ounce of soy-based meat substitute, e.g., soy crumbles
- 1 ounce of fish or shellfish
- ¼ cup fat-free cottage cheese
- 1 egg, 2 egg whites or ¼ cup of fat-free, cholesterol-free liquid egg substitute (or the equivalent in dried egg white powder)
- 1 ounce of canned flake meat or fish, such as chicken, tuna, or crab
- 1 one-ounce slice of deli meat (high in sodium, though, so do not choose too often)

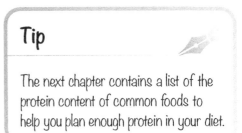

Tip

The next chapter contains a list of the protein content of common foods to help you plan enough protein in your diet.

These foods have extra calories from carbohydrates and/or fat in addition to their protein, but they are great choices because of their extra nutrients:

- 1 ounce of low-fat cheese, 2 tablespoons of fat-free or low-fat ricotta or grated cheese, such as parmesan, or ¼ cup of shredded cheese, such as cheddar or jack.
- ½ cup of yogurt (fat-free, no sugar-added or plain)
  ½ cup of pudding (fat-free, no sugar-added, calcium-fortified)
- 1 tablespoon of creamy (smooth) peanut butter—It is a small serving size because it is so high in calories.
- Four to six almonds, cashews, or pecans; or about 2 tablespoons of peanuts, walnuts, or other nuts. Chew them well and avoid them until you are sure you are comfortable on the solid foods diet
- 1 ounce of dry tofu (e.g., veggie burger) or 2 ounces (one-quarter cup) of silken tofu
- ½ cup of cooked beans or lentils. Add beans to your diet very slowly. You might start with just 1 or 2 tablespoons and gradually work up to ½ of a cup after a few days or weeks if they do not make you gassy
- ¼ cup of hummus or garbanzo bean dip

Non-starchy Vegetables: Great Choices for Weight Loss and Life

Vegetables are low in calories and high in fiber, making them perfect for reducing hunger without interfering with your weight loss. When you can handle them, include a serving or two with most meals and snacks so you can take advantage of their vitamins and minerals. Start with cooked vegetables, and be patient as you add raw vegetables back into your diet. Always make sure you peel them, avoid stringy vegetables, and chew them thoroughly. The serving size for vegetables is bigger than for other groups because they are so low-calorie and healthy. Eat them after eating your protein.

- ½ cup of cooked vegetables, such as cooked, canned, or frozen carrots; green beans; broccoli and cauliflower florets; zucchini; green peas; onions; artichokes; mushrooms; eggplant; and turnips.
- 1 cup of raw vegetables, such as peeled cucumbers, carrot sticks, radishes, or lettuce
- ¼ cup of tomato sauce or salsa
- 6 ounces (¾ cup) of tomato or vegetable juice

Carbohydrate Foods: Fruits

Full of vitamins, minerals, and antioxidants, fruits deserve their reputation as healthy sweet treats. They have no protein and they contain carbohydrates in the form of sugars, but they are good choices because of their nutrients and low amount of calories. As you progress from Phase 3, the semi-solid foods phase, you can incorporate more raw fruits into your diet. Ask your nutritionist about adding specific types of fruit back into your diet and how to prepare them. Choose softer, riper fruits at first. Seeds and scratchy peels can irritate your surgery wounds before they are completely healed. Be sure to chew your fruit very thoroughly.

- ¼ cup of cooked, peeled fruit or canned fruit (in its own juice, not in heavy syrup)
- ½ cup of grapes (avoid grapes until you are deep into the solid foods phase because their skins are difficult to chew thoroughly and they can get lodged in an unhealed seam of your stomach pouch)
- ½ of a regular fresh fruit, such as a medium apple, orange, pear, or peach
- 1 piece of small fruit, such as an apricot or plum
- ¾ cup berries
- ½ cup of fruit juice (remember to dilute with water)
- ½ cup of canned mashed pumpkin

Carbohydrate Foods: Nutritious Grains and Starches

Carbohydrates' reputation for ruining diets is not entirely fair. High-carbohydrate foods can be healthy if you choose the right ones and eat limited quantities. Fortified whole grains, such as whole-wheat, whole grain, multi-grain, and oats, are usually the best choices because of their fiber, antioxidants, and essential vitamins and minerals. Starchy vegetables are also nutritious.

- ½ slice of regular bread or toast
- 1 slice of low-calorie bread or toast
- ½ of an English muffin

- ¼ of a bagel
- ¼ cup of cooked grains, such as rice or pasta, or hot cereal, such as cream of wheat, farina, or oatmeal
- ¼ cup of cooked starchy vegetables, such as potatoes, acorn squash, sweet potatoes, or butternut squash
- ¾ ounce hard pretzels
- ½ cup of puffed cereal or one-quarter cup of bran cereal or granola
- four crackers, e.g., four saltines, four Ritz crackers, or four quarters of a graham cracker (one large graham cracker)
- ¼ cup of canned or cooked corn

Choose High-Fat Foods Wisely and Measure Your Portions

Fat is necessary for absorbing certain nutrients, and nutritious sources may have other health benefits as long as you limit your intake. Some sources of fats, such as oils, salad dressings, and avocados, are great choices. In contrast, butter is a poor choice because of its high amount of unhealthy saturated fat. High-fat foods are very high in calories, so always measure your serving size of these "extra" foods to avoid eating more calories than you intend to. These are some healthy choices for fat:

- 1 teaspoon of olive oil or vegetable oil, such as canola or sunflower—yes, that's a *teaspoon*, not a tablespoon. A teaspoon is only one-third of a tablespoon.
- 1 teaspoon of mayonnaise
- 1 teaspoon of trans fat-free margarine
- 1 tablespoon of low-fat mayonnaise (such as Miracle Whip), salad dressing, cream cheese, sour cream, or tahini (sesame seed paste)
- 2 tablespoons of mashed avocado or guacamole—Avocados are high in heart-healthy monounsaturated fats that made the Mediterranean diet famous as well as vitamin C, vitamin E, and dietary fiber.

Foods to Postpone

Some foods are nutritious, but it is better to postpone them until you are well into Phase 4, the solid foods diet. These foods may be particularly hard or difficult to chew or have small pieces that can get into your surgery seams. You should not eat them until you are certain that your surgery wounds are completely healed. These are some examples:

- Nuts and peanuts
- Seeds, such as sunflower and pumpkin
- Dried fruit
- "Sneaky" foods that may have nuts, seeds, or dried fruit in them. Multi-grain bread with nuts and raisin bran are two examples.
- Popcorn

- Celery—it is very fibrous, and the strings can irritate your stomach. Asparagus and broccoli stalks are also fibrous.
- Citrus fruits and pineapple—besides being acidic, they have pulp that can be irritating.

Foods to Avoid

The long-term gastric bypass diet allows for a varied, healthy diet as you gradually widen your choices, but there are some foods that should be limited or avoided indefinitely. They may be unhealthy, high in calories, and/or low in nutrition. High-sugar, high-fat foods can cause dumping syndrome. Some patients have trouble tolerating certain nutritious foods too.

Sugary Foods

Sugary foods are high in calories and not very filling. Letting them creep into your diet can derail your weight loss. They can also cause dumping syndrome. These are some high-sugar foods to avoid:

- Full strength fruit juice (dilute it 50–50 with water)
- Sugar-sweetened fruit drinks and fruit punch
- Other sugar-sweetened beverages: lemonade, ice tea with sugar, coffee beverages
- Chocolate and other flavored milk
- Sugar-sweetened flavored soy milk
- Sugar-sweetened flavored yogurt
- Regular frozen yogurt and ice cream
- Canned and frozen fruit in syrup
- Sugary breakfast cereal
- Pastries and doughnuts
- Cakes, cookies, and pies
- Jams and jellies
- Sugar, syrup, honey, and molasses
- Dried fruit

Need a Sweet Treat?

Sometimes you may want something sweet, but too much sugar can cause dumping syndrome. Sticking to foods with under five grams of sugar can help prevent dumping syndrome. That cuts out many of your old standbys.

- A half-cup of rich ice cream, a brownie, a candy bar, and a piece of cheesecake can each have over 20 grams of sugar.
- A 20-ounce bottle of soda has 50 grams of sugar, and a 12-ounce mocha or other flavored coffee beverage made with milk has 45 grams.

You still have many options to satisfy your sweet tooth. Sugar substitutes such as aspartame, sugar alcohols, sucralose and stevia are not likely to cause dumping syndrome. Many sugar-free and no sugar added products are okay on the RYGB diet. You can also add sweeteners to make your own sweet foods.

- Frozen whipped topping, better known by the brand name Cool Whip, has 4 grams of sugar per ¼ cup. Fat-free Cool Whip has 2 grams of sugar in a ¼ cup, and sugar-free Cool Whip has 0 grams of sugar.
- Other sugar-free options include pudding, beverages, cookies, and candies.
- A half-cup of no sugar added ice cream has 5 grams of sugar.
- A half-cup of plain Greek yogurt with cinnamon and calorie-free sweetener has 3 grams of sugar.
- Hot cocoa made with cocoa powder and sweetener is nearly sugar-free.

High-Fat Foods

Over half of gastric bypass patients have dumping syndrome shortly after surgery, but most get over it within a few months or a year. You will quickly learn which foods can cause dumping syndrome. High-fat foods can trigger it. Eat only small portions of healthy fats, and spread your servings throughout the day instead of having them at one meal. Limit unhealthy fats.

Healthy fats include:

- Nuts, peanuts, and nut and peanut butters
- Avocados
- Olive oil and olives
- Vegetable oil
- Trans-fat free margarine

Foods with fats that you do not need include:

- Butter
- Full-fat dairy products, such as whole milk and full-fat yogurt and cheese
- Fatty meats, including fatty steaks, regular ground beef, bacon, sausage, and poultry with skin
- Fried foods, including French fries, onion rings, and doughnuts

Foods That You Cannot Tolerate

Everyone has a different set of foods that they can tolerate. Some patients have to avoid certain foods, even though they are nutritious, because of symptoms of vomiting or regurgitation. You are more likely to tolerate a wider variety of foods when you follow the post-surgery diet progression very carefully and have a good post-surgery care program.[2] These are some foods that might unexpectedly cause symptoms:

- Red meat
- Poultry
- Salad
- Vegetables
- Bread
- Rice
- Pasta
- Fish

The list is pretty broad, but you are not going to have trouble with *all* of these foods. More likely is that you will have trouble with only one or two foods in just one or two categories.

Other Poor Choices

Other foods and beverages may be poor choices because they are unhealthy or because they can cause complications with the gastric bypass. These are a few examples of foods and beverages to avoid or at least limit:

- *Carbonated beverages:* These can make you feel unpleasantly full, and sugar-sweetened choices can give you dumping syndrome, especially if you choose sugar-sweetened ones. Both regular and diet soft drinks can stretch your stomach pouch so it does not restrict your food intake as much.

- *Alcoholic beverages:* Alcoholic beverages should be avoided or strictly limited for several reasons.

  - They are high-calorie. A 12-ounce can of beer has 180 calories; a 5-ounce can of beer has 130 calories; a 1.5-ounce shot of whisky has 100 calories.

  - Alcohol relaxes you. When you are under the influence of alcohol, you are more likely to give in to high-calorie temptations.

  - Your tolerance decreases after RYGB. Your blood alcohol concentration increases faster and more than before surgery when you have the same amount of alcohol.[3]

- *Tough meat:* Dry, stringy, tough meat can wreak havoc on your seam lines. Swallowing an unchewable piece of meat can be irritating. Avoid tough meats as well as sausage and ground beef with gristle.[4]

- *Foods high in saturated fat:* Saturated fat is not an essential nutrient, and it is unhealthy for your heart because it raises your blood cholesterol levels. It is bad for weight loss because it is high in calories, and it is often in high-calorie foods, such as cakes made with shortening, full-fat cheese, and fatty meats, such as steak and bacon.

- *Fried foods:* Fried foods contain extra calories that slow down weight loss; for example, a cup of steamed onion rings has 92 calories, while a cup of onion rings fried in

1 tablespoon of oil has 212 calories. Fried foods often have breading; a cup of breaded and fried onion rings has over 300 calories. Fried foods contain trans fats, which are even worse for your health than saturated fats. Finally, fried foods are often high in refined carbohydrates (think about doughnuts, fried breaded chicken, and French fries). Why take something healthy and delicious and fry it?

- *Caffeine:* Caffeine may increase your risk of ulcers, but there is not much evidence either way.[5] Caffeine is a trigger for heartburn for many people. One clear reason to avoid caffeine after RYGB is that too much caffeine can harm your bones—and RYGB patients are already at risk for weaker bones because of low nutrient intakes and rapid weight loss.

Tips for Phase 4

As you transition from Phase 3, the semi-solid or soft foods diet, to Phase 4, solid foods, following a few tips can lower your risk of side effects from new foods.

- *Start with the solid foods that seem easiest, and gradually work your way to a full diet.* There are no hard-and-fast rules for the order to introduce foods, but a good guideline is to start with softer foods. For example, for your first raw fruit, you might choose cut ripe cantaloupe, which is soft, instead of a hard apple. Or you might go with oatmeal, a soft food, before moving to dry breakfast cereal.

- *Have only tiny quantities of new foods.* Add, for example, only a single bite of a cracker with your meal just to make sure that you can tolerate it before having a whole serving of crackers the next day.

- *Chew your food well.* Solid foods are solid—and you need to chew them thoroughly before swallowing them so that they do not make you nauseous or sick. Eating more slowly reduces your risk of complications.

- *Try hard to meet recommendations for protein, or about 60 to 85 or more grams per day.*[6] This amount of protein can reduce the amount of lean muscle mass that you lose as you are losing body fat. If you do not get enough protein, your body will break down your muscle, and your metabolism will slow down. You can increase your protein intake by choosing protein first at each meal and by loading the front of your day with protein.

- *Aim for at least five servings of vegetables and fruits.* Eat them right after your protein because they are high priorities in your diet.

- *Drink no sooner than a half an hour before or after a meal or snack.* Having liquid with meals can make them less filling. It can also stretch your stomach pouch and lead to leaks. The recommended minimum fluid intake is 1.5 liters (6 or 7 cups) per day. You can meet this by continuing to drink throughout the day in between meals.

Help with Meal Planning on the RYGB Diet

Now you know which foods you can eat, but you still need to know how to put together a balanced meal plan for weight loss and health. This section will guide you through the general meal plan so you can start to plan your own menus. Meal planning will become easier and faster as you practice more.

Sample Menus

Table 27 displays two sample menus to try. They have a variety of different foods to provide a range of nutrients and prevent boredom. Each of these days has three small meals and three snacks; do not forget to drink your water in between your eating times!

The sizes of these meals and snacks are maximums. Stop eating if you feel full before you eat everything that you had planned. Also, your surgeon or dietitian might recommend skipping the snacks and sticking to three meals per day.

Sample Meal Patterns

Meal or Snack	Day 1 Sample	Day 2 Sample
Breakfast	1 packet of plain instant oatmeal made with fat-free milk (cinnamon and/or artificial sweetener optional) ¼ medium banana 6 almonds	2 scrambled egg whites or one-quarter cup of liquid egg substitute made with skim milk and 1 tsp. canola oil 1 ounce low-fat cheddar cheese melted into eggs 1 slice of toast spread with 2 teaspoons trans-fat free margarine ½ of a medium orange
Snack 1	1 cup cucumber sticks (peeled) ¼ cup hummus	½ apple 1 tablespoon peanut butter
Lunch	½ whole grain English muffin 1 ounce turkey breast slice 1 ounce low-fat cheese ½ cup applesauce	½ cup canned tuna in water 1 cup of salad made with greens and other raw vegetables 1 tablespoon of salad dressing ½ of a whole-wheat bagel
Snack 2	4 crackers 1 hard-boiled egg	½ cup plain Greek yogurt (optional cinnamon and sweetener)
Dinner	2 ounces chicken breast ½ cup cooked carrots ½ cup cooked brown rice (or white if you are just starting the solid foods diet)	Burger made with 2 ounces of extra lean ground beef, turkey, chicken, or soy crumbles 1 light whole-wheat hamburger bun ½ to 1 cup cooked cauliflower 1 tablespoon light mayo (Miracle Whip)
Snack 3	½ cup sugar-free chocolate pudding	½ cup fat-free cottage cheese

Table 27: Sample Meal Patterns for Phase 4

Making Your Own Daily Menu from a Standard Meal Pattern

But what happens if you want to make your own meal plans? After all, you are going to be on this diet for years, and you do not want to get bored! A good meal plan meets your nutrient needs and has tons of flexibility so that you can pick and choose the foods you feel like eating each day. It has to be bypass-friendly and lead to weight loss too. Each day should include:

- 60 to 120 grams of protein
- At least five servings of fruits and vegetables
- 130 grams of total carbohydrates
- 20 grams of fat
- At least 1.5 liters of fluid (drank between meals and snacks)

You will come close to your protein, carbohydrate, and fat recommendations if you get these servings:

- Six to 10 proteins
- Two to three fruits
- Three to five vegetables
- Five to seven grains
- Three to six healthy fats (remember, these are *small* serving sizes!)

One-for-One Swaps

One way to make your own food plan is to make one-for-one substitutions. That means exchanging a fruit for a fruit, a grain for a grain, a protein for a protein, and so on. So if you decide you want fish and peas instead of chicken and carrots, take a look at the food lists. On the protein list, you would just swap one serving (2 ounces) of fish for one serving (2 ounces) of chicken. From the vegetable list, you would switch a ½ cup of peas for a ½ cup of carrots. That is pretty simple, right? Just by substituting, you can make your diet completely personalized.

Are you ready to give it a try? *Table 28* is a basic plan that will keep up your protein and provide a balanced diet. Aim for about one cup of food at each meal and one-half cup of food per snack. Remember to drink between meals but not immediately before or after as well as during them.

Meal or Snack	Meal Pattern	Sample Day Based on the Patten
Breakfast	2 proteins 1 grain	1 hard-boiled egg ½ cup whole-grain breakfast cereal 1 cup fat-free milk
Snack 1	1 protein 1 grain 1 fat	2 ounces canned tuna in water with 1 tablespoon light mayo 4 saltine crackers
Lunch	1 protein 2 vegetables 1 fruit	½ cup cottage cheese 1 cup cooked green beans ½ cup diced melon
Snack 2	1 fruit	1 plum
Dinner	1 protein 1 grain 1 vegetable 1 fat	2 ounces chicken breast grilled with 1 teaspoon olive oil ½ cup whole-wheat pasta
Snack 3	1 protein	1 cup yogurt (no sugar added)

Table 28: Basic Meal Plan (to help keep up you protein intake and provide a balanced diet)

The plan has plenty of flexibility. If you want fruit for breakfast, for example, have your "lunch" serving of fruit at breakfast. Or if you want a sandwich for lunch, have your "Snack 1" serving of grain at lunch. In that case, you might consider having one of your "Lunch" servings of vegetables at Snack 1 so that your lunch does not get too big.

Strategies for Reducing Hunger

If the meal plan leaves you feeling hungry, try adding some vegetables because they are filling and low-calorie. Increasing your protein intake can also help. Protein is slow to digest, so it staves off hunger for longer. Be sure that you are drinking enough water throughout the day because it can help suppress hunger. Your nutritionist or dietitian may have additional strategies for reducing hunger.

Keeping Your Menus Nutritious and Adequate

Select a variety of foods to get a full range of nutrients. Also, remember to take your daily supplements as recommended by your surgeon or dietitian. Another caution is that the above meal patterns are for a very, very low-calorie diet, which is safe only under medical supervision.

Do You Need Help with the Measurements?

Measuring your serving sizes is critical. Chapter 13 introduced measuring cups and spoons as some of the indispensible kitchen tools for success on the RYGB diet. If you do not have any cooking experience, though, the various measurements may be difficult at first. This is a conversion table to help with serving sizes. Knowing how to convert lets you read recipes and instructions from any source and measure them using your own set of cups and spoons.

These are some of the most common measurements that you might see in recipes and diet plans.

Converting Volumes

Unit	Equals	Also Equals:	In Metric
1 teaspoon (1 tsp.)	1/3 tablespoon (1/3 tbsp.)		5 milliliters (5 mL)
1 tablespoon (1 tbsp.)	3 tsp.	½ fluid ounce (½ fl. oz.)	15 ml
2 tbsp.	1/8 cup	1 fl. oz.	30 ml
4 tbsp.	¼ cup	2 fl. oz.	60 ml
8 tbsp.	½ cup	4 fl. oz.	120 ml
16 tbsp.	1 cup	8 fl. oz.	240 ml
2 cups	1 pint	16 fl. oz.	480 ml (about ½ liter)
4 cups	1 quart	32 fl. oz.	960 ml, or just under 1 liter
1 liter		33 fl. oz	1000 ml

Keep this chart handy toward the beginning of your RYGB journey when you are first starting to measure everything. If you measure all of your foods diligently, you will soon find that converting becomes natural.

A diet with so few calories is considered an extreme diet, and its risks include nutritional deficiencies and loss of bone mineral density. You can minimize the risk by working closely with your dietitian and surgeon and following their instructions for eating and taking your dietary supplements.

Guidelines for Success on the Gastric Bypass Diet

Following these guidelines can help you lose weight faster and reduce your risk for complications.

Daily Tips

These tips are the basis for success. We suggest putting this list on your fridge so you see it when you are ready to eat or drink.

- *Take small bites.* Using a small teaspoon instead of large soup spoon is an effective strategy. Another tip is to cut your food into small pieces. Focus on spearing a small piece of food with your fork instead of piling food onto your fork.

- *Chew each bite 30 times before swallowing.* This prevents hard pieces of food from irritating your stomach shortly after surgery, and it prevents you from eating too quickly as you try to lose weight. Although it may be tiresome, literally count 30 chews before swallowing. Do this until you are used to thorough chewing. You will be in the habit within days.

- *Stop eating when you are full.* That keeps you from overeating. Since you may need to retrain yourself to recognize hunger signals, for the first several weeks or months you may need to stop eating *before* you think you are full.

- *Eat your protein first.* It is an essential nutrient for maintaining lean body mass, and it helps decrease hunger. Choose it first at meals and be especially careful to get a high-protein breakfast and morning snack.

- *Separate solids from liquids.* Eat solid foods at least 30 minutes apart from when you drink liquids. This helps you take full advantage of the RYGB procedure because solid foods stay in the stomach pouch for longer when you do not have fluids with them. If you drink beverages while you are eating solid food, your stomach pouch may stretch and you will eventually have less restriction.

- *Be patient.* Only eat the foods that are in your allowed foods list, and introduce new foods gradually. Eating other foods can cause long-term trouble after gastric bypass. Always stop to think about how you feel before you eat more. It is better to stop eating if you feel full than to force yourself to continue eating your planned meal. Also be careful to avoid trouble foods if you discover them.

- *Measure your food.* Keep your meals and snacks small by measuring each portion and choosing only the type and amount of foods on your plan. A typical daily plan includes three small meals and up to three snacks.

- *Do not "munch."* Munching means eating and drinking bits of foods here and there. You might take a few tastes while you are in the kitchen cooking, grab a couple of nuts from the bowl on the secretary's desk, or have just a few tastes of your spouse's meal when you are out at dinner. Everything you eat counts, and these small bites of food can really add up to interfere with your weight loss. A single one-inch square piece of brownie and a tablespoon of peanut butter each have about 100 calories. Eating the crumbs while you are scraping the pan of brownies and licking the knife after you spread your peanut butter are just two examples of mindless munching that can add hundreds of calories without you even noticing it. To avoid this, only eat foods that you measure and plan, and only eat them at the table. Do not eat in your car, while in the kitchen, or when walking around at work.

- *Do not drink your calories.* Liquid calories can quickly derail weight loss. They make the gastric bypass less effective. Soft drinks, juices, sweetened coffee and tea, and other beverages with calories can add hundreds of calories to your day without reducing hunger. They can also cause dumping syndrome because of their sugar. Fat-free milk and vegetable juice are likely to be the only caloric beverages that your dietitian recommends. Fat-free milk has 80 calories and 8 grams of protein per cup. Tomato and mixed vegetable juice have about 50 calories per cup each and count as servings of vegetables.

- *Stay hydrated.* The minimum goal is 1.5 liters of fluid per day. You need more water if you sweat heavily or the weather is especially hot or dry. With some practice, you can make a habit out of drinking water and other non-caloric beverages in between meals and snacks to stay hydrated and prevent headaches and fatigue related to dehydration.

The Benefits of Eating Slowly

Many of the above guidelines help you eat more slowly to promote successful weight loss. Eating slowly has a variety of benefits:

- *It lets you get full before you eat as much.* Remember how we mentioned that it takes a while for your brain to realize that you are full? If you wolf down your food, you might finish your food and go back for more because you still feel hungry. Eating slower gives your stomach a chance to send fullness signals to your brain before you have eaten too much.

- *It is more pleasant.* Eating slowly lets you savor your food. Before surgery, enjoying food might have been the same as eating more food. With the RYGB and your new eating habits, you start to notice and appreciate the flavors in food. You might feel a healthier satisfaction from the act of eating.

- *It reduces your risk of complications.* Eating too quickly can give you dumping syndrome, leading to vomiting, diarrhea, or shakiness. Eating too quickly can stretch your stomach pouch and make weight loss more difficult.

✍ **Summary**

- ☞ This chapter gave you tools for successful weight loss after RYGB by covering the RYGB diet that you will be following long term. You now know what to eat on your daily diet. The chapter provided a few sample meal plans and a basic menu that you can tweak to create varied menus for yourself day after day.

- ☞ This chapter also talked about making nutritious choices, but you might not yet know how to do that.

- ☞ The next chapter provides an overview of basic nutrition and gives some guidelines on selecting a balanced and healthy diet. By the end of the next chapter, you will be an expert nutritionist!

Time to Take Action: Practice Making Some Menus!

This chapter provides a template for your daily menus. We came up with two sample menus based on the template, but you are going to need more menus than that if your meal plan is going to stay interesting! Why not try making your own menu based on the template? In *Table 29*, you can see the template in the left column. In the column on the right, write in foods and their serving sizes that match up with the template.

Meal or Snack	Meal Pattern	Sample Menu	Your Own Menu
Breakfast	2 protein 1 grain 1 fat 1 fruit	½ cup cottage cheese 1 slice reduced-calorie whole-wheat bread ½ apple 1 tablespoon peanut butter	
Snack 1	1 protein 1 grain 1 fat	½ whole-grain bagel 1 ounce low-fat cheese	
Lunch	1 protein 2 vegetables 1 fruit 1 fat	1 ounce low-sodium deli meat ½ cup cooked green beans 1 cup salad with 1 tbsp. salad dressing ½ orange	
Snack 2	1 fruit	1 apricot	
Dinner	1 protein 1 grain 1 vegetable 1 fat	2 ounces grilled chicken with 1 tsp. olive oil ½ cup cooked zucchini with 1 tsp. olive oil	
Snack 3	1 protein	1 cup fat-free yogurt, no sugar added	

Table 29: Create Your Own Menu – Template1

Now, try a different meal pattern in *Table 30*. Like the first one, this meal pattern meets the general recommendations for servings from each group. Having an alternative meal pattern to work with gives you even more options for menus so you never have to get bored.

Meal or Snack	Day 1 Sample	Sample Menu	Your Own Menu
Breakfast	2 protein 2 grain 1 fat 1 fruit	2 packets instant oatmeal 1 tablespoon peanut butter 1 cup fat-free milk ½ grapefruit	
Snack 1	1 protein 1 vegetable 1 fat	1 hard-boiled egg 1 cup red pepper strips 2 tablespoons guacamole	
Lunch	1 protein 1 fruit 1 fat 1 vegetable	½ cup cooked kidney beans ½ cup cooked orange squash 1 cup cut melon 16 pistachio nuts	
Snack 2	1 protein 1 grain	1 cup fat-free yogurt 1 ounce whole-grain cereal	
Dinner	2 protein 1 grain 1 vegetable	2 ounces grilled salmon ½ cup brown rice ½ cup Brussels sprouts with 1 tsp. olive oil	
Snack 3	1 fruit	½ mashed banana	

Table 30: Create Your Own Menu – Template 2

1   Rosenthal RJ. International Sleeve Gastrectomy Expert Panel consensus statement: best practice guidelines based on experience of > 12,000 cases. Surgery for Obesity and Related Diseases. 2012;8(1):8-19.

2   Aills L, Blankenship J, Buffington C, Furtado M, Parrott, J. ASMBS Integrated health nutritional guidelines for the surgical weight loss patient. Surgery for Obesity and Related Diseases, 2008;S73-S108.

3   Woodard GA, Downey J, Hernandez-Boussard T, Morton JM. Impaired alcohol metabolism after gastric bypass surgery: a case-crossover trial. J Am Coll Surg, 2011;21(2):209-214.

4   Realize. Bariatric surgery recovery expectations. Web site. http://www.realize.com/bariatric-surgery-recovery-expectations.htm. 2012, August 1. Accessed October 16, 2012.

5   Aills L, Blankenship J, Buffington C, Furtado M, Parrott J. ASMBS Allied Health nutritional guidelines for the surgical weight loss patient. Surg Obes Relat Dis. 2008;4(5Suppl):S73-S108.

6   Ziegler O, Sirveaux MA, Brunaud L, Reibel N, Quillot D. Medical follow-up after bariatric surgery: nutritional and drug issues. General recommendations for the prevention and treatment of nutritional deficiencies. Diabetes Metab. 2009;35(6 Pt 2):544-547.

15

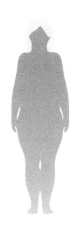

The RYGB Diet & Nutrition

The last chapter included the essentials of the RYGB diet. After reading it, you know what to eat and how much to eat. You saw some sample menus and practiced making your own gastric bypass meal plan. The chapter presented several tips for success with the RYGB diet.

Your weight loss journey is also about health, and a bit of nutrition knowledge can help you make choices that will greatly improve your health. This chapter provides a lesson on basic nutrition and covers these topics:

- Calories, energy, and weight control
- Protein, fat, and carbohydrates: their roles and choosing the best ones
- Vitamins and minerals and which are of concern to you as a RYGB patient
- Water: why you need it and how to get enough
- Making sense of nutrition labels
- Keeping condiments from sabotaging your diet
- Alcoholic beverages and how they can harm your weight loss and health

A lot of this chapter's content is common sense. For example, you probably already know that lean proteins, vegetables, whole grains, and fruits are healthier choices than sweets and fried foods. But you may also learn a few things, such as which high-fat foods are healthy choices.

If you are not interested in all of the details right now, you can just skim this chapter. Later, when you are more comfortable with the gastric bypass diet, you might want to use it as a reference.

Calories and Weight Loss

You have already heard a lot about calories—it is impossible to avoid them! Calories come up almost everywhere, from nutrition labels on food packages to weight loss guides to calorie counts on restaurant menus. Calories are the single most important factor in weight loss. What are calories? They are units of energy.

Your body converts some of the nutrients in food into energy. The amount of energy you get is measured in calories. Your body uses energy too. The amount of energy you use is also measured in calories.

These concepts are critical:

- You must burn off, or expend, more calories than you consume in order to lose weight.
- Your body weight will be stable if you eat the same number of calories that you burn off.
- You will gain weight if you eat more calories than you burn.

Weight Change	Energy Balance	Calories in versus out	Eating versus
Lose weight	Calorie (or energy) deficit	Calories in < calories out	eat < burn
Maintain weight	Calorie (or energy) balance	Calories in = calories out	eat = burn
Gain weight	Calorie (or energy) excess	Calories in > calories out	eat > burn

Table 31: Calories & Weight Change

Energy balance is fundamental to weight control. Surgery or not, you can only lose weight if you consume fewer calories than you burn. This is called creating a calorie deficit. You can create your calorie deficit by eating less, exercising more, or doing both. The gastric bypass helps reduce your calorie consumption by helping you eat less and absorb fewer calories.

3,500 Calories per Pound of Body Fat

A pound of body fat is worth about 3,500 calories. So you have to create a calorie deficit of 3,500 calories to lose a pound of body fat. In other words, you must expend 3,500 calories more than you consume.

To lose one pound per week, you need to burn off an extra 3,500 calories per week or have an average deficit of 500 calories per day. To lose two pounds of fat per week, you have to burn off 7,000 calories or have an average daily calorie deficit of 1,000 calories. Let's break down some numbers.

- *Calorie expenditure*: An obese man who weighs 240 pounds and is 5 feet, 9 inches tall needs about 2,700 calories per day before adding in any exercise that he may do. That is according to the Harris-Benedict equation, which is a famous and impressively accurate equation to estimate daily calorie needs.[1]
- *Calorie intake*: Many bariatric surgery diet plans have you eating only about 1,000 or 1,200 calories per day or even less right after surgery. The menus in the previous chapter are within that approximate range.

At an intake level of 1,200 calories per day, the man would be creating a calorie deficit of 1,500 calories per day — or an average weight loss of three pounds per week! You can see that a very low-calorie diet, such as the one you follow after the gastric bypass, will lead to substantial weight loss.

Plenty of online calculators can estimate your daily calorie needs. Most of them ask for your height, weight, age, and gender. As you lose weight, your energy needs, or metabolic rate, will decrease. Your weight loss will slow down if you do not make any changes, but you can make up for your slower metabolism — and improve your health — by increasing your physical activity.

Do You Have to Count Calories?

And so you can see that the calorie contents of your foods and beverages affect your weight loss. Luckily, you do not have to count calories if you stick to the meal plan. Having the recommended number of servings and proper portion sizes should ensure that you hit the right number of calories each day. You can also compare the calorie content per serving of food when you are at the grocery store or about to prepare a meal and choose the option with fewer calories. Making low-calorie choices will help you lose weight faster.

Nutrient-Dense versus Empty Calories: How Do They Affect Weight Loss?

When it comes to your weight, a calorie is a calorie is a calorie. Eat 3,500 calories too many, and you will gain a pound of body fat. Cut out 3,500 calories from your diet or burn off an extra 3,500 calories from exercising more—or any combination of eating less and exercising more—and you will lose a pound. That is true no matter where your calories come from, whether it is junk food or healthy food.

So does it matter where your calories come from when you are talking about controlling your weight? In theory, it should not. A calorie is always a calorie. In reality, though, healthy foods can help you lose weight because they are more filling than junk food. That means you can get fuller from eating the same number of calories of a healthy food rather than junk food. Think about these examples. Would you be less hungry after eating:

- 1 cup of cucumber sticks and 1 cup of fat-free yogurt or 10 potato chips (both are about 100 calories)?
- 1 packet of instant oatmeal or two scrambled egg whites and half an apple?
- 1 ounce of cheese and two strips of bacon fried in 1 tablespoon of butter (both are about 200 calories)?
- 2 ounces of grilled chicken breast, ½ a cup cottage cheese, 1 cup of cauliflower, and ½ a cup rice or 4 ounces of ground beef (both are about 300 calories)?

The U.S. Department of Agriculture and Department of Health and Human Services use a term called "nutrient-dense" to describe foods that are high in nutrients. These are the foods you should focus on. "Empty calories" come from foods that do not have health benefits—they are "empty" of essential nutrients. Foods with empty calories are foods with saturated fat, trans fats, added sugars, refined grains, or high amounts of sodium.

In the following table are some nutrient-dense foods and foods with empty calories. Your diet should be based mostly on the left column. You can see that most, but not all, of the nutrient-dense foods are low in calories. Some healthy foods, such as nuts, peanuts, and avocados, are high in calories and fat. But since their fats are heart-healthy and they have other important nutrients, such as dietary fiber and vitamin E, they make good choices. Just make sure to eat them in moderation.

Nutrient-Dense Foods (Choose These)	Empty Calories (Limit These)
• Lean meats (e.g., extra-lean ground beef and sirloin tip)	• Fatty cuts of meat, such as fatty steak, bacon, and sausage
• Tofu and soy products	• Fried foods, including French fries, onion rings, fried chicken, and banana chips
• White-meat poultry (e.g., chicken and turkey breast) without the skin	• Unenriched refined grains, e.g. (unenriched white bread, pasta and rice, and refined sugary breakfast cereals)
• Seafood, including fish and shellfish	
• Reduced-fat milk, yogurt, and cheese	• Full-fat dairy products
• Egg whites	• Sweets, such as candy, ice cream, and milk chocolate
• Beans, lentils, and split peas	
• Unsalted nuts, peanuts, and seeds	• Sugar-sweetened beverages
• Avocados and olive oil	• Baked goods, such as pies, cookies, sweet rolls, and cakes
• Fruits	• Processed snack foods, such as crackers and potato chips
• Vegetables	
• Whole grain products, such as oatmeal, whole-wheat bread and pasta, and brown rice	• Prepared foods, such as fast foods
	• Salty, fatty, or sugary sauces, dressings, gravies, and other condiments

Source:[2]

Protein, Fat, and Carbohydrates

Proteins, fats, and carbohydrates are called the macronutrients because you need larger amounts ("macro") of them compared to the small amounts ("micro") that you need of the micronutrients, or vitamins and minerals. Protein, fat, and carbohydrates all provide calories, or energy. However, they have different functions and affect your health in different ways.

Protein

All proteins are made of amino acids. When you think about protein metabolism, start with the proteins in food. Your body breaks down these food proteins into amino acids and then into even smaller components. Then your body rearranges these components and builds them back up into amino acids and proteins that come together to form tissues and organs and structures. Proteins are not only part of your regular muscles but also your bones, skins, lungs, heart, and blood vessels. Proteins are necessary for a strong immune system to fight infections, for carrying nutrients and oxygen around your body, and for pretty much every reaction that occurs in your body.[3]

Protein as an Energy Source

Proteins from food provide energy. Each gram of protein has four calories. Your body is very good at using protein for energy. However, getting most of your energy from carbohydrates and fat lets you use protein for other functions, such as preventing muscle breakdown. Using carbohydrates and fat instead of protein for energy lets your body "spare proteins."

Complete and Incomplete Proteins and Vegetarianism

Proteins in food can be complete or incomplete. *Complete*, or high-quality, proteins have each of the essential amino acids that you need to get from your diet. *Incomplete* proteins are missing one or more of the amino acids, but you can still meet all of your amino acid needs by eating a variety of incomplete protein foods.

These are some good sources of protein:

- Complete proteins include all proteins from animal sources, such as meat, poultry, fish, eggs, and dairy products. Soy and quinoa are plant-based sources of complete proteins.

- Incomplete protein sources include most other plant-based foods. Legumes, or beans, split peas, and lentils are highest in protein. Nuts, grains, vegetables, and seeds also provide protein.

A common myth is that vegetarians cannot meet their protein needs. That is not true. Vegetarians can meet their protein needs without trouble. Lacto-ovo vegetarians can get complete proteins from eggs and dairy products. Strict vegetarians, such as vegans, can get complete proteins from soy products such as soybeans, veggie burgers, tofu, and other soy-based products provide complete protein. You can get complete proteins by combining incomplete protein sources. To do this, eat a variety of incomplete proteins. These are some examples of complete proteins:

- Beans and rice
- Crackers and hummus
- Bean and pasta soup
- Peanut butter and whole-grain bread

How much protein do you need while you are losing weight? Aim for at least 60 to 85 grams of protein per day. This amount of protein can be challenging when your total food intake is so low, but you can do it if you make protein your priority. Eat your protein first at meals, and start your day off with a high-protein breakfast.

Protein Content of Common Foods

Getting your 65 or more daily grams of protein supports recovery from surgery and helps maintain lean muscle tissue to keep up your strength and metabolism. More than one-third of bariatric patients do not consistently get enough protein throughout their first year post-surgery,[4] but you can when you know how much protein is in your food options.

These Tables Can Help You Translate Grams of Protein into Food

These handy charts/tables can help you consume enough protein each day. Each chart/ table contains foods that are divided into categories based on their protein content.[5] They are divided into high-protein *(Table 32)*, medium–protein *(Table 33),* and low-protein foods *(Table 34).* Foods are listed alphabetically within each category.

- High-protein foods are nearly pure protein with very little carbohydrate or fat.
- Medium-protein foods have a high amount of protein and also some carbohydrates and/or fat.
- Low-protein foods mostly have carbohydrates and/or fat, but they provide some protein.
- Foods without protein are not listed in these tables, although many of them still have important roles in your RYGB diet. Healthy options include oils, fruit, and many vegetables, and other less healthy choices include butter, fruit juices, and most condiments.

Food	RYGB Diet Serving Size	Protein per Serving in Grams
Beef, ground, extra lean	2 ounces	11
Beef, sirloin, lean only	2 ounces	16
Chicken breast, skinless, roasted	2 ounces	18
Chicken, canned	2 ounces	11
Chicken, ground, raw	2 ounces	13
Cod, fresh	2 ounces	11
Cottage cheese, fat-free or low-fat	½ cup	14
Crab, canned	2 ounces	10
Egg	1 large	6
Egg white	2 large	12
Egg substitute, fat-free substitute	½ cup	6
Halibut	2 ounces	10
Protein powder, unflavored/sugar-free	10 grams	5–8
Ricotta cheese, fat-free	¼ cup	7
Salmon, fresh	2 ounces	11
Tuna, canned light in water	2 ounces	11
Turkey, ground	2 ounces	15
Turkey breast, deli meat	1 ounce	7
Turkey, white meat, skinless, roasted	2 ounces	16

Table 32: High-protein foods

Medium-Protein Foods

Food	RYGB Diet Serving Size	Protein per Serving in Grams
Almonds	2 tablespoons (6–8)	3
Beans, canned or boiled (e.g., pinto, kidney, garbanzo, navy)	½ cup	7
Cheese, hard, fat-free	1 ounce	9
Cheese, hard, low-fat	1 ounce	7
Cheese, hard, regular (e.g., Swiss or cheddar)	1 ounce	7
Lentils, cooked	½ cup	9
Milk	8 ounces (1 cup)	8
Peanuts	¼ cup	3
Peanut butter	1 tablespoon	3
Pecans	2 tablespoons (6–8)	1
Seeds, sunflower	2 tablespoons	3
Soybeans, roasted	1 ounce	9
Tofu, silken, hard or soft	½ cup	6–10
Walnuts	2 tablespoons	4
Yogurt, fat-free	8 ounces (1 cup)	8–12
Yogurt, Greek, fat-free	8 ounces (1 cup)	23

Table 33: Medium-protein foods

Low-Protein Foods

Food	RYGB Diet Serving Size	Protein per Serving in Grams
Bread, reduced-calorie	1 slice	3
Bread, white	½ slice	3
Bread, whole-wheat	½ slice	3
Cauliflower, cooked	½ cup	2
Carrots, cooked	½ cup	1
Corn, canned or cooked	½ cup	3
Green beans, cooked	½ cup	1

Food	RYGB Diet Serving Size	Protein per Serving in Grams
Oatmeal, dry	1 packet	2
Pasta, cooked, enriched white	½ cup	3
Pasta, cooked, whole-grain	½ cup	3
Rice, cooked, brown	½ cup	3
Soybeans, raw (green) – edamame	1 ounce	4
Spinach, cooked	½ cup	1

Table 34: Low-protein foods

These charts can help you choose high-protein foods. They can also help you monitor your protein intake so you know that you are getting enough. If you are not getting enough protein, your dietitian can help you with strategies, such as having an extra snack (high-protein snack) or including a protein supplement in your diet. Many members of BariatricPal.com, an online community dedicated specifically to the weight loss surgery community, can give you their own tried-and-true tips for increasing protein intake.

Fat

Fat is a great source of energy—which unfortunately also means that it is very high in calories. A single gram of fat has nine calories or more than twice the amount of calories in a gram of protein or a carbohydrate. That is why a high-fat diet is often linked to obesity, and it is why following a low-fat diet is a recommendation to help people lose weight.

You Need Fat for Nutrient Absorption

Fat is not all bad though. You need it to be able to absorb nutrients from your diet. That is especially challenging after the gastric bypass, which decreases absorption of the fat-soluble vitamins A, D, E, and K. RYGB patients are also at risk for deficiencies of these vitamins because of a very low-fat diet.

Not All Fats Are Equal

All fats provide nine calories per gram, but they have different effects on your health.[6] Solid fats, such as butter, shortening, and animal fat, are generally unhealthy. They mostly contain saturated fats and may have trans fats. Liquid fats, or oils, are usually healthier. They contain mostly monounsaturated and polyunsaturated fats. Often foods with unhealthy fats are low in other nutrients, while foods with healthy fats are high in other essential nutrients. *Table 35* shows you the different categories of fat, recommendations for healthy intake, and which foods they are in.

Type of Fat	Effects on Your Body and Recommendations	Food Sources
Saturated Fat	• Raises LDL cholesterol • Increases your risk for heart disease • Should provide at most 7 to 10% of total calories, or 9 to 14 grams per day on a 1,200-calorie diet.	• Butter • Fatty meats, such as fatty beef and pork, sausage, and bacon • Dark-meat poultry with skin • Full-fat dairy products • Coconut and palm oil
Trans Fats	• Raise LDL cholesterol levels • Lower levels of healthy HDL cholesterol • Raises risk for heart disease • Minimize intake by aiming for less than 1 gram a day on a low-calorie diet.	• Fried foods, such as French fries, fried chicken, fried fish, and doughnuts • Partially hydrogenated oils found in many processed snack foods, such as crackers, cookies, and snack cakes
Monounsaturated Fats (you will also see them referred to as MUFA)	• Lower blood pressure • Improved cholesterol levels • Heart-healthy Mediterranean diets have high levels of MUFA. • 10 to 20% of total calories, or 14 to 25 grams per day on a 1,200 calorie diet	• Nuts and peanuts • Most vegetable oils, such as canola, sunflower, safflower, and soybean • Seeds • Flaxseed oil and flaxseed
Polyunsaturated fats (sometimes they are called PUFA)	• Lower cholesterol if chosen instead of saturated fats • 10% of your total calories from PUFA, or 14 grams per day on a 1,200-calorie diet.	• Olive oil, olives • Peanut and canola oil • Avocados • Peanuts • Almonds and other nuts
N-3 fatty acids (these are specific types of polyunsaturated fats that have important health benefits)	• Lower blood pressure • Lower triglycerides • At least two servings of seafood per week or a fish oil supplement • N-3s in vegetarian sources are not quite as powerful, but they are still healthy.	• Fatty fish, such as salmon, herring, mackerel, and tuna • Shellfish, such as oysters, shrimp, crab, lobster, and mussels • Cod liver oil and fish oil supplements • Vegetarian sources include flaxseed, flaxseed oil, walnuts, and canola oil.

Table 35: Different types of fat & the general recommendations for healthy intake

Does Low-Fat Mean Low-Calorie?

No, not necessarily. Fat has nine calories per gram compared to only four calories per gram in carbohydrates and proteins. Many low-fat and fat-free foods are lower in calories than their regular, full-fat versions.

- *Non-fat and low-fat milk, cheese, and yogurt*
- *Lean and extra-lean ground beef*
- *Most reduced-fat salad dressings*

But low-fat or fat-free does not always mean low-calorie. Fat adds flavor, volume, and texture to many foods. When manufacturers take out the fat, they often add carbohydrates, such as sugars or starches, to replace the taste, volume, and texture that fat normally provides. The result can be a low-fat or fat-free product with as many as or more calories than the original one. These are some low-fat foods that have similar amounts of calories in their reduced-fat and regular versions:

- *Peanut butter*
- *Baked goods (e.g., cookies, cakes, pies, and pastries)*
- *Some condiments (but some reduced-fat versions are also reduced-calorie)*
- *Ramen noodles*
- *Canned tuna (i.e., oil-packed versus water-packed)*
- *Granola*

This is quite a varied list, so how can you make the best choices? Read the nutrition facts panels on food labels. Place the regular, full-fat version of the food next to the reduced-fat option, and compare their calories per serving. Make sure you are looking at the same serving size so you do not get tricked!

Carbohydrates

Each gram of carbohydrates supplies four calories. Providing energy is the only function of dietary carbohydrates. When you eat carbohydrates, your body breaks them down into small units of a simple sugar called glucose. The glucose goes into your bloodstream. Your brain depends on glucose for energy.[7] Other organs, such as your muscles, kidneys, and liver, valso are good at using glucose when it is available. For most people, carbohydrates are the major source of energy, providing 45 to 65% of calories.

> **Tip**
>
> See **Chapter 1, "Obesity – A Widespread Disease,"** to read about how your body breaks down carbohydrates from foods. See **Chapter 13, "Post-Surgery Diet: From Liquid Diet to Solid Foods,"** for information on the nutritional differences between added sugars versus natural sugars.

Caloric Carbohydrates and Dietary Fiber

There are two main categories of carbohydrates: carbohydrates with calories and those with dietary fiber. Fiber does not provide calories, because your body does not process it the same way as other carbohydrates. The kinds of carbohydrates with calories include sugars and starches.

- *Sugars are simple carbohydrates.* They include added sugars, used for sweetening foods and adding volume to food products, and natural sugars, such as lactose in milk and fructose in fruit. Sugars can cause dumping syndrome.

- *Starches are complex carbohydrates.* Foods with refined starches, such as white bread, are generally less healthy than other sources of starch, such as whole grains and starchy vegetables. Starchy grains are generally high-calorie and should be eaten last at each meal.

Dietary Fiber and Your Health

Dietary fiber is a different kind of carbohydrate. It is made up of the same small units as other carbohydrates, but fiber does not have calories; your body cannot break down the big pieces of fiber into small enough pieces to get energy. When you eat a food with fiber, your body digests and absorbs sugars and starches, fats, and proteins. The fiber stays behind in your gastrointestinal tract—and provides multiple health benefits! These are some of them:[8]

- *Helps control your weight.* Dietary fiber ties in very well with RYGB.
  - Many high-fiber foods, such as fruits and vegetables, take a long time to chew. They help you slow your eating so you can eat less and lose weight.
  - Another reason why dietary fiber helps control your weight is that it makes food take longer to empty from your stomach. You will stay full for longer after a high-fiber meal or snack.

- *Helps prevent constipation.* The undigested fiber helps add bulk and water to your stool so bowel movements are softer and more regular. Keep drinking your water, too, to prevent constipation.

- *Helps control blood sugar.* Since fiber slows absorption of carbohydrates, sugar is slower to enter your bloodstream as blood glucose. Your blood sugar does not spike as high after a meal, and it does not drop as quickly. That is great news if you have pre-diabetes or diabetes. It is also good because it helps prevent hunger that occurs when your blood sugar drops.

- *Lowers your cholesterol levels.* Fiber lowers the amount of cholesterol that you absorb from food so blood levels of unhealthy LDL cholesterol drop. That is good for your heart.

- *Lowers blood pressure and reduces inflammation.* Scientists are not quite sure how fiber helps with these, but the evidence for these two heart-healthy benefits looks pretty clear.

Dietary fiber is in plant-based foods, not animal products. These are some good sources:

- *Whole-grain cereal:* oatmeal, whole-wheat cereals, bran cereals
- *Whole-grain breads and crackers*
- *Other whole grains:* brown rice, whole-grain multi-grain pasta, barley, bulgur
- *Vegetables:* Fibrous is not necessarily the same as *high-fiber.* While you may need to avoid very stringy vegetables like asparagus stalks and raw celery, there are plenty of high-fiber choices, such as butternut squash, onions, and carrots, on the RYGB diet.
- *Fruit:* fresh or frozen. Canned fruit has some fiber, and fruit juice is not a good source of fiber.
- *Legumes:* peas, beans, and lentils, including dips and soups
- *Nuts and peanuts:* Of course, chew them very well and watch your portion sizes because they are high-fat and high-calorie!

The recommended intake of fiber is based on the amount of calories that you eat. The general recommendation is to get at least 14 grams for every 1,000 calories that you eat. You do not have to count fiber grams to be sure that you are getting enough. On the RYGB diet, you are probably not going to be counting calories, and you are almost certainly not going to be counting grams of fiber. Instead, follow RYGB diet rules, such as eating vegetables and fruits right after protein and choosing whole grains instead of refined.

Food Sources of Carbohydrates

Which foods have caloric carbohydrates? This list contains some of the foods that provide sugars, starches, or both. They have varying amounts of carbohydrates, fat, and protein. Foods with sugars can be healthy OR unhealthy, and foods with starches can be healthy OR unhealthy. Foods marked with * provide dietary fiber.

- *Grains*: (contain starches) whole grain and white bread, cereal, pasta, rice, oatmeal, bulgur, barley, popcorn
- *Legumes*: (contain starches) split peas, black-eyed peas, lentils, and all kinds of beans, such as black, pinto, and garbanzo
- *Fruit*: (contain sugars) fresh, frozen, canned, dried, and juice
- *Nuts*, *seeds*, *soy nuts*, and *peanuts*: (contain starches)
- *Dairy products*: (contain sugars) milk, yogurt, cheese, frozen yogurt
- *Starchy vegetables*: (contain starches) potatoes, sweet potatoes and yams, acorn and butternut squash, corn, beets
- *Non-starchy vegetables*: green beans, broccoli, cauliflower, eggplant, lettuce, carrots
- *Sweets*: (contain simple sugars) candy, ice cream, pudding, chocolate, fudge
- *Sugar-sweetened beverages*: (contain simple sugars) soft drinks, coffee with sugar, energy drinks, smoothies

- *Baked goods*: (contain starches and simple sugars) cakes, cookies, pies, pastries
- *Condiments*: (contain starches and simple sugars) ketchup, salad dressing, sauces, gravies, jams and jellies
- *Mixed foods*: (contain starches and simple sugars) battered fried chicken and fish, pizza, sandwiches

What does not have carbohydrates? Some healthy foods, and some unhealthy foods, are carbohydrate-free:

- Eggs
- Meats, such as beef and pork
- Poultry
- Fish and most shellfish
- Pure fats, such as butter and oil

The Micronutrients: Vitamins and Minerals

Vitamins and minerals are called "micronutrients" because you only need small amounts of them ("micro") compared to the macronutrients, which include carbohydrates, proteins, and fats. You might eat hundreds of grams per day of macronutrients, but you only need a gram, a milligram (one one-thousandth of a gram), or even just a few micrograms (one one-millionth of a gram) per day of each micronutrient. Vitamins and minerals do not have calories, but they are just as important as the calorie-providing nutrients.

An Overview of the Micronutrients

Thirteen vitamins and at least 15 minerals are essential. Most of them are not of concern; you are to get enough of them if your diet is adequate and balanced. Some micronutrients are of greater concern for RYGB patients, though, because of your limited food intake and nutrient malabsorption.

Meeting Your Vitamin and Mineral Requirements

You can minimize micronutrient deficiencies by:

- Eating a balanced diet
- Taking your supplements as recommended
- Getting tested regularly for deficiencies so you can be sure to catch them early, before they become serious

You may become deficient in several vitamins and minerals without supplements.[9] *Table 6* includes some of the most likely nutrients of concern. It includes their functions in your body—why you need them—as well as why you might be deficient and which foods you can get them from.

You definitely *do not* need to memorize *Table 6*! These are some of the main points to get:

- Eating a variety of foods will help you get the nutrients you need.
- Choosing healthy foods will help you get the nutrients you need. You already know that healthy, nutrient-dense foods include meat and poultry, seafood, legumes, vegetables, whole grains, dairy products, and fruit. These come up a lot on the table.
- *Table 36* does not include junk foods—they are not your best sources of nutrients.

When in doubt, choose healthy! Go for unprocessed foods instead of processed. Even without thinking about calories, saturated fat, and sugar, you can see that unprocessed foods are healthier—most of the good sources listed are foods that we think of as "healthy."

Do Not Forget Your Supplements!

A balanced, nutritious diet is a healthy foundation, but you will probably still need vitamin and mineral supplements to prevent nutritional deficiencies after gastric bypass surgery. A daily multivitamin providing 100 to 200% of the daily value for most nutrients is common. These specific supplements are also common:[13]

- Iron (likely with vitamin C to increase absorption)
- Vitamin B12
- Calcium
- Vitamin D
- Folic acid (most likely if you are a woman who may become pregnant)

Your surgeon and dietitian might also recommend taking supplements of one or more of these if they think you are at risk for developing deficiencies:

- Zinc
- Selenium
- Thiamin or vitamin B1
- Vitamin A, E, or K

Anemia and Roux-en-Y Gastric Bypass

Anemia is common after weight loss surgery, with 25 to 50% of patients having it. Premenopausal women are at highest risk, with close to three-quarters of them developing anemia.[14]

Anemia is a lower-than-normal level of healthy red blood cells. As shown in **Table 6**, it can result from deficiency of iron, vitamin B12, or folic acid, or it can have other causes. Inadequate levels of healthy red blood cells can result from one or more of the following problems:

- Your red blood cells are not formed correctly. They can be immature or deformed; this

Vitamin or Mineral and Requirement	Why You Need It and Other Background Information[10]	Reasons for Potential Deficiency	Food Sources
Thiamin (vitamin B1) (1.7 milligrams per day)	• Allows your body to metabolize energy from fat, protein, and carbohydrates • Normally absorbed from jejunum (upper part of small intestine) • Early detection of deficiency can prevent serious permanent consequences.	• Less absorption after RYGB, especially with postoperative vomiting • Lower intake on RYGB diet	• Legumes (beans, peas, lentils) • Pork • Yeast • Fortified grains, such as bread, cereal, pasta, and rice
Iron (8 milligrams per day for men and postmenopausal women; 18 milligrams per day for menstruating women)	• Lets your red blood cells carry oxygen to the cells in your body • Iron deficiency is the most common micronutrient deficiency in the world. • Iron deficiency is widespread in the U.S., too, especially among women and teenage girls. • Deficiency leads to anemia, with symptoms of fatigue and weakness. • May require higher-dose iron supplement than in multivitamin and mineral pill.	• Lower intake of iron because of restricted diet (low-calorie diet) • Increased losses if you have bleeding from complications during or after surgery • Lower intake of vitamin C, which increases iron absorption from vegetarian foods • Menstruating women, especially those with a heavy menstrual cycle and high blood losses	• Red meat, including beef, liver, and pork • Seafood, such as oysters and tuna • Legumes, such as kidney beans and lentils • Fortified grains, such as bread, breakfast cereal, rice, and pasta • Potatoes, tofu, and nuts • Raisins and prunes (although high in sugar and limited on the RYGB diet)
Calcium (1,000 to 1,500 milligrams per day)	• Forms a major part of bone mineral • Necessary for strong bones • Prevents osteoporosis later in life • Losing bone mineral density is nearly irreversible.	• Rapid weight loss, as with RYGB, increases calcium loss from your body and bones. • Inadequate intake from diet, which is likely if you are having less than three servings per day of high-calcium dairy products (often occurs because of lactose intolerance and low dietary intake) • Decreased absorption from food after RYGB	• Milk, cheese, and yogurt • Fortified breakfast cereals and breads—check the label to see if it has at least 10% of the daily value (DV) for calcium • Canned fish, such as salmon and sardines, because it has bones in it • Fortified tofu, soymilk, and other soy products

Vitamin or Mineral and Requirement	Why You Need It and Other Background Information[10]	Reasons for Potential Deficiency	Food Sources
Vitamin D (400 to 4,000 International Units [IU] per day)	• Helps your body absorb calcium from food • Helps your body regulate calcium so you can have strong bones • Deficiency can lead to bone problems such as osteoporosis and osteomalacia. • Deficiency may increase your risk for heart disease.	• Low dietary intake, which is common because it is not in many foods. • Reduced absorption due to very low-fat diet • Not enough exposure to high-intensity sun (common in northern climates and if you stay indoors) • Older adults • Dark-skinned individuals	• Vitamin D-fortified milk • Fish oil and fatty fish • Some fortified products (e.g., some breakfast cereals, orange juice, and yogurt [read the label])
Zinc (15 milligrams per day)	• Supports a healthy immune system • Needed for proper wound healing[11]	• Low dietary intake, especially if you avoid red meat and shellfish • Low fat intake on the RYGB diet reduces zinc absorption	• Shellfish (e.g., oysters and crab) • Dark-meat chicken and turkey • Beef and pork • Beans • Nuts • Milk and yogurt
Potassium (at least 4,700 milligrams per day)	• Needed to maintain a healthy (lower) blood pressure • Can prevent muscle cramps	• Diet low in fruits and vegetables, which can occur if you are not careful to eat them right after protein • Diet high in processed foods and sodium increase potassium needs	• Potatoes • Beans, lentils • Winter squash • Most fruits, including bananas • Most vegetables • Meat and fish • Potassium supplements are rare.
Vitamin E (15 milligrams, or 22.5 international units, per day)	• Has heart-healthy antioxidant functions • May reduce your risk of developing cataracts and macular degeneration • Severe deficiency is rare, but lower-than-optimal levels are common.	• Low-fat diet and decreased fat absorption lead to reduced vitamin E absorption. • Low intake of vitamin E because it is mostly in high-fat foods, which are limited on the RYGB diet	• Avocados • Nuts and peanut butter • Seeds (be sure you chew them well!) • Vegetable oils and salad dressings • Whole grains • Carrots • Spinach

Vitamin or Mineral and Requirement	Why You Need It and Other Background Information[10]	Reasons for Potential Deficiency	Food Sources
Vitamin C (60 milligrams per day)	• Strong immune system • Antioxidant functions • Supports heart health • Necessary for proper wound healing • Increases your absorption of iron from plant-based foods • Deficiency is rare, but higher intake can be healthy.	• Low intake of fresh fruits and vegetables • Diet high in processed foods	• Citrus fruits, such as oranges and tangerines • Vegetables, such as red peppers, tomatoes, broccoli, and kale • Many other fruits, such as papaya, pineapple, kiwis, cantaloupe, and berries • Potatoes
Vitamin A (900 micrograms, or 3,000 international units, per day for men; 700 micrograms, or 2,333 international units, per day for women)	• Antioxidant functions • Night vision and maintaining eye health • Deficiency can cause night blindness. • Toxicity from supplements can lead to liver damage. • A high amount of beta-carotene, the form of vitamin A in plant foods, is not dangerous.	• Very low fat intake, reduced fat absorption, and lower vitamin A absorption • Low intake of fruits and vegetables • Toxicity can result from unnecessary vitamin A supplements.	• Orange vegetables, such as carrots, sweet potatoes, yams, and acorn squash • Orange fruit, such as cantaloupe and mangos • Green leafy vegetables, such as spinach • Butter (should be limited on RYGB diet) • Liver and cod liver oil
Vitamin K (120 micrograms per day for men; 90 micrograms per day for women)	• Normal blood clotting • Supplements can interfere with blood-thinning medications (anti-coagulants, such as warfarin).	• Very low fat intake, reduced fat absorption, and lower vitamin K absorption • Low dietary intake of vitamin K from limited diet	• Leafy green vegetables • Other vegetables • Fruits • Vegetable oils

Vitamin or Mineral and Requirement	Why You Need It and Other Background Information[10]	Reasons for Potential Deficiency	Food Sources
Folic Acid (vitamin B-9) (400 micrograms per day)	• Adequate intake needed for preventing neural tube birth defects such as spina bifida • May be heart-healthy • May lower your risk for some cancers • Healthy red blood cells • Deficiency can cause anemia.	• Low intake of folate or folic acid from the diet • The RYGB diet emphasizes proteins, but meats and poultry do not have folate. • Medications, such as oral contraceptives, can increase deficiency risk.	• Fortified grains—the same ones as for iron • Legumes, such as lima beans, garbanzo beans, and lentils • Orange juice • Leafy green vegetables, such as kale, and spinach
Vitamin B-12 (12 micrograms per day)	• Good nerve functioning—deficiency can cause permanent nerve damage. • Only naturally in animal-derived products • Needed for healthy red blood cells; deficiency can cause anemia.	• Plant-based diet—avoiding animal foods • Low intake from limited RYGB diet • Decreased digestion and absorption from protein foods • Medications used to treat esophageal reflux, ulcers, and bowel inflammation[12]	• Seafood, such as clams, mussels, crab, salmon, and tuna • Meat and poultry, such as beef and chicken • Eggs and dairy products • Fortified foods, such as some breakfast cereals—read the label
Other B vitamins: Riboflavin (B2), Niacin (B3), Pantothenic acid (B5), Vitamin (B6)	• Needed for energy production with many food sources and most Americans get plenty. You need these B vitamins for proper metabolism of nutrients.	• Low dietary intake from limited amount of food on a low-calorie RYGB diet	• Whole grains and fortified grains • Protein foods • Nuts and beans • Milk • Potatoes • Vegetables

Table 36: Vitamin/Mineral and Requirement

can happen with a folic acid or vitamin B12 deficiency, since your body needs those vitamins for making red blood cells.

- You do not have enough red blood cells, which happens if you lose a lot of blood. This can happen during or after surgery, and is a greater problem for menstruating women.
- Your red blood cells do not do a good job of carrying oxygen to the cells in your body, including your muscles and brain—this can happen with iron deficiency because iron is what allows your red blood cells to carry oxygen.

You are always at risk for anemia after gastric bypass. Anemia makes you feel tired and irritable and can interfere with concentration. More severe anemia can cause shortness of breath, brittle nails, and lightheadedness.[15] To prevent serious effects of anemia, follow your physician's and dietitian's recommendations for choosing nutritious foods and taking your dietary supplements. Also, go in for your recommended blood tests to monitor your nutritional status.

Long-Term Consequences of Nutrient Deficiencies

You are almost certain to need supplements for life because of your limited diet and reduced nutrient absorption after gastric bypass.[16] Nutrient deficiencies can cause serious consequences and should be taken seriously. Some nutrient deficiency symptoms go away when you get your nutrient levels back to normal. Other nutrient deficiency symptoms are irreversible. Unless you get tested regularly, you may not know that you are deficient until it is too late. Osteoporosis, peripheral neuropathy, and heart disease are some of the potential long-term consequences of certain nutrient deficiencies.[17]

Osteoporosis

Osteoporosis is a condition with lower-than-normal bone mineral density and a higher-than-normal risk for fractures or broken bones. We tend to think of this as an old lady's disease because they are at highest risk for fractures, but your bones can become thinner and more brittle for years before you break a bone and learn that you have osteoporosis. Your risk for osteoporosis increases even more if you do not get enough calcium, vitamin D, and physical activity.

- There is no easy blood test to tell whether you are getting enough calcium. The best way to ensure that you are is to emphasize high-calcium foods, such as yogurt, and take your supplements consistently.
- Taking vitamin D supplements, eating fortified foods and fatty fish, and getting plenty of sunshine help you meet your vitamin D needs.
- Weight bearing activities include walking, dancing, lifting weights, and playing tennis.

Peripheral Neuropathy

Peripheral neuropathy is damage to one or more nerves that connect your brain to your spinal cord or your spinal cord to other parts of your body.[18] Peripheral neuropathy has many possible causes, and as a RYGB patient, you are at risk for peripheral neuropathy caused by deficiency of vitamin B12. Symptoms may become permanent, and they include the following:

- Tingling or numb feet or hands
- Confusion or memory loss
- Dizziness
- Lack of coordination

Fortified Foods: What Are They and What is in Them?

We have already mentioned fortified foods several times because they are great ways to get certain nutrients. Fortification means that the manufacturer adds extra vitamins or minerals to food. Certain foods are required to have certain nutrients. For example, fortified milk in the United States always contains vitamin D and vitamin A. Fortified grains, including bread, flour, cereal, rice, and pasta, contain extra amounts of these nutrients:

- Vitamin B1 (thiamin)
- Vitamin B2 (riboflavin)
- Vitamin B3 (niacin)
- Folic acid
- Iron

Fortified foods may also contain additional nutrients. They are not required by law, though, so you need to check the label to see whether your food contains them. These are some examples of common nutrient-food combinations, but you need to read the label to make sure that these foods contain the nutrients you are looking for.

- Calcium and vitamin D in fortified breakfast cereals, orange juice, and soy milk
- Vitamin B12 in breakfast cereals and vegetarian meat substitutes
- Vitamin D in yogurt
- Calcium in pudding
- Many vitamins and minerals in breakfast cereals

Source:[20]

Following these steps can reduce your risk for peripheral neuropathy:

- Eat animal-based proteins: meat, fish, poultry, dairy products, eggs
- Choose breakfast cereals and other foods that are fortified with vitamin B12 (check the label)
- Get your levels of vitamin B12 tested regularly
- Take dietary supplements if recommended by your surgeon and/or dietitian

What Is the Scoop on Sodium?

Sodium is an essential nutrient because it is necessary for life. Like potassium, sodium is a mineral and an electrolyte. Both help maintain water balance in your body. So why are you always hearing that you should lower your sodium intake? While potassium helps lower blood pressure by letting your body get rid of extra water, sodium is linked to high blood pressure because it encourages your body to hold onto water.

You already know that salt makes you retain water if you have ever felt bloated after eating a salty meal! Water retention does not just make you feel uncomfortable. It is actually unhealthy. The extra water that you retain gives you an extra high volume of blood, which raises your blood pressure and strains your kidneys.

The average American gets 3,400 milligrams of sodium per day. That is more than the recommended maximum of 2,300 milligrams and far more than the amount you really need to survive, which is probably slightly over 500 milligrams per day. You can get about that much by having a cup of milk, an egg, and two slices of bread. You can get to 500 milligrams just by eating three ounces of canned salmon, or a half-cup of canned soup! You are only going to be deficient if you have some sort of health problem, such as severe dehydration.

Another reason to keep your sodium intake in check is because high amounts of sodium make your RYGB experience more difficult. A high-salt diet makes you thirstier so that you want to drink more, but drinking extra fluid can be a challenge when you are already struggling to hit your 1.5 liters of water per day on the gastric bypass diet. You cannot drink within 30 minutes of eating solid food, so it is hard to increase your fluid intake when you are trying to make up for extra sodium consumption.

Most high-sodium food sources are prepared and processed foods because they are salty. A single teaspoon of salt has more than 2,300 milligrams of sodium! These are some foods that are high in sodium:

- Canned soups; broth and bouillon powders and cubes; dry soup mixes
- Other canned foods, such as canned beans, vegetables, tuna, and chili
- Frozen meals and appetizers
- Bread: Surprisingly, bread is the single biggest source of sodium for Americans!
- Ready-to-eat foods, such as pasta dishes, pizza, and Chinese food
- Salty snack foods, such as peanuts, pretzels, popcorn, crackers, and potato chips
- Salty sauces and dressings, such as soy, teriyaki and spaghetti sauces, and salad dressings
- Cheese
- Cured foods, such as pickles, olives, ham, and sauerkraut

A general guideline for when you are trying to limit your sodium intake is to choose less processed options. The more processing steps and the further the food is from its natural source, the more sodium it is likely to have. Yes, many kinds of foods naturally have a small amount of sodium. Meat, fish, celery, and tomatoes are examples. But fresh meat is far lower in sodium than sausages or cold cuts; fresh fish is lower than canned, and celery and tomatoes are lower in sodium than vegetable juice.

You can also lower your sodium intake by choosing low-sodium or reduced-salt options, such as low-sodium canned vegetables and unsalted pretzels. Using herbs, spices, and low-sodium dressings can also help you reduce the amount of salt and salty seasonings you use while still enjoying flavorful foods.

Do Not Let Vitamin and Mineral Supplements Turn into Too Much of a Good Thing

Overdoses and chronic toxicity from high levels of vitamins and minerals from supplements can be just as dangerous as deficiencies. For that reason, only take supplements that your surgeon or nutritionist recommends. The likelihood and consequences of toxicity depend on which vitamins and minerals you are taking, how much extra you are taking, and how long you have been taking more than you need. They can include liver disease, an increased risk for heart disease, higher risk of kidney stones, and/or other nutrient deficiencies because of blocked absorption.[19]

Condiments on the RYGB Diet

Condiments should not be afterthoughts, because they can throw off your weight loss if you are not careful. Condiments include the sauces, spreads, spices, dips, and garnishes that can make your food taste better or make your meal feel complete. Some condiments are benign, but others threaten your weight loss. Many condiments are also low in essential nutrients.

How Many Calories Can Condiments Contribute?

Take a look at the following table to get an idea of how many calories you can get from what seems like just a few condiments. The table shows a day on the RYGB diet with just one or two "extras" at each meal.

Table 37: Sample day on the RYGB diet with a few condiments. Notice how quickly just a few small amounts of condiments can add up!

Meal or Snack	Foods with Condiments	Extra Calories from Condiments
Breakfast	Toast with 1 tablespoon jam (50 calories) and 2 teaspoons butter (70 calories)	120 calories
Snack 1	Tuna salad with 1 tablespoon mayonnaise (90 calories)	90 calories
Lunch	Deli turkey with 2 tablespoons cream cheese (100 calories); green beans with 1 teaspoon butter (30 calories)	130 calories
Snack 2	½ cup pasta with 2 tablespoons pesto sauce (110 calories)	110 calories
Dinner	Ground turkey burger with 2 tablespoons Thousand Island dressing (120 calories)	120 calories
Snack 3	Fruit salad with 2 tablespoons sweetened whipped cream (30 calories)	30 calories
Beverages	Coffee with 1 container creamer (30 calories) and 2 sugar packets (60 calories)	90 calories
Total		690 calories

Table 37: Sample day on the RYGB diet with a few condiments

This example is slightly exaggerated, but it gets the point across. Adding just one or two "extras" to each meal or snack can add up to several hundred — in this case, 690 — calories! If you add an extra 690 calories per day to your RYGB diet without realizing it, your weight loss will slow by more than a pound a week. If you are trying to maintain your weight loss or you have hit a plateau, you might even gain weight because of extra condiments.

Tips to Keep Condiments in Check

So what can you do to maintain a tasty, satisfying diet while you prevent condiments from sabotaging your weight loss? These suggestions may help:

- Measure and record your condiments — do not just let them sneak into your diet.

- Limit your portion size. Using a ½ tablespoon of mayo instead of 1 tablespoon in your tuna salad saves you 50 calories, and you probably will not even notice the difference.

- Use fewer condiments at a time. Instead of butter *and* jam to make your toast less dry, try using butter *or* jam. This strategy can be twice as effective because it will make your toast slightly drier. It will help you eat slower because it will take longer to chew.

- Make better choices. Substitute more nutritious, lower-calorie choices for regular high-calorie options. In general, try to avoid high-fat, high-calorie, high-sugar condiments.

Condiment Substitutions to Try

Table 38 compares some poorer condiment choices with some substitutes that can be healthier or lower-calorie choices. Regularly choosing better options will eventually show up on the scale.

Instead of...	Consider...
1 tablespoon of butter on a baked potato or vegetables: 100 calories and high saturated fat	Melted low-fat cheese: 60 calories, including some protein and calcium
2 tablespoons full-fat salad dressing: 200 calories	2 tablespoons reduced-calorie dressing: 20 calories
1 tablespoon of regular mayonnaise: 90 calories	1 tablespoon of fat-free mayonnaise: 15 calories
1 teaspoon of yellow, Dijon, or deli mustard: 5 calories	2 tablespoons of hummus (garbanzo bean dip): 60 calories, high in protein 2 tablespoons salsa: 20 calories, fat-free
2 tablespoons of ranch, French onion, and other regular dips: 120–200 calories, high-fat	2 tablespoons of hummus (garbanzo bean dip): 60 calories, high in protein
2 tablespoons salsa: 20 calories, fat-free	½ cup applesauce or half mashed banana: 50 calories
2 tablespoons of low-calorie salad dressing: 10 to 50 calories	¼ cup tomato or pizza sauce: 50 calories
1 tablespoon flavored coffee creamer: 35 calories	1 tablespoon fat-free milk: 5 calories
1 tablespoon of fruit preserves, jam, or jelly: 50 calories, high-sugar	½ cup applesauce or half of a mashed banana: 50 calories
1 ounce (2 tablespoons) pesto sauce: 110 calories	½ tablespoon sugar or honey plus cinnamon and cloves (25 calories)
¼ cup alfredo sauce: 100 calories	¼ cup tomato or pizza sauce: 50 calories
1 tablespoon of butter or margarine: 100 calories	1 tablespoon reduced-fat margarine: 50 calories
Salt and salty seasonings	Herbs and spices, e.g., oregano, thyme, rosemary, black pepper, marjoram, caraway, dill, garlic
1 tablespoon of sugar or honey (50 calories)	½ tablespoon sugar or honey plus cinnamon and cloves (25 calories)

Table 38: Condiment Substitutions to Try

Good Condiment Choices Can Promote Success

Well-chosen condiments can encourage good choices on the RYGB diet. These are a few examples:

- Add lemon juice instead of butter to your fish.
- Use teriyaki sauce or fat-free marinade, such as a lemon-pepper or Italian herb marinade, to prevent dryness and persuade you to grill or bake chicken breast instead of frying it.
- Instead of choosing high-fat ground beef, choose lean ground turkey and add soy sauce or tomato sauce to prevent dryness.
- Liven up vegetables with curry powder or other herbs and spices instead of drowning them in butter.
- Dip vegetables into fat-free salad dressing for a low-calorie snack.

Balance the benefits you get from the extra taste and change in texture from condiments with the possible disadvantages of the extra calories. You can still have great-tasting food on the RYGB diet. Just be as mindful of your condiments as you are with your other food

Water

Water is the sixth nutrient; the other five are protein, carbohydrates, fat, vitamins, and minerals. You need about 8–13 cups of fluid per day.[21] Water not only keeps you hydrated but also helps you lose weight. It is calorie-free and naturally suppresses hunger.

Alternatives to Plain Water

Some people do not like drinking water. You might be able to train yourself to like water, but some weight loss surgery patients find that they are not able to stomach plain water. Plenty of other options are acceptable alternatives to plain water. These are some suggestions for calorie-free or low-calorie beverages:

- Ice water – Ice-cold water can be more palatable than room-temperature.
- Water with a slice of lemon or lime or a sprig of fresh mint (you can find it in your grocery store's produce section with the other fresh herbs)
- Diet drinks – diet fruit drinks, diet iced tea, (avoid carbonated beverages—they will increase your risk of stretching your stomach pouch and causing leaks.)
- Calorie-free flavored waters (still water; not sparkling or carbonated)
- Hot or iced coffee, green tea, or black tea – without cream or sugar. You can use artificial sweeteners, such as saccharin in the pink packet, aspartame in the blue packet, or sucralose in the yellow packet. They have almost no calories. Caffeine-free coffee and tea are safer than caffeinated versions shortly after surgery.
- Low-sodium broth or bouillon

Milk is high in protein, calcium, and vitamin D, but it does have calories. If your surgeon and dietitian allow fat-free or 1 percent reduced-fat milk, they are likely to suggest having only one or two servings per day. Better choices for weight loss might be a calorie-free beverage for your fluid and fortified, fat-free yogurt and reduced-fat cheese to fill you up and provide protein, calcium, and vitamin D.

Caffeine and Roux-en-Y Gastric Bypass

Many people worry that caffeine is dehydrating. It is true that caffeine is a diuretic; it increases the amount of water that your body loses in urine. However, the effect is very small, and caffeinated beverages, such as coffee and tea, still count toward your daily water requirements. Avoid caffeine if you notice that it keeps you up at night or gives you heartburn.

Plan Your Fluid Intake Carefully!

Your weight loss and health will be better if you take your hydration as seriously as you take your diet. These are a few reminders and tips to help you plan your fluid intake:

- Aim for six to seven cups per day. You can meet this goal by drinking one to two cups between each meal and snack.
- Stick to water or other non-caloric (or low-calorie) beverages.
- Keep water handy so you remember to drink it. Have a water bottle in your car and desk and keep a pitcher of water in the fridge.
- Do not drink within 30 minutes before or after eating solid foods.

Alcohol and RYGB

Moderate consumption of red wine may have some benefits for your heart. It may raise your levels of healthy HDL cholesterol and help protect your blood vessels against damage.[22] Alcohol also helps you relax. However, alcohol is not an essential nutrient, and drinking alcoholic beverages can throw off your weight loss and cause health problems.

Calories, Alcohol, and Your Weight

Alcoholic beverages are high in calories. Each gram of alcohol has seven calories, and that is not even counting the carbohydrates that are in some alcoholic beverages.

- A 5-ounce serving of wine has 130 calories; an 8-ounce cup has 200 calories, or about twice as many as a glass of juice.
- A 1.4-ounce shot of vodka has 103 calories, or nearly 600 calories in an 8-ounce cup.
- A 12-ounce can of beer contains 164 calories.

Drinking alcohol can cause you to take in more calories than you intended. Beyond the calories in the alcoholic beverage, alcohol relaxes you and decreases your inhibition and the ability to say "no." You are more likely to give into temptations to eat high-calorie foods. You are also more likely to eat without planning for it or writing it down. Drinking alcohol with RYGB is not worth it. You are working so hard to lose weight that it would be a shame to counteract your efforts just because you drank too much and lost your good judgment.

Other Concerns with Alcoholic Beverages

Alcohol, even in moderation, can cause problems in addition to interfering with weight loss:[23]

- It can make your blood sugar levels spike.
- It interferes with memory.
- It can increase blood pressure.
- It can damage your liver.

Alcohol Metabolism and the Gastric Bypass

You may be more susceptible to the effects of alcohol after RYGB.[24] With the same amount of alcohol, your blood alcohol content (BAC) may rise higher, and alcohol may stay in your body for longer than before your gastric bypass surgery.

Food Labels Can Help You Lose Weight and Make Healthy Choices

Luckily, the U.S. has relatively strict food labeling laws. If you grew up in the U.S., you probably take detailed food labels for granted. They are relatively complete and standardized. Almost every food item that you can find has a label with these required components:

- The weight of the package
- The number of servings in the package
- A nutrition facts panel with nutrition information per serving
- A list of ingredients
- Any common allergens

The Nutrition Facts Panel: One of Your New Best Friends

The nutrition facts panel can look confusing at first, but it is easy to use once you learn how. By law, nutrition facts panels must look very similar and have certain information.[25] Once you learn your way around one label, you will be able to navigate your way around any food label.

The nutrition facts panel is required to contain information on the nutrients that are most likely to be of concern; that is, the nutrients that Americans eat too much or too little of on average. A typical nutrition facts panel looks like this.

It is relatively easy to use food labels to your advantage once you know how. Each food has a required set of information that must be listed, and in many cases, the information must be listed in a certain order so that it is easy for you to find. In this section, you will learn your way around the food label so you know how to make the best choices.

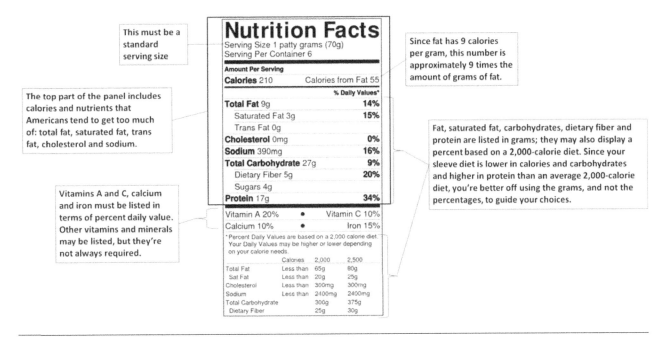

Figure 3 : Standard Nutrition Label

The nutrition label can make your weight loss journey easier and more successful. Nearly all packaged foods are required to have nutrition labels with certain information.

The List of Ingredients Is Full of Useful Information

The ingredients list is not just "fine print" to ignore. It can provide extra information that is not on the nutrition facts panel. The ingredients are listed in order of weight. That means that the first ingredients that are listed are the main ingredients, and the ones listed toward the end are only there in small amounts. This information can help you make healthier choices:

- A grain product whose first ingredient is a "whole" grain or flour has more whole grains than a product whose first ingredient is "enriched or "refined."
- A product with sugar, corn syrup, honey, or another kind of sugar listed first has more sugar than any other ingredient and is probably not very healthy.

You can also use the list of ingredients to avoid certain ingredients to protect your health:

- Ingredients that you might be allergic to, such as soy or egg whites
- Partially hydrogenated oils, which contain trans fat
- Additives that you are sensitive to, such as monosodium glutamate (MSG)
- Foods that are not allowed on your current diet, such as nuts and raisins when you are still recovering from surgery and you are not yet on a fully solid foods diet.

Food Regulation in the U.S.

The Food, Drug and Cosmetic Act, or FDCA, is the groundbreaking legislation that governs most food products in the U.S. The Food and Drug Administration, or FDA, and the U.S. Department of Agriculture, or USDA, are the two main federal agencies that carry out the FDCA and regulate food in the U.S. They are responsible for food safety and for helping consumers make informed decisions about the food they eat.

- *The FDA* regulates most food products, including fish and mixed dishes containing meats and poultry, such as frozen dinners. Most of the food products and labels that you see in stores are regulated by the FDA. The nutrition label that we discussed above is the label required by the FDA on these products. If you are choosing unpackaged foods like raw fish, fruits, and vegetables, the nutrition information might be posted in the section of the grocery store right near the food product, but it is not yet required by law.

- *The USDA* regulates raw meat, poultry, and egg products. Some of the nutrition labeling requirements are the same as the FDA's, but some are not. The USDA does not require small businesses to provide nutrition information about their products. The USDA also administers the National Organic Program (NOP). Foods that are USDA-certified organic are produced without synthetic pesticides, fertilizers, or other chemicals. They are all-natural.

- The Bureau of Alcohol, Tobacco and Firearms regulates alcoholic beverages. That is why the information you see on bottles of beer, wine, and liquor is a little different than labels on foods and other beverages.

Source:[26,27,28,29,30,31]

☞ Summary

- ☞ By now, you are not only an expert with RYGB but you are also becoming an expert nutritionist. You know what it means to make nutritious choices that will promote weight loss and your health. This chapter has the information you need to select the healthiest foods and meet your nutrient needs. You now have the tools you need for a nutritious diet to lose weight:

  - ☞ Which foods to select

  - ☞ How much to eat

  - ☞ How to create a daily menu

  - ☞ Which nutrients to emphasize

  - ☞ Vitamin and mineral supplements to consider

  - ☞ How to stay hydrated

  - ☞ Pitfalls to avoid

- ☞ Now that you know all about your RYGB diet, it is time to look at another part of your new lifestyle: exercise. It is not as scary or difficult as you might think. The next chapter goes over the basics of starting an exercise program from the very beginning—even if you are not used to exercising at all.

Time to Take Action: Keeping a Detailed Diet Record

The diet record (*Table 39*) may become a key to your weight loss success with the RYGB. It helps you stay truthful to yourself about your diet intake. This is some information that should go in a diet record—give it a try! Be very specific about quantities and condiments to make sure you do not forget anything.

Meal or Snack	What did you eat?	Describe the meal setting and how it affected you.	Record other notes here. How hungry were you before and after the meal or snack? Did you eat what you planned?
Sample	3 ounces lean ground turkey, 1 tablespoon ketchup, one-half whole-wheat English muffin, half-cup cooked carrots	Family dinner with the wife and kids. I focused on talking to them rather than wolfing my food.	Pleasant meal. Chewed everything well and felt satisfied (but could have eaten more) by the end. Ate exactly what I had planned.
Breakfast			
Lunch			
Dinner			
Any snacks			

Table 39: Maintain a detailed diet record

1   Critical Care Pediatrics. Basal energy expenditure: Harris-Benedict equation. Joan and Sanford I. Weill Medical College, Cornell University. Web site. http://www-users.med.cornell.edu/~spon/picu/calc/beecalc.htm. 2000, October 3. Accessed February 28, 2013.

2   U.S. Department of Health and Human Services and U.S. Department of Agriculture. Dietary guidelines for Americans, 2010. http://www.health.gov/dietaryguidelines/dga2010/DietaryGuidelines2010.pdf. 2011. Accessed October 19, 2012.

3   Gropper, S.S., & Smith, J.L. Advanced Nutrition and Human Metabolism (5th ed.). 2008;Wadsworth Publishing: Belmont, California.

4   Andreu A, Moize V, Rodriguez L, Flores L, Vidal J. Protein intake, body composition and protein status following bariatric surgery. Obes Surg. 2010;20(11):1509-15.

5   Agricultural Research Service, National Agricultural Library. Nutrient Data Library Foods List. US Department of Agriculture. Web site. http://ndb.nal.usda.gov/ndb/foods/list. December, 2011. Accessed October 17, 2012.

6   Harvard School of Public Health. Fats and cholesterol: out with the bad, in with the good. The Nutrition Source. Web site. http://www.hsph.harvard.edu/nutritionsource/what-should-you-eat/fats-full-story/index.html. 2012. Accessed October 19, 2012.

7   Berg, J.M., Tymockzo, J.L., & Stryer, L. (2002). Biochemistry. 5th edition. New York, W.H. Freeman.

8   Mayo Clinic Staff. Dietary fiber: essential for a healthy diet. Mayo Clinic. Web site. http://www.mayoclinic.com/health/fiber/NU00033/METHOD=print. November 9, 2009. Accessed October 19, 2012.

9   Aills L, Blankenship J, Buffington C, Furtado M, Parrott J. ASMBS Allied Health nutritional guidelines for the surgical weight loss patient. Surg Obes Relat Dis. 2008;4(5Suppl):S73-S108.

10 Gropper, S.S., & Smith, J.L. Advanced Nutrition and Human Metabolism (5th ed.). 2008;Wadsworth Publishing: Belmont, California.

11 Dietary supplement fact sheet: zinc. Office of Dietary Supplements, National Institutes of Health. Web site. http://ods.od.nih.gov/factsheets/Zinc-HealthProfessional/. Reviewed September 20, 2011. Accessed October 20, 2012.

12 Aills L, Blankenship J, Buffington C, Furtado M, Parrott J. ASMBS Allied Health nutritional guidelines for the surgical weight loss patient. Surg Obes Relat Dis. 2008;4(5Suppl):S73-S108.

13 Ziegler O, Sirveaux MA, Brunaud L, Reibel N, Quillot D. Medical follow-up after bariatric surgery: nutritional and drug issues. General recommendations for the prevention and treatment of nutritional deficiencies. Diabetes Metab. 2009;35(6 Pt 2):544-547.

14 Aills L, Blankenship J, Buffington C, Furtado M, Parrott, J. ASMBS Integrated health nutritional guidelines for the surgical weight loss patient. Surgery for Obesity and Related Diseases, 2008;S73-S108.

15 Chen YB, Zieve D. Anemia. Medline Plus. Web site. http://www.nlm.nih.gov/medlineplus/ency/article/000560.htm. Updated 2012, February 7. Accessed October 20, 2012.

16 Ziegler O, Sirveaux MA, Brunaud L, Reibel N, Quillot D. Medical follow-up after bariatric surgery: nutritional and drug issues. General recommendations for the prevention and treatment of nutritional deficiencies. Diabetes Metab. 2009;35(6 Pt 2):544-547.

17 Ziegler O, Sirveaux MA, Brunaud L, Reibel N, Quillot D. Medical follow-up after bariatric surgery: nutritional and drug issues. General recommendations for the prevention and treatment of nutritional deficiencies. Diabetes Metab. 2009;35(6 Pt 2):544-547.

18 Zieve D, Eltz DR, Dugdale DC. Peripheral Neuropathy. Medline Plus, US National Library of Medicine and National Institutes of Health. Web site. http://www.nlm.nih.gov/medlineplus/ency/article/000593.htm. Updated 2011, April 26. Accessed October 22, 2012.

19 Dietary supplement fact sheet: calcium. Office of Dietary Supplements, National Institutes of Health. Web site. http://ods.od.nih.gov/factsheets/Calcium-HealthProfessional/. Reviewed August 1, 2012. Accessed October 20, 2012.

20 Agricultural Research Service, U.S. Department of Agriculture. USDA national nutrient database for standard reference, release 18: sodium, Na (mg) content of selected foods per common measure, sorted by nutrient content. http://www.nal.usda.gov/fnic/foodcomp/Data/SR18/nutrlist/sr18w307.pdf. 2011. Accessed October 20, 2012.

21 Myklebust M, Wunder J. Healing foods pyramid: water. University of Michigan Health System. Web site. http://www.med.umich.edu/umim/food-pyramid/water.htm. 2010. Accessed October 20, 2012.

22 Cordova, A.C., et al. The cardiovascular protective effect of red wine. Journal of the American College of Surgeons. 2005;200:428-438.

23 Beyond hangovers: understanding alcohol's impact on your health. National Institute on Alcohol Abuse and Alcoholism, National Institutes of Health. Web site. http://pubs.niaaa.nih.gov/publications/Hangovers/beyondHangovers.pdf. Accessed October 22, 2012.

24 Woodard GA, Downey J, Hernandez-Boussard T, Morton JM. Impaired alcohol metabolism after gastric bypass surgery: a case-crossover trial. J Am Coll Surg. 2011 Feb;212(2):209-14

25 Guidance for industry: a food labeling guide. Center for Food Safety and Applied Nutrition. Food and Drug Administration. Web site. http://www.fda.gov/Food/GuidanceComplianceRegulatoryInformation/GuidanceDocuments/FoodLabelingNutrition/FoodLabelingGuide/default.htm. Revised 2009, October. Accessed October 22, 2012.

26 U.S. Congress. (2010). Food, Drug and Cosmetic Act. U.S. Code of Federal Regulations. *Government Printing Office*, Washington, D.C

27 U.S. Congress. (2011). Title 21, U.S. Code of Federal Regulations. *Government Printing Office*, Washington, D.C

28 National Organic Program. US Department of Agriculture. Web site. http://www.ams.usda.gov/AMSv1.0/nop. 2012, June 6. Accessed October 22, 2012.

29 Nutrition information for raw fruits, vegetables and fish. U.S. Food and Drug Administration. Web site. http://www.fda.gov/Food/LabelingNutrition/FoodLabelingGuidanceRegulatoryInformation/InformationforRestaurantsRetailEstablishments/ucm063367.htm. 2009. Accessed October 22, 2012.

30 U.S. Congress. (2011). Title 9, U.S. Code of Federal Regulations. *Government Printing Office*, Washington, D.C.

31 Bureau of Alcohol, Tobacco and Firearms. Web site. http://www.fsis.usda.gov/PDF/Nutrition_labeling_Q&A_041312.pdf. 2012. Accessed October 22, 2012.

16

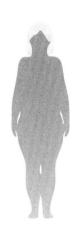

Physical Activity to Control Weight Loss

Safe recovery from surgery and the RYGB diet are essential for losing weight and staying healthy. After reading the past few chapters, you know how to take care of yourself to minimize complications and to eat a nutritious diet for weight loss.

A healthy lifestyle is not just about diet. Starting an exercise program can improve your health and promote weight loss and maintenance. You might have avoided exercise for years because it was uncomfortable, you felt self-conscious, it felt useless, or you simply did not like it. Maybe you did not even know what to do!

This chapter can change all that by covering the following topics:

- Why exercise is good for your weight and health
- Recommended types and amounts of exercise
- How a complete beginner can safely and gradually start a physical activity program when you still have a lot of weight to lose
- How to make your program more advanced as you progress
- How to stick to your exercise program for the long term

Exercise and physical activity are used interchangeably in this chapter, so do not worry about which term is used. Now, let's get moving!

The Importance of Physical Activity

Exercise is good for you for an almost unlimited number of reasons. Most people think of weight loss first when they think of exercise; next, you might think about heart health. Exercise has other physical and mental benefits, and of course, exercise makes you look pretty good too! At any weight, a firmer, more toned body is more attractive!

Physical Activity Burns Calories to Help You Control Your Weight

Physical activity helps you control your weight because it burns calories. You burn calories while you are actually exercising, and physical activity boosts your metabolism so that you burn additional calories throughout the day. Plus, building muscles is good for your weight because muscles use more calories than your body fat whether you are exercising or resting.

In general, the more you exercise, the more calories you burn and the faster you lose weight. The National Weight Control Registry, which follows individuals who have lost weight and kept it off for at least a year, reported that more than 90 percent of its members included physical activity in their successful weight loss and weight maintenance programs.[1]

So how many calories does exercise burn? It depends on which activity, how long you work out, how hard you exercise (your intensity), and how much you weigh.

How Many Calories Can You Burn with Exercise?

Online calculators provide fairly accurate information on your calorie burn. The U.S. Department of Health and Human Services suggests one from the Calorie Control Council.[2] Many other calculators are also available online.

For a quick reference, just so you can get an idea of how many calories different types of activities burn, refer to *Table 40,* which is a table of calories burned doing different activities at different weights.[3] These numbers are for an hour of exercise.

Activity	Your Weight			
	160 pounds	200 pounds	250 pounds	300 pounds
aerobics, low-impact	364	455	568	682
basketball, shooting baskets	327	409	511	614
bicycling, stationary, easy effort	255	318	398	477
bicycling, stationary, vigorous effort	495	618	773	927
circuit training	313	391	489	586
dancing, average	291	364	455	545
elliptical trainer	436	545	682	818
frisbee or catch	218	273	341	409
golf, walking, carrying clubs	313	391	489	586
Pilates	218	273	341	409
run and walk combination	436	545	682	818
running/jogging, 6.0 mph (10 minutes per mile)	713	891	1114	1336
stretching	167	209	261	314
swimming	423	528	632	737
tennis, doubles	327	409	511	614
walking, slowly, 2.0 miles per hour (mph)	204	255	318	382
walking, medium, 3.0 mph	255	318	398	477
walking, fast, 4.0 mph	364	455	568	682
walking, uphill at 3 percent grade, 3.5 mph	385	482	602	723
water aerobics	385	482	602	723
weight lifting, 8 to 12 repetitions per set	255	318	398	477
yoga, Hatha	182	227	284	341
yoga, power	291	364	455	545

Table 40: Calories burned doing different activities at different weights

Keeping Your Calorie Burn High

Doing the same activity, heavier individuals burn more calories per hour than lighter ones. That is discouraging because, as you lose weight, you will burn calories slower doing the same activities as when you were heavier.

On the other hand, you are going to be in much better shape as you exercise and lose weight. You will be able to exercise for longer and at a higher intensity. So you can still keep your calorie burn up pretty high. As an example, you might walk slowly for 20 minutes when you weigh 300 pounds and burn about 182 calories.[4] Let's say that you keep your exercise program up for a while and lose a lot of weight. Let's say that you get down to 200 pounds. You would only burn 85 calories if you walked slowly for 20 minutes. More likely, though, you will be more comfortable working out longer and harder. You might be able to jog for 40 minutes and burn 242 calories without feeling as tired as you did when you were walking slowly at a weight of 300 pounds.

> **Tip**
>
> Chapter 2, "Options for Losing Weight: Diets, Exercise, Weight Loss Drugs, and Surgery," talks about burning calories through exercise and the fact that exercise on its own is not enough to get you to lose weight and keep it off. You also need to follow your RYGB diet.

You lose a pound of body fat every time you burn off an extra 3,500 calories. Exercise helps, but it is just a small component of the lifestyle changes that you are making in order to lose weight as quickly as you had hoped. At 300 pounds, you would have to burn 500 calories per day, which is the equivalent of walking for an hour a day, to lose an extra pound per week. Sticking to the RYGB diet, even if you are pretty active, is necessary to keep shedding the pounds.

Physical Activity Helps Prevent or Manage Obesity-Related Diseases

We have already talked about the numerous diseases that are related to obesity. Having some of these conditions or being afraid of developing them might have influenced you to get the gastric bypass. Losing weight can reduce your risk of developing many health conditions or make them less severe. Exercise not only helps you lose weight but also improves your physical health.[5]

Exercise Improves Your Heart Health

Heart disease is the top killer of Americans. Your obesity likely caused risk factors for heart disease, such as high blood cholesterol levels and blood pressure. Exercise has many positive effects on your heart health:[6]

- It lowers your risk of developing heart disease.
- It raises levels of your HDL cholesterol, which is the healthy kind.
- It lowers your blood pressure. That means that your heart does not have to work so hard, so you are less likely to get a kind of heart disease called congestive heart failure. Lower blood pressure also lowers your risk of stroke.
- It lowers your LDL cholesterol, which is the bad kind of cholesterol.
- It lowers your levels of unhealthy triglycerides in your blood.
- It reduces your chances of developing atherosclerosis, or hardening of the arteries.
- It makes your lungs stronger, so your blood flow is more efficient and your heart does not have to work as hard.

Physical Activity May Lower Your Risk for Certain Cancers

Cancer is the second leading cause of death in the U.S., right behind heart disease. While scientists do not know everything about cancer, they think exercise can protect you against certain kinds. The American Cancer Society recommends regular physical activity to lower your risk for breast, colorectal, kidney, pancreatic, prostate, stomach, and lower esophageal cancers.[7]

Physical Activity May Improve Your Blood Sugar Control

Exercise helps your body regulate blood sugar to help prevent or manage pre-diabetes or diabetes.[8] Better blood sugar management is great news because it helps prevent diabetes complications such as heart disease, kidney disease, blindness, infections, and amputations. Exercise helps keep blood sugar low by helping your working muscles use glucose (sugar) for energy instead of letting it sit in your blood. Physical activity also fights type 2 diabetes by reducing dangerous insulin resistance.[9]

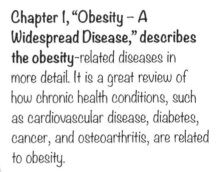

Tip

Chapter 1, "Obesity – A Widespread Disease," describes the obesity-related diseases in more detail. It is a great review of how chronic health conditions, such as cardiovascular disease, diabetes, cancer, and osteoarthritis, are related to obesity.

Physical Activity Often Helps Relieve Osteoarthritis

You may have osteoarthritis if you have chronic pain in your knees, hips, and other joints. Obesity may be to blame for your osteoarthritis, which is described as wear and tear on your joints. Extra body weight really increases the strain. Sometimes all you want to do when you have osteoarthritis is sit or lie down, but exercising is more likely to help than avoiding activity.

Surprisingly, most kinds of gentle or moderate physical activity can reduce your pain and swelling. This may be because physical activity increases your blood flow to the injured joint, helping to soothe and heal it. Exercise may increase your flexibility and range of motion so that you can start to feel like you are *moving* your body instead of *straining* it. People with arthritis that exercise have more mobility and higher quality of life. Stick with exercises that do not cause pain, and ask a physical therapist or your doctor if you are not sure about what to do.

If you have osteoarthritis because of your obesity, you can probably start exercising sooner after your gastric bypass surgery than you might expect. You do not have to lose hundreds of pounds before you can exercise. In one study, bariatric surgery patients had significantly less pain and better mobility after only three months.[10]

Exercise Helps You Live Longer!

By the way, you are more likely to live longer if you exercise regularly than if you avoid physical activity. That is a pretty good reason to start exercising!

Exercise Supports Healthy Bones

Some kinds of exercise are good for your bones. That is important for everyone but especially for you as a RYGB patient. Many bariatric surgery patients develop low bone mineral density, or osteoporosis, and are at a high risk for bone fractures.

- Your intake of bone nutrients, such as vitamin D, calcium, and vitamin K, may be low because of your restricted diet.
- You can have lower absorption of bone nutrients.
- Rapid weight loss can cause rapid loss of bone mineral density. You cannot regain much bone mineral density back after you are about 30 years old.

How Physical Activity Can Improve Bone Health

Physical activity can be a powerful weapon in your collection of tools to prevent osteoporosis. Your bones are constantly changing. Their bone mineral is always breaking down and building back up in a process called remodeling. When you are under 30 years old, you gain bone mineral density (BMD) faster than you lose it so that your bones are getting stronger.[11] You hit your peak bone mineral density around 30 years old. Then you lose bone mineral faster than you gain it. For the rest of your life, your goal is to slow the loss of bone mineral density and keep your bones as strong as possible. Getting plenty of calcium and vitamin D is one important strategy to preserve your bones. Exercise is another.

This is how it works. Exercise stresses your bones. Your bones' response is to compensate by growing stronger. It is a lot like how your muscles work—when you lift heavy weights, your muscles compensate by growing stronger.

Choosing the Best Exercises for Your Bones

The exercises that help your bones are known as *weight-bearing activities*. You can choose to do high-impact or low-impact weight-bearing activities to help your bones out.[12]

Low-impact activities: In low-impact activities, at least one foot is always on the ground. These are good ones to start with when you are not that experienced with exercise. They do not burn as many calories as high-impact activities, but they are not as likely to cause injuries. These are some examples:

- Strength or resistance training. You can lift weights, do exercises that use your own body weight, or use a resistance loop. We will talk more about strength training later in the chapter.
- Using the elliptical machine at the gym, especially when you increase the resistance and use the handlebars to work your arms and back as well as your legs
- Dancing or low-impact aerobics
- Walking or hiking
- Stair climbers or step machines
- Downhill skiing

High-impact activities: These usually involve leaving the ground. They can be high-intensity and fun, but they are not for beginners. High-impact activities are challenging and can cause injuries if you are not ready for them. Save them for when you are in good shape and you have lost a good amount of weight.

Here are some examples of high-impact activities that can help your bones:

- High-impact aerobics
- Jogging or running
- Dancing
- Basketball, soccer, and tennis
- Jumping rope
- Cross-country skiing
- Dancing with a lot of jumping

You will notice that some activities are on both lists. A lot of activities, such as dancing and aerobics, can be modified to be high-impact or low-impact.

Some Exercises Have Other Health Benefits but Do Not Strengthen Your Bones

Swimming, water aerobics, rowing, and biking are examples of activities that are non-weight-bearing. These exercises provide many of the other great benefits of exercise, such as burning calories, helping with arthritis, reducing stress, and improving your cardiovascular fitness. But they do not have much effect on your bones. You also need to regularly include weight-bearing activities in your exercise program if you want to protect your bones.

Keep Exercising to Maintain Strong Bones

Staying active is just as important as *getting* active because you can lose bone density quickly when you stop exercising. This can happen within just a few weeks, and the effects can last for months. Here is the information:

- People that are confined to a few weeks of bed rest lose some bone mineral and continue to have lower bone density for more than five months after their hospital stays.[13]
- Being in outer space is a lot like skipping weight-bearing activity because of the lack of gravity that makes astronauts feel weightless. Astronauts can lose their bone mineral density 6 to 12 times as fast as the average adult on Earth.[14] What is the take-home message? Start an exercise program and stick with it—consistency really pays off!

The Psychosocial Benefits of Physical Activity

Physical activity is not just good for your physical health. It is also great for your psychosocial health—your mental and emotional health. These benefits are very well-documented, and many of them have biological explanations—so they are not just in your head!

Exercise Relieves Stress

Physical activity reduces stress.[15] Exercise might help you relax through a variety of possible ways:

- Repetitive motions such as walking can be calming. Taking a walk is a far healthier repetitive motion than emotional eating if you are trying to handle stress!
- The regularity of your exercise sessions can be comforting. You get to look forward to your exercise, and once you start, the familiar activities let you feel in control instead of anxious.
- Your mind gets a chance to wander. You can think through your day without interruptions or the pressure of coming to any conclusions immediately.
- Exercise changes your hormone levels to improve your mood.

Exercise Improves Your Energy Levels

Morning exercisers find that they are sharper and more alert throughout the day. Some people find that they like exercising in the evening because it takes the fatigue away after a long day at work. And still others like to exercise on their lunch hour—because they say it prevents them from wanting to take a mid-afternoon nap. Experiment to find the time that is best for you.

Regular exercise is also good for your energy because it improves sleep. You will sleep more deeply and wake up more refreshed when you get into a regular exercise routine. Starting an exercise program can reduce insomnia too.[16]

Exercise Is Good for Your Brain

Exercise can even make you smarter! Activity increases your blood flow to your brain so your brain gets more oxygen and nutrients. Physically fit adults have more active brains and better performances on cognitive tests[17] and are mentally sharper[18] than adults that do not exercise. Better yet, the effects do not stop when you are done exercising for the day. Adults that exercise have more white matter, which is the thinking part, in their brains.[19] So keep exercising and becoming smarter! Nobody will believe you when you tell them why you are suddenly being even sharper on the job!

Exercise Makes You Happier

Plenty of anecdotal and scientific evidence show that exercise improves your mood. One reason is related to what is known as the "runner's high." It is the release of chemicals, called opioids or endorphins that activate different parts of your brain to make you happy.[20] Luckily, the "runner's high" is not just for runners. Anyone that exercises can get the same effects!

Exercise Improves Your Confidence

The victories that you achieve during an exercise program increase your confidence in the rest of your life. Exercise provides so many opportunities for you to succeed. You can be proud of yourself for:

- Getting up early and going to the gym even though you did not want to
- Going a minute longer or 0.1 mph faster on the treadmill than you ever had before
- Trying a new fitness class that you never would have dared to do before getting your surgery
- Finishing what is now "just a regular workout" — because in the old days, you would not have even started

When you succeed at these challenges, you start to realize that you can succeed at challenges in your everyday life.

Exercise Can Improve Your Social Life

You have many opportunities to meet people through exercise:

- *At the gym:* Everyone at the gym has the same basic goals that you do — to control weight and improve health and fitness. A workout partner or small workout group can keep you company on the cardio equipment and while lifting weights. Do not be shy about asking people to work out with you, and do not take it personally if they prefer to work out alone. Just ask someone else.
- *In group fitness classes*: Strike up a conversation before or after class. You might want to schedule a workout together for the next day or ask someone to join you for coffee after class. You might find a new workout partner or even a good friend.
- *Online:* Use search engines to see if you can join up with individuals or groups in your area. Many groups are specifically started for obese adults that want to lose weight, and you can make unbelievably deep connections if you are able to exercise your way through your weight loss journey with someone that is in the same boat as you. Members that attend your gastric bypass or bariatric surgery support group meetings are great candidates because you know they live in your area.
- *In the park:* Tag along with walkers — you will be surprised at how many of them are looking for company too.

Exercise does not just help you make new friends. You can take advantage of your new exercise program to strengthen your old relationships with friends and family. Getting through workouts together is one of the most supportive things you can do for each other.

Even if you prefer to exercise alone, your exercise program can improve your social life because of the way you carry yourself. Instead of being ashamed of yourself, you will be proud of that body of yours that is capable of doing the physical activity that you have demanded of it. People will respond better to you when you are proud of ourself.

Help! I Am Afraid That People Are Making Fun of Me When I Am Exercising!

You walk into the fitness center. To the right, heavily muscled men are pumping iron. To the left, skinny women in tank tops are using treadmills, stationary bikes, and elliptical trainers. And in the group exercise room, there are about 20 highly fit and coordinated people following their aerobics instructor in perfect synch. The whole scene makes you want to turn around and run out of there as fast as you can before anyone sees your imperfect body and questionable fitness skills. But wait!

A huge concern for many obese people is that other people will look down on them. It can be such a strong fear that it can threaten your fitness program, but you can overcome it. Yes, it is tough to walk into a gym full of strangers that look like they are confident and that are in great shape when you are not feeling so confident in yourself. They might even come off as snobbish or arrogant. But you know what? In most cases, it is all in your head.

Most of the people at the gym are just like you. They have careers and families too, and the gym is just one part of their busy lives. They have the same reasons for exercising that you do—they want to be healthy, control their weight, and relieve stress. They have their good workouts and bad workouts, just like you, and they have to drag themselves out of bed or away from the couch to get to the gym, just like you. They are focused on their own workouts and lives and may not even notice you. If they do, these regular exercisers are far more likely to admire than disrespect you because they know how much effort you are putting in.

Remember we said that "in most cases, it is all in your head"? Well, we admit that occasionally you will run into gym snobs, just like you run into snobs occasionally in the rest of your life. There are the clothing snobs that judge your lack of designer clothing, the car snobs that think your car is not worth driving, the coffee snobs that would not be caught dead drinking anything other than their favorite brand of coffee and…well, you get the point. At the gym, just like in every crowd, there is that someone that tries to ruin it for everyone else. So keep in mind that it is in their head, not yours, and let it be their problem if they do not like the way your biceps look. You have just as much right to the dumbbells as they do.

So what do people think about you when exercising? These are some likely possibilities:

- "Who cares?" (They barely notice you because they are wrapped up in their own workouts.)

- "You are the best." (They recognize the challenges you are overcoming and are inspired by your dedication.)

- "You are not good enough." (These are snobs that do not think anyone is good enough, so do not take it personally. In fact, take it as a compliment because, really, who would wants the approval of snobs?)

How Much Should You Exercise?

How much do you need to exercise to get the benefits? The ASMBS guideline for bariatric surgery patients is to aim for 30 minutes on most days.[21] Only one-quarter of patients tend to hit that amount though.[22]

The 30-minute-per-day recommendation is consistent with national guidelines from the Centers for Disease Control and Prevention, or CDC, for healthy adults to aim for at least 30 minutes on most days of the week.[23] Later in this section, we will break down the types of exercise that you should include to get to your 30 minutes per day.

Do Not Limit Yourself!

Extra exercise may have additional benefits. You will still get a lot of the benefits of exercise if you hit your 30 minutes per day on most days of the week, and you will be way ahead of the average American. In fact, only half of Americans meet CDC recommendations to exercise at least 30 minutes for five times a week at a moderate intensity or for at least 20 minutes three times a week at a vigorous intensity.[24]

You can get even more benefits if you increase your exercise beyond these goals. The Weight-Control Information Network, or WIN, is part of the National Institutes of Health. The organization states that aiming for about 60 minutes per day can help you lose weight.[25] And you have heard—and maybe even experienced for yourself in a previous yo-yo diet cycle—that keeping the weight off is even harder than losing it in the first place. The WIN suggests aiming for 60 to 90 minutes per day of exercise to maintain significant weight loss—which is what you will achieve within years of gastric bypass if you stick to the diet.

Exercise Like the Weight Loss Pros:
The National Weight Control Registry

The National Weight Control Registry, or NWCR, is a list of people nationwide that have successfully lost weight and kept it off. It was started by doctors at Brown Medical School in Rhode Island and the University of Colorado. You can only sign up to join the registry after you have lost at least 30 pounds and kept it off for at least a year, and there are currently more than 10,000 members.

The goal of the NWCR is to discover how people lose weight and keep it off. The NWCR gathers data through questionnaires that ask members about their diet, physical activity, and other health habits that may be related to their weight loss success. The results have been interesting!

Sources:[26, 27, 28, 29]

Habits That Prevent Weight Regain

Just under half of participants lost their weight on their own; the other half used a program. Two-thirds of these role models keep their weight off by limiting themselves to no more than ten hours of television per week. Three-quarters of them eat breakfast every day and weigh themselves at least weekly. They follow low-fat, low-calorie diets, and compared to average Americans, their diets tend to be more nutritious, with a higher amount of calcium, vitamin C, and vitamin A.

Exercise and Weight Maintenance

The NWCR has found that nine out of every ten NWCR members exercise for at least an hour per day. They burn, on average, about 400 calories per day through a variety of activities, such as running, aerobics, bicycling, and weight lifting. This amount and intensity of exercise is a little more than the CDC's minimum recommendation to get at least 30 minutes per day on most days of the week, but it is doable. It is very motivational to know that your hard work can pay off, just like it does for members of the NWCR.

Aerobic Exercise: What it is and How Much to Do

Aerobic exercise is often called "cardio" because of its effects on your cardiovascular system, or your heart and blood vessels. Aerobic exercise is what a lot of us just think of as "exercise." It gets your heart rate up for a continuous period of time. You breathe a little deeper and faster to get more oxygen into your lungs and to your blood. Your heart pumps harder and faster so you can circulate more blood and get enough oxygen to your working muscles.

Recommendations for how much aerobic exercise to get depend on intensity. National recommendations for healthy adults are to get at least 150 minutes of moderate-intensity aerobic exercise per week, or at least 75 minutes of vigorous intensity aerobic exercise per week, or a combination of the two.[30] You can do any combination of moderate or vigorous activity. Here are some examples:

- 30 minutes of moderate intensity physical activity on five separate days
- 15 minutes of moderate intensity on five separate days
- 30 minutes of moderate intensity physical activity on two days and 15 minutes of vigorous intensity physical activity on three days
- An hour of moderate intensity physical activity on two days and 15 minutes of vigorous intensity physical activity on one day
- 25 minutes of vigorous physical activity on three days

Moderate versus Vigorous Physical Activity

To help you determine whether you are doing moderate or vigorous physical activities, the National Heart Lung and Blood Institute provides several examples of common lists of activities and their intensities.[31]

Moderate physical activities

- Walking
- Dancing
- Leisurely bicycling
- Water aerobics
- Mowing the lawn and other gardening activities
- Washing the windows
- Shooting hoops, non-competitively
- Using a rowing machine at the gym

Vigorous physical activities

- Jogging or running
- Walking uphill
- Swimming laps quickly
- Playing full-court basketball, soccer, or an intense game of tennis
- High-impact step aerobics
- Elliptical machine at the gym

Moderate and vigorous physical activity can change depending on how fit you are and how much effort you put into it. At the beginning of your weight loss journey, you might sweat buckets and be huffing and puffing just by walking slowly around the block. That is vigorous physical activity. By the time you have lost some weight and you are fitter, slow walking might be moderate physical activity. To raise the intensity so that walking counts as a vigorous activity, you might speed up or walk uphill.

You Can Break Up Your Exercise Sessions

On some days, setting aside 15 to 60 minutes for a single workout might not be possible. You can always break up your exercise into smaller sessions. Instead of a 30-minute walk, for example, you can squeeze in a quick 10-minute walk during your lunch break, another 10 minutes before coming home from work, and your final 10 minutes after dinner.

Breaking it up can make your exercise easier mentally too. If you are feeling tired after dinner, you might end up not doing anything if you feel obligated to commit to a full 30 minutes. Instead, you might find it easier to get moving for 10 minutes. Everything you do counts, so do not let an all-or-nothing attitude turn your exercise routine into "nothing." In general, when it comes to exercise, some is better than none, and more is better than less.

How Hard Should You Exercise?

Exactly how do you know if you are exercising at the right level for the maximum benefits when you are in the middle of a cardio workout? Your perceived exertion is the simplest method. Aerobic exercise should be tough enough to make you feel like you are working but not so hard that you think you are going to collapse. A general way to tell if you are in your aerobic zone is to do the talk test. You should be able to talk in short sentences but not have enough breath to sing a song.

You can also use your heart rate as a guide if you know your maximum heart rate. If you do not, you can use the standard formula of 220 minus your age to estimate your maximum heart rate, but keep in mind that individual maximum heart rates can vary a lot. Once you get your maximum heart rate, multiply it by 0.5 to get the target by getting the value of 50 percent of your maximum heart rate, which is the low end of an aerobic workout. Multiply your maximum by 0.8 to find out 80 percent of your maximum heart rate, which is about the high end of your aerobic workout zone.

Here is an example. Let's say you are 42 years old:

- Your estimated maximum heart rate is 220 minus 42, or 178 beats per minute.
- Your lower end goal is 0.5 times 178, or 89 beats per minute.
- Your upper end goal is 0.8 times 178, or 142 beats per minute.
- You want to keep your heart rate between 89 and 142 beats per minute. That is a pretty big range. It gives you plenty of room for easy days, hard days, and everything in between.

Here are a few tips for keeping it simple:

- Online calculators can save you trouble. Organizations like the American Council on Exercise, American Cancer Society, and National Institutes of Health, along with a bunch of other websites, have calculators that will tell you your goal heart rate. You can just put in your age and get the guidelines.
- You can use a heart rate monitor that consists of a chest strap and a wrist watch or just a wrist watch. Most sporting goods stores sell them, and a sales associate can help you out when you are choosing one.
- You can take your pulse by yourself if you do not want to buy or wear a heart rate monitor. Place your index and middle finger (not your thumb) on your carotid artery on either side of your Adam's apple in your neck. Count the beats for 6 seconds, multiply by ten, and that is your heart rate. So if you count to 13 in six seconds, your heart rate is 13x10, or 130 beats per minute.

- It is not a precise science. It is okay if your workout ends up harder or easier than you had intended. Over time you will figure out the zones that work best for you, and you will not even have to consciously think about staying in your aerobic zone.

- Give yourself a while to warm up before thinking about your heart rate. Your heart rate will take at least five minutes to increase from resting up to your aerobic zone.

Sources:[32, 33]

Strength or Resistance Training: What It Is and How Much to Do

Strength training is also known as resistance training or weight training. This portion of your exercise program is good for your muscles and bones as well as your looks. Strength training is not just for body builders and men. It is for anyone that is interested in a well-rounded exercise program, a tight and toned appearance, faster metabolism, and increased confidence from being stronger.

Aim for Two Sessions per Week for Each Major Muscle Group

Your major muscle groups are your hips, legs, shoulders, back, abdomen, and arms. Try to include exercises that target each of these groups at least twice per week.[34] You do not have to hit all the major muscle groups each time you do your strength training. You can break up your workouts however you want. Here are some examples:

- You can do all of your muscles in one workout, and do that twice per week.

- You can do your legs and hips two days a week, and your back, shoulders, abdomen, and arms on two other days.

- You can do your hips and legs on two days, your core (back and abdomen) on two days, and your arms and shoulders on two days. That is a great schedule if you just want to get in a quick strength-training session after your cardio workouts but you do not want to set aside too long for your resistance training.

When you do your strength training, you should choose activities and weights that get you tired after 8 to 12 repetitions.[35] Those 8 to 12 repetitions count as one set, and you should be tired and want to rest after them. To count as a strength training session, you only have to do one set for each muscle! You can do two sets if you want though. Just rest for a little bit after the first set before you start your second set of 8 to 12 repetitions. If 8 to 12 repetitions becomes too easy, increase the weight until it becomes challenging again.

Ask for Help if You Need It

Proper form, or technique, reduces your risk for injuries from strength training, and it gives you better results. Resistance training is not as natural as, say, walking, so it is a good idea to ask an expert to show you good form when you are first starting your resistance training program. A physical therapist or a trainer at the gym can give you beginner modifications and watch to correct your form and technique. Group fitness class instructors demonstrate proper form and can give you pointers. You can also look online for descriptions, photos, and videos of various exercises for more guidance.

You Have Many Different Options for Strength Training Equipment

Familiar weights, such as dumbbells and barbells, are just the start of your options for your strength training sessions. These are some traditional and less traditional choices for improving your strength.

Traditional options:

- *Dumbbells:* These are great to have at home or to use at the gym. Just hold them in your hands and get your workout in.
- *Barbells*: These include a bar with weights in the shape of disks at the end. Barbells can be pretty heavy, so you probably will not be using them for a while.
- *Big resistance machines:* Weight benches and exercise-specific weight training machines at the gym are designed to target certain muscles. They work pretty well, but they may be uncomfortable for you to use when you are still very overweight.
- *Multi-Gyms: These* are available at most gyms, and they come in home-designed models in case you get very enthusiastic about your weight-training program. You can work out each major muscle group on a multi-gym.
- *Kettlebells:* These are round, steel balls that have a handle. A lot of workouts are designed using one kettlebell. Kettlebells are pretty fun to use and give you some variety. Kettlebell workouts often double as cardio workouts because they can get your heart rate up in a hurry.

Other options:

- *Body weight:* Many exercises do not require any equipment at all! Pushups (start on your knees, not your toes, when you are a beginner), sit-ups and crunches, arm raises, calf raises, squats, dips, and lunges do not require any equipment. Your own body weight is great resistance.
- *Resistance band or loop*: These elastic bands come in different sizes and resistance levels, and you can use them to work your whole body.
- *Stability ball*: These big balls look like giant beach balls. They are good for challenging your whole body because you have to work on balancing while you are using them for exercises.[36] You can use them for almost anything, such as crunches, push-ups, squats, and planks.

- *Medicine ball*: These are heavy balls that you can use to work your arms, shoulders, back, and abdominals. You can even use them to strengthen your legs if you hold one while doing lunges.
- *Soup cans*: Each one weighs about a pound, so soup cans are great for making the transition from no weights to heavier weights.

Strength Training Can Help You Lose Weight

Most strength training exercises burn fewer calories per minute than most aerobic exercises, but strength training can play an important role in your weight loss. Strength training builds and maintains your muscle mass. Muscle tissue is *metabolically active*; it burns more calories at rest than fat does. Strength training can keep you from losing muscle mass and having a slower metabolism, which is especially important for RYGB patients that are losing weight rapidly. You cannot avoid losing a small amount of muscle mass when you lose weight, but strength training can greatly reduce the amount of muscle mass that you lose.

Strength training can do double duty as an aerobic workout. We just talked about aerobic exercise as being physical activity that keeps your heart rate up for a continuous period of time. You can turn strength training into an aerobic workout by moving without stopping. Here are a couple of ideas for getting your heart rate up while strength training:

- Progress to the next set of repetitions as soon as you finish one set. The first set will make your muscles tired, so the next set of repetitions should target a different muscle group. For example, if you just worked your arms, do some leg exercises for your next set of 8 to 12 repetitions. Then move on to your back and then back to your arms. Think about moving on to the next muscle group as soon as one becomes tired. The first portion of your workout might consist of:
  - 8 to 12 reps of bicep curls
  - 8 to 12 reps of lunges
  - 8 to 12 reps of chest presses
  - 8 to 12 reps of bicep curls
  - 8 to 12 reps of lunges
  - 8 to 12 reps of chest presses
  - Then you would move on to another set of exercises, such as tricep dips, squats, and seated rows.
- Keep moving in between sets instead of sitting still to recover. Walking or marching in place can keep your heart rate up as your muscles recover for the next set of 8 to 12 repetitions.

When you turn your strength training into an aerobic workout, you burn more calories and do not have to spend as long on your exercise. This is how you can turn resistance training into an aerobic workout.

You will know that you are getting a good cardio workout in if your heart rate is in your zone (that is 50 to 80 percent of your maximum heart rate), if your breathing is heavy, and if you can talk but not sing. You are getting a good resistance training workout if your muscles are burning at the end of each set of 8 to 12 repetitions.

Flexibility

Many people think of this as an "extra," but it is essential to fitness. Stretch at each workout or at least three times per week. Stretching improves your flexibility, which makes you less likely to get injured. It lengthens your muscles and helps them recover better from your workouts so that you are feeling ready to go again by the next day or the next time you have a workout scheduled. Other potential benefits of stretching include reducing stress and improving your posture.[37]

When you stretch, think about working the same muscle groups that you do when you lift weights. That is, try to hit each of the major muscle groups. A physical therapist or staff member at a gym can get you started with effective stretches. Traditional stretching, yoga, and stretching with a rope can improve your flexibility.

Build Up Slowly to Prevent Injuries

The above goals for the amount of exercise you should do are long-term goals for more experienced exercisers. Do not worry about hitting these goals for exercise when you are first starting your program. Instead, just focus on getting in the amount that is comfortable for you. That might be just one or two minutes at a time to start with. You have plenty of time to build up the time you spend exercising as your weight continues to come off and your physical fitness improves.

Everyone Needs Regular Rest Days

Rest is a crucial part of an exercise program for beginners and world-class athletes:

- It lets your body heal so you are less likely to get injured
- It lets your muscles build up so they are stronger than before
- Gives you a mental break so you are eager to get back in the game the next day

Just as you have been learning to listen to your body as you follow the gastric bypass diet, you need to learn to listen to your body when you are starting an exercise program. Learn to recognize the difference between being lazy and truly needing a day off. A general rule of thumb when you are not sure is to try your warm-up. If you finish your warm-up and still feel more tired than you should, you need a day off. However, if you feel good after warming up, you probably do not need a day off right now.

Restrictions after the RYGB

Such a life-changing experience as getting the RYGB naturally can make you wonder whether you need to avoid certain activities. As long as your surgery wounds are fully healed and you start new activities only slowly and gradually, the RYGB should not interfere with your workout routine. Just be sure to get your physician's approval before starting any new activity. RYGB patients can successfully participate in a range of activities, such as the following:

- Water activities, such as swimming, water jogging, and water aerobics
- Weight-lifting, as long as you don't strain yourself
- Walking, running, and hiking
- Dancing and aerobics
- Sports, such as basketball and tennis

The main precaution that you can take is to warm up well before exercising, which is what everyone should do anyway. Warming up helps prevent you from straining your abdominal muscles and taking the risk of splitting seams from surgery. Your surgeon can advise you on any restricted activities, but there will not be many of them.

Everything Counts!

As you develop your exercise program and count your minutes of exercise, try to keep your ultimate goals in mind: you want to lose weight and get healthy. Each bit of movement that you do takes you a step closer to achieving your goals.

- It helps you develop new lifestyle habits as part of a new lifestyle. Walking an extra minute or two to cool down after your workout, parking farther away from the store, and taking the stairs at work can all become habitual.
- A few extra minutes of exercise can translate into measurable calories and noticeable weight loss. Every bit helps you lose weight and improve your health, even if you are not logging it as part of your exercise for the day.
- It keeps you motivated. It is easy to get discouraged if you think that you have to do a lengthy workout just to benefit from exercise. Instead, you can be confident that walking to the corner after dinner and doing knee bends during commercial breaks are absolutely worth the effort.

Everything counts, so keep moving!

Starting and Developing Your Exercise Routine

The first part of the chapter covered why exercise is beneficial and how much you should eventually aim for. You know the *what, why,* and *when.* Now it is time to get down to the nitty-gritty — the *how* of exercise. Starting an exercise can be almost overwhelming if you have never exercised before or if it has been a while, but this section will walk you through it step by step.

Getting Active after the Roux-en-Y Gastric Bypass

Your body is not ready for a complete exercise program right after the gastric bypass surgery. You will need a few weeks before you can be medically cleared for most activities. By that time you will be into the solid foods diet phase, so it is a great time to develop a regular exercise routine that fits into your new lifestyle.

Activity after RYGB Surgery

Even though you cannot do vigorous exercise right after surgery, you can start some light activities. Light exercise will make the transition easier as you shift to more intense exercises later. It also might speed your recovery from surgery. Any gentle, painless movements you make increase blood flow and can help your wounds heal faster.

Small movements around the house can give you the benefits of exercise. You will be surprised about how much activity you can easily add to your daily life once you start trying. Here are a few possibilities:

> **Tip**
>
> Chapter 12, "Aftercare: Your Post-Surgery Care Program," talks about the slow return to activity after surgery. The chapter talks about avoiding heavy weights and water activities until you have healed a little bit and also about the benefits of keeping your body moving even during your recovery period.

- Walking around the house
- Folding the laundry (being careful not to carry a heavy, full laundry basket!)
- Standing up instead of sitting
- Cooking, setting the table, and washing the dishes
- Playing with children (without lifting them up, if you are still close to surgery)
- Light housecleaning, such as making the beds and washing the windows (but avoid carrying or pushing a heavy vacuum cleaner or scrubbing the floors if you are still close to surgery)
- Playing golf

You can start these activities as soon as you feel comfortable after getting home from the hospital. They are not formal parts of a specific exercise program, but they help you prepare for your planned exercise that will start about six weeks after surgery. Until then, slow walking is probably a safe option until you get your surgeon's go-ahead to add in aerobics or other, more intense activities.

Getting Medical Support and Clearance

People should check with their doctors before starting exercise programs if they have certain conditions. These include being overweight or obese, having heart disease, diabetes, arthritis, or asthma or other respiratory problems and if you have not exercised regularly for a while.[38] That almost certainly describes you! Seek medical clearance before starting your program because you are starting off at an obese weight, and you might have other medical conditions that you need to be careful of. Plus, you want to be absolutely certain that you are fully healed from your surgery so that you do not reopen wounds and risk infections or leakage. Your surgeon or your primary care physician can give you the go-ahead for an exercise program.

Take Advantage of Expert Help

We recommend taking advantage of any physical therapy services that you are entitled to through your insurance plan or as part of the aftercare package that your surgeon provides. Physical therapists and physical therapist assistants are trained to evaluate your physical abilities and limitations and design an appropriate exercise program to meet your goals.[39] They are skilled at designing pain-free, interesting exercise programs that let you make progress and eventually take charge of your own fitness.

Even without a physical therapist, you likely have access to helpful resources. Here are a few ideas:

- *A personal trainer at a local gym:* You might not want to pay the fees for a personal trainer, but many gyms and fitness centers provide free services to help you plan a program.

- *Your own friends, family members, and coworkers, if they know a bit about exercise*: Most regular exercisers are rightfully proud of their routines and are happy to share the knowledge they have gained.

- *A coach at a local high school or community college:* Some will be too busy to help you, but many will be glad to let you participate in practice and give you a few pointers.

- *Online resources:* The American Council on Exercise has an assortment of articles for beginning exercisers on goal-setting and performing various exercises.[40] It also provides links to additional resources.

- *This book:* We will guide you through a basic program starting at the beginning.

Online communities are great for advice too. BariatricPal.com, for example, is an online community whose members include thousands of weight loss surgery patients. They can share their own experiences with you so you have some ideas of what kind of exercises and progressions work for them. The forum is encouraging and has a zero tolerance for rudeness, and new members are always welcome and warmly greeted.

A medical professional should approve any new exercise that you plan to try. It is safest to inform your doctor or surgeon about your plans before you try anything new just to be sure you are ready.

Start Slowly after You Get Medical Clearance

Medical clearance to start your exercise program is permission to start slowly, not to jump into an intense Olympic training schedule. Starting out conservatively has a few benefits:

- It gives you a chance to find out what it feels like to exercise after gastric bypass.
- It reduces your risk of injuries.
- It prevents burn-out or mental fatigue from feeling obligated to do too much.
- It increases your motivation as you hit realistic goals.

Sample Plan for Starting a Workout Plan

Table 41 is an example of how you can get from being sedentary—doing almost no regular

	Monday	Tuesday	Wednesday	Thursday	Friday	Saturday	Sunday
Week 1	5 minute warm-up 5 minute cool down	5 minute warm up 5 minute cool down	Day off	5 minute warm-up 5 minutes medium-speed walking 5 minute cool down	5 minute warm-up 5 minute cool down	5 minute warm-up 5 minutes medium-speed walking 5 minute cool down	Day off
Week 2	5 minute warm-up 10 minutes medium-speed walking 5 minute cool down	5 minute warm-up 5 minutes medium-speed walking 5 minute cool down	Day off	5 minute warm-up 10 minutes medium-speed walking 5 minute cool down	5 minute warm-up 5 minutes medium-speed walking 5 minute cool down	5 minute warm-up 5 minutes brisk walking 5 minute cool down	Day off
Week 3	5 minute warm-up 15 minutes medium-speed walking 5 minute cool down	5 minute warm-up 5 minutes brisk walking 5 minute cool down	Day off	5 minute warm-up 15 minutes medium-speed walking 5 minute cool down	5 minute warm-up 5 minutes medium-speed walking 5 minute cool down	5 minute warm-up 10 minutes brisk walking 5 minute cool down	Day off
Week 4	5 minute warm-up 20 minutes medium-speed walking 5 minute cool down	5 minute warm-up 10 minutes medium-speed walking 5 minute cool down	Day off	5 minute warm-up 20 minutes medium-speed walking 5 minute cool down	5 minute warm-up 10 minutes medium-speed walking 5 minute cool down	5 minute warm-up 15 minutes brisk walking 5 minute cool down	Day off
Week 5	5 minute warm-up 20 minutes medium-speed walking—can add in 15 seconds of jogging if you feel good—can do this up to 5 times during the 20 minutes and walk in between each one 5 minute cool down	5 minute warm-up 10 minutes medium-speed walking 5 minute cool down	Day off	5 minute warm-up Same as Monday—jogging is optional. 5 minute cool down	5 minute warm-up 15 minutes medium-speed walking 5 minute cool down	5 minute warm-up 15 minutes brisk walking—can run up to 5 times but only if you feel great! 5 minute cool down	Day off

	Monday	Tuesday	Wednesday	Thursday	Friday	Saturday	Sunday
Week 6	5 minute warm-up 25 minutes of brisk walking alternating with up to six short jogs 5 minute cool down	5 minute warm-up 15 minutes of medium-speed walking 5 minute cool down	Day off	5 minute warm up 20 minutes of brisk walking with up to 6 short jogs 5 minute cool down	5 minute warm-up 20 minutes of medium-speed walking. 5 minute cool down	5 minute warm-up Same as last Friday—you can jog up to five times if you feel good. 5 minute cool down	Day off
Week 7	5 minute warm-up 25 minutes of brisk walking with as many as 10 short jogs 5 minute cool down	5 minute warm-up 15 minutes of medium-speed walking 5 minute cool down	Day off	5 minute warm-up 15 minutes of brisk walking with up to 5 jogs 5 minute cool down	5 minute warm-up 20 minutes of medium-speed walking 5 minute cool down	5 minute warm-up 20 minutes of brisk walking with up to 6 jogs. 5 minute cool down	Day off
Week 8	5 minute warm-up 30 minutes of brisk walking with jogs as you feel like it! 5 minute cool down	5 minute warm-up 20 minutes of medium speed walking 5 minute cool down	Day off	5 minute warm-up 20 minutes of brisk walking with short jogs 5 minute cool down	5 minute warm-up 25 minutes of medium-speed walking 5 minute cool down	5 minute warm-up 20 minutes of brisk walking and/or jogging 5 minute cool down	Day off
	Saturday	Sunday	Monday	Tuesday	Wednesday	Thursday	Friday

Table 41: Sample Plan for Starting a Workout Plan

physical activity—to becoming a regular walk-jogger. It is closer to your grasp than you probably think! This chart provides an example of an eight-week progression that is gradual and safe to follow with the supervision of your physician. Do not forget to include your warm-up, your cool down, and some stretching!

Here are a few additional tips for the program:

- Feel free to "start" your week on any day that works for you—you do not have to start on Mondays and take your days off on Wednesdays and Sundays. You could, as you see on the bottom row of the chart, "start" your weeks on Saturdays and take days off on Mondays and Fridays.

- Take as long as you need to get through the program. For example, if you get to Week 3 and struggle with it, go back to Week 2 and repeat it one or more times. When you feel ready, try Week 3 again. This strategy is similar to the strategy you used during your post-surgery dietary progression from liquid foods to solid foods. When a new food was too much for you to handle, you had to step back a bit to the liquid, pureed, or soft foods diet that you were already comfortable with. Then, when you felt better, you could try the new food again. That is how it is with exercise too. When a week makes you especially tired or sore, just go back a week and repeat it until you feel better. Try the new week again when you are ready. There is no need to hurry—you are trying to develop an exercise program for life, not to rush through a specific exercise plan that ends after a few weeks.

- Warm up, cool down, and stretch. You will feel better.

- Invite a friend along whenever you can. The time will fly by.

All about an Exercise "Workout"

We have mentioned "workout" a few times. A "workout" is a single exercise session. It goes from when you get off the couch (or step into the gym) to when you hit the showers. A workout includes your main cardio and/or strength-training components as well as additional components. In this section, you will learn exactly how to get started and get through an entire workout so that you get the most out of it.

Components of a Workout

A standard workout includes these components in this order:

- Warm-up
- Stretching (here and/or after cool-down)
- Main physical activity session: cardio and/or resistance training
- Cool down
- Stretching (here and/or after warm-up)

Start Off Right with a Good Warm-Up: Before you start exercising, your body is at rest, whether you are a morning exerciser who is just getting out of bed or an afternoon exerciser who has been sitting at a desk all day. The warm-up is your bridge between resting and getting into the full swing of your exercise. It slowly raises your heart rate, gets you breathing a little faster and deeper, and may even have you breaking a sweat by the end. Your warm-up should be some light aerobic activity, such as one of the following:

- Slow walking, gradually speeding up to brisk walking by the end
- Deep knee bends and lunges
- Swinging and lifting your arms
- Kicking your legs forward and to the sides, one leg at a time
- You can use almost any light aerobic physical activity as a warm-up. Just go slower and easier than you would during the middle of a hard workout. Slow cycling before a hilly ride, walking in the pool before lap swimming, and shooting free throws or easy lay-ups before a basketball game are some examples.

Your warm-up should be five to 10 minutes. Start slowly and comfortably and gradually pick up the intensity so that by the end, you are about ready to get into the main activity for the day. Warming up properly not only makes it mentally easier to start your workout, but it also lowers your risk of injuries.[41] In addition, a good warm-up can reduce the amount of soreness that you feel over the next day or two.[42]

A Good Cool Down Can End Your Workout on a Strong Note: The cool down is almost a mirror-image of your warm-up. It takes you from a high-intensity exercise to a resting state—but gradually. If you skip your cool down, you can get blood pooling in your legs and risk feeling light-headed or dizzy. Any activity that you did for a warm-up can also serve as a cool down.

The cool down should be about five to 10 minutes. It gradually goes from the intensity of your main physical activity down to a very light effort. You know when you have cooled down enough when your heart is not pounding any more, your breathing feels relaxed and normal, and your face is no longer beet red.

Stretch When Your Body Is Warm: There is no single best time to stretch.[43] The key to remember is that it is very important to only stretch after your muscles are warmed up. You can stretch after your warm-up or after your cool down, but do not try to stretch before you are warmed up. Stretching cold muscles is similar to trying to stretch an old rubber band that is no longer very elastic. The rubber band can break if you force it—and your cold muscles can be pulled or strained if you force them.

How do you stretch? These are a few tips:

- *Be sure to hit each major muscle group.* You will get your calves (back of your lower legs), hamstrings (back of your thighs), quadriceps (front of your thighs), shoulders and neck, biceps (front of upper arms), triceps (back of upper arms), groin, hip flexors (front of hips), and outside of hips.
- *Ease into each stretch and hold it for at least 15 to 30 seconds.* Do not bounce; instead, stay still or gradually go deeper into the stretch.

- *Stretching should never be painful.* Deepen each stretch until you feel gentle pressure but no pain.
- *Everyone is at a different level of flexibility.* Ask your physical therapist or look online for beginners' modifications if you need them.
- *Continue to breathe as you stretch.* Do not hold your breath.

As long as you are warmed up, it is really up to you to decide when you want to stretch — as long as you make sure that you *do* stretch! Stretching after your warm-up and before the main part of your workout gives you a chance to get revved up for your upcoming workout.[44] Stretching after your workout and cool down lets you focus on your accomplishment and reduce the tightness in your muscles. Some people like to stretch after the warm-up *and* before the cool down.

Cross-Training Should Be a Regular Choice: Cross-training just means doing something different. Hard-core runners might cross-train by swimming; tennis players might cross-train with running, and triathletes, who compete in swimming, bicycling, and running, might cross-train by lifting weights. Cross-training can be as simple as doing at least two or three different types of activities per week. Cross-training has many mental and physical benefits.[45]

Injury Prevention: Cross-training reduces your risk for injuries, such as overuse injuries. These injuries come from repeatedly doing the same motions over and over again. Tendinitis, muscle strains, joint pain, and stress fractures in your bones are examples of overuse injuries. Cross-training provides a break from the same motions.

Preventing Muscle Imbalances: If you always bicycle but never lift weights, you will have strong legs but not strong arms. If you are a right-hander who is always playing tennis, you might get a very strong right arm but not a strong left arm. A balanced strength-training program in addition to playing tennis will make you stronger in both arms and give you extra strength in your legs, hips, back, and core to improve your game. Cross-training promotes balanced muscles to not only look more proportioned but also prevent injuries.

Improved Fitness: Cross-training improves your overall fitness. If you always work on cardio, you will have a strong heart and lungs but might not have the strong muscles and bones that you can get from including strength training. If you regularly walk, adding some dancing to your schedule can improve your balance and agility. Often, increasing the variety of activities that you do can lower your resting heart rate and increase your metabolism.

It Gives You a Mental Break: You get to look forward to doing different activities so you do not get bored doing the same thing every day.

How to Cross-Train: Include one or more different activities in your schedule in a typical week. These are some examples of fitting in some cross-training:

- If you normally walk five days a week, consider cutting back to three days and bicycling on one day and swimming one day instead.

- Join a weekly sports league so you can practice or compete once a week, and do your regular cardio and strength workouts on the other days.

- Take new group fitness classes, such as Latin dancing, aerobics, or yoga.

- Try circuits at the gym. Pick 10 to 15 different exercises, such as squats, bicep curls, lunges, and treadmill walking. Do each exercise for about 30 to 60 seconds. When you are done, you can repeat the circuit. This counts as cross-training because you are doing so many different activities. Try to vary your circuits regularly so that you do not get stale.

As you plan your fitness program to include cross-training, be sure your schedule includes aerobic activities, resistance training, and flexibility exercises. [46]

Goal-Setting: Goal-setting is an important part of planning an exercise program. Goals give you a sense of purpose. They let you know where you are going, and they help you recognize the progress you have made.

Examples of Possible Goals

You can have several goals at once. You might have some goals related to types of activities to try, how often you want to exercise, or specific achievements. They can be short-term or long-term. These are some examples:

- To start with, your plan can be as simple as having a short-term goal of walking up and down the driveway twice, with a medium-term goal of walking to the end of the block and back. Your long-term goal might be to jog around the block.

- Your goal might be to do one strength-training exercise and one aerobic activity in the first week. You might plan to increase your amount most weeks until you reach your final goal of three strength-training days and five aerobic activity days each week (yes, you can do strength-training and aerobic activity on the same day if you want!).

- Your immediate goal might be to stay on the treadmill for five minutes at a slow walking pace at 0% incline. You might work up to 30 minutes at an incline of 3% within a month.

- Your goal might be to do two sessions of cardiovascular, strength training, and stretching exercises every week for the next four months so that when you get to Colorado for your vacation, you will be ready for anything your snowboarding instructor hits you with.

- Your goal might be to find a new exercise buddy to meet you at the gym once a week.

Keep Yourself Accountable

Specific goals are better than general goals. That way, you can know whether you have achieved them or not. That keeps you accountable to yourself so that you work harder, and it makes you feel prouder when you accomplish them. Having interim goals, such as walking to the end of the block in between going up and down the driveway and jogging around the block, guides you and lets you know that your goal is attainable. These interim goals keep you motivated because you see progress. Recording your workouts is a great way to track your progress toward your goals. It is a lot like recording your food intake because you hold yourself accountable.

Sticking to the Exercise Program: Problems and Solutions

You are gung-ho at the beginning. You are right on time for each exercise session. The time flies by, and you nail each workout. Then your exercise program does not seem as fun. You cut a few workouts short because you are bored, and you sleep through a few workouts because you do not want to work out. Pretty soon, you are feeling more like your old sedentary self than the fit person you want to be. You have gone down the exercise-quitting road before, and you are afraid you are going to do that again.

This Time Is Different

This time, you are going to stick to your program. Why? This time, you are committed. You invested in the gastric bypass surgery, and your commitment to a healthy lifestyle includes exercise. The same persistence and dedication that you use for your diet can carry through to your exercise program.

Keeping your exercise program on track is all about figuring out what is wrong and fixing it. This section helps you work through some common barriers to exercise to help you stick to your own program.

Problem: Disliking Your Exercise

If you do not like calculus, do not major in math; if you do not like reading, do not become an English major. If you do not like swimming, do not limit yourself to the pool. Sticking to an exercise program that you do not like is unnecessary and nearly impossible. Exercise should, and can, be fun. Consider the following factors to help you design an exercise program that you like instead of dread.

Choose Activities That Match Your Personality

People have different likes and dislikes for foods, clothing, and hobbies — so why not for exercise, too? Choose the wrong activities, and you'll be bored out of your mind. Choose the right ones, and you will not be able to stop working out! And just like in other areas of your life, your physical activity preferences probably include a range of options.

Since you are just beginning an exercise program, you may not already know your exercise personality. You may need to try several different options before you find some activities that you like. As you try different activities, think about these questions, and remember that you can have more than one answer to each of these questions:

- Do you want to work out alone, with one partner, with a group of friends, on a team, or with a group of strangers?
- Do you want to be indoors, in an air-conditioned and clean building, or outdoors, in the fresh air and changing scenery?

- Do you want to do a competitive sport, non-competitive activity, or something in between? You can find leagues and teams of all skill levels, gender combinations (all male, all female, co-ed), age ranges, and time commitments to match your preference.

Do Not Count Yourself Out!

Give all activities a try, even if you did not like something the last time you tried it. For example, your last experience with weight lifting might have been 30 years ago, in your physical education class during your freshman year of high school. Maybe it was the most miserable thing you have ever done if the football jocks teased you about your weight and ridiculed you for being weaker than them. Now, though, you might discover that lifting weights makes you feel strong and powerful, and you do not have to take showers in a locker room with 100 of your closest 14-year-old enemies.

Keep It Interesting!

Boredom is about the quickest and most preventable reason for wanting to quit an exercise program. If you are not feeling motivated anymore, take a step back and ask yourself whether you are simply bored. These are a just a few ways you can keep individual workouts and your entire exercise program more interesting and motivating:

- *Vary your workouts.* Try doing two or three different aerobic activities one to three times a week each. You might walk with your spouse on Mondays and Saturdays, go to an aerobics class on Tuesdays, and play tennis with your friends on Sundays. That way, you always get to look forward to something fun and different.
- *Try a circuit.* If you tend to get bored quickly, break up your workout by doing a circuit workout at the gym. Divide your workout into short segments of about three to five minutes each. Do one activity per segment, then move quickly to the next activity for the next segment. If you are just working on cardio, you can get in a quick twenty-five minutes by doing the treadmill, stair-climber, stationary bike, elliptical trainer, and rowing machine for five minutes each. Another option is to alternate segments of cardio with segments of weight training. Your heart rate will stay up, and you will get in a great resistance training session. The time flies by on these kinds of workouts because you do not have a chance to get bored before it is time to go to the next exercise.
- *Take a class.* Group fitness classes help prevent boredom because no two classes are the same, even if you have the same instructor teaching the same kind of class each week. There will be minor changes mixed with the familiarity of the class. Group fitness classes give you the chance to challenge yourself even while you are getting more comfortable with the moves.
- *Vary the intensity.* Alternate fast cycling with slow cycling, uphill walking on the treadmill with level walking, and swimming laps with water calisthenics in the pool. Varying the intensity makes the time fly by because you are focusing on your hard and easy intervals. This type of training can get your heart rate up and burn more calories

than a steady intensity workout.

- *Go social.* Surrounding yourself with fun people can prevent boredom. You never know exactly how the workout is going to go or what you will get to talk about during it. You will often find yourself exercising for longer because you are deep in conversation.

Challenge Yourself with New Activities

New activities give you more options for your exercise. The more new activities you try, the more options you have for enjoyable activities. Set a goal to regularly try a new activity. You might resolve to try one new exercise each month, or you can even tie your new activities to weight loss after RYGB. Here is a sample progression of adding new activities when you hit certain weight loss goals:

- You might start your exercise program with walking.
- At 50 pounds, your next goal might be to go to a yoga class at the gym.
- At 100 pounds of weight loss, you might decide to add some running to your walking routine.
- At 150 pounds, you might start training to surf.
- At 200 pounds, you might take your dream trip to Hawaii and be ready for whatever your surf teacher throws at you.

Keep Trying

Whatever you do, do not give up. You may start to wonder if you are ever going to find the exercise that works for you. Walking is too boring, you are not coordinated enough to enjoy dance classes, aerobics is too old-school, you live in an apartment so you cannot garden outside, you do not like team sports…and then a last-ditch effort leads you to meet up with a hiking group and you fall in love with the scenery and your new best friends! Or maybe you feel as though you have tried and disliked everything…until you pick up your son after school and realize that you do not want to leave because you love being a referee for the children. So many different scenarios can lead to finding the exercise or exercises to keep you healthy and losing weight. Do not give up until you find them!

Give It a Second Chance

A good rule of thumb is to always try something twice or more before deciding you do not like it. There is a good chance that you will find the dance moves easier to follow, that you will be able to build the mental strength to prevent boredom on a treadmill, and that you will feel like a strong fish instead of a drowning landlubber.

Problem: No Time

This is probably the most common excuse that people give for not exercising. You probably are extremely busy and may even believe that this excuse is the truth, but it is just an excuse. You can get the physical activity you need if you try hard enough.

First, take a good hard look at your schedule. Make sure that you are truly short on time—and not that you are finding ways to fill your time so that you do not *have* to exercise. If that is what you are doing, it is time to find some activities that you genuinely enjoy and look forward to. That is what the above section is about.

When There Is a Will, There Is a Way

Making time is possible if you want to badly enough. We are all busy. Ask anyone who is exercising at your local gym or park, and they will tell you that they are busy too. You may be shocked at how busy some of the regular exercisers that you see are. Okay. Now that we have established that everyone is busy, it is time to think about *how*, not *whether*, you are planning to fit in your exercise.

You Are Worth It

Some RYGB patients feel guilty because they think that their exercise commitments are taking away from the family. That is just not true. You are losing weight and following a healthy lifestyle so that you can be a better family member. You are gaining more energy and on the path to being a better contributor to the family. Compared to the 30 daily minutes you are dedicating to exercise, your family is going to get a ton more benefits from your health and happiness—and the possibility that you will live longer. You need to remember every second of every day that *you are worth it*. You are on this weight loss journey because you chose to get healthy, so take advantage of every second of it.

A Few Way to Make Time

These are a few more ideas for making time in your schedule for exercise:

- *Include your family.* Instead of having family time in front of the television, ask your kids about their school days while you are shooting hoops in the driveway. Walk them to school instead of driving them.
- *Walk around the field instead of sitting in the stands while your children are at soccer practice.* You will still get to watch the action as you burn calories.
- *Write down your exercise plans in your planner.* You will be amazed that treating it like a firm appointment will allow you to leave time available.
- *Exercise on your lunch break.* Invite a coworker to walk or go to the gym with you, and you might gain a new friend as you get fit.
- *Bike to work.* You would be surprised at how many workplaces support employees biking to work. You might be able to shower and store your clothes at work. If not, another option is to join a gym close to your workplace and shower there.
- *Keep your exercise gear handy and ready to use so that you can grab it whenever you have a few minutes to work out.*
- *Cut down your food prep time to make more time for exercise by preparing multiple servings at a time.* You can do a few days' worth of mixing and measuring at once so that on other

days your food is ready and you have extra time for exercise.

Each Small Change Helps

Some days you will not be able to fit in a full, uninterrupted workout, but small changes in your lifestyle can add up to extra calories burned and better fitness without taking too much time. These are a few ideas that can get you moving without eating into your time. They are good not only for busy days but also for your daily routine.

- Park a few blocks away or at the far end of the parking lot instead of within feet of building entrances — and when parking lots are crowded, this can actually save time because you will not have to drive in endless circles looking for a parking spot.

- Take the stairs to get from floor to floor instead of using the elevator. This one is sometimes a time-saver, too, when elevators are slow or crowded.

- Stand up periodically when you are working at your desk. Stretch and do a few arm swings, deep knee bends, and lunges.

- Pace back and forth while talking on your cell phone instead of sitting down. If you are on a landline, buy a cordless phone so you can walk around the house or office.

- Walk to the other side of your workplace to talk to your colleagues instead of sending an email or phoning them. They will probably appreciate seeing you anyway.

- Do knee lifts while you are waiting for the microwave to go off, calf raises while you are washing the dishes after dinner, and squats during television commercials (of course, you can always skip the television program altogether and head off for a full exercise session…).

Problem: Self-Consciousness

Many new exercisers, especially obese ones, worry what others think of them. As mentioned earlier in this chapter, you have nothing to worry about as long as you know deep down that you are doing the best you can for your health. But if you are so worried about what people think of you that you just cannot face the thought of exercising in public, then do not. You have other options. Exercise in the privacy of your own home using your own equipment. Alternatively, some people choose to exercise before dawn or after dark to avoid being seen by others. You might make the eventual change from being a shy, dark-only exerciser to an outgoing, anytime exerciser! If you do choose to exercise in the dark, stay in well-lit areas, wear reflective clothing, and be alert.

Problem: The Weather Will Not Cooperate

You plan an outdoors workout, but it is too hot, cold, windy, wet, humid, or icy. Maybe you do not want to go outside in the snow during the winter or face the heat of summer. What do you do when the weather is not on your side?

Get Used to It

Your body is a lot tougher than you might think. If you never tried walking in the drizzle or cross-country skiing, you might not have realized that you can. Tons of exercisers brave the elements and continue with their planned workouts. Another option is to change your workout time—so if you normally work out at lunchtime, try getting up super early in the summer to beat the heat. Or in the winter, if you know that the roads will be cleared of snow later in the day, postpone your workout until lunchtime, when it is light and the streets are cleared. Do not ever try to exercise in dangerous conditions, such as thunderstorms, freezing rain, heavy snowfall, or an excessive heat warning.

Modify Your Workout

If you just cannot beat the weather, do not let it beat you. Change your workout so it is appropriate. Swim or go to an air-conditioned gym or recreation center in the summer; go to the gym or use an exercise DVD at home during the winter.

How Should I Change My Diet When I Start a Physical Activity Program?

Your exercise program burns calories and builds muscle. You need the right nutrition to support your activity, but your diet does not need to change much from your prescribed diet. That is especially true when you are near the beginning of your weight loss journey. At that time, you are already losing weight quickly, and one of your primary goals is to keep up your calorie deficit. That is, you want to keep a big difference between the calories you eat and the calories you burn. Exercise increases the deficit and supports weight loss.

In the beginning, the gastric bypass diet is also appropriate for your physical activity program for these reasons:

- It is nutritious. The protein and other nutrients that the RYGB diet emphasizes are the same ones you need to support physical activity.

- You are not exercising too intensely at the beginning. You do not need a lot of extra calories to support intense exercise.

- You eat frequently. The small, frequent meals and snacks on the gastric bypass diet keep your energy levels up so you can be ready for exercise and recover from each workout.

Water is the biggest concern with exercise, especially if you are a heavy sweater or are exercising in hot conditions. In addition to your regular six to eight cups of water throughout the day, drink about 16 extra ounces of water about an hour before you work out. Then drink another 16 ounces afterward. During exercise, drink water when you are thirsty. You almost never need a sports drink during regular exercise.

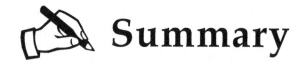 # Summary

- This chapter has the information you need to go from being a sedentary person to an active, fit one.

- First, get your doctor's approval.

- Then start with easy activities in short exercise sessions. Only gradually increase the intensity and length of your workouts.

- Most of all...enjoy your new freedom to find activities that you love and that will make you healthier and happier at the same time!

Time to Take Action: Keeping Your Exercise Log

An exercise log helps you plan and record your physical activity. Some people like to keep a weekly calendar; others prefer a monthly calendar. Keeping an exercise log can motivate you to keep going because you get to fill it in each day and watch it fill up. Include what you did, how long you did it for, how you felt, whether other people were involved, and any other details, such as hitting a goal or extreme weather conditions.

Table 42 is a four-week log for you to start. You can photocopy the blank one and use it again once you fill up the first one.

	Sunday	Monday	Tuesday	Wednesday	Thursday	Friday	Saturday
Sample	30 minutes hiking with Betty. Hard but so fun! Sunny—we took water bottles.	Planned day off. Needed it badly; sore from weekend	Normal gym day. 20 minutes on treadmill, 15 minutes weight lifting. Nothing exciting.	Boot camp in the park! First class. I was nervous, but people were nice. They are something for me to strive for!	Sore everywhere from yesterday! Aqua aerobics at the gym 50 minutes. Good workout.	Walked 20 minutes moderate with Bill, then 10 minutes at home with dumbbells. Tired, not into it. Glad to finish.	Off. Needed rest after yesterday and want to be ready for tomorrow's hike with Betty!
Week 1							
Week 2							
Week 3							
Week 4							

Table 42: Four-week exercise log

RYGB Patient Story: Christie

Christie from Arkansas started with the laparoscopic adjustable gastric band (lap-band), but as you'll read in her story, the band didn't work out for her. The Roux-en-Y gastric bypass was her second weight loss surgery. Concerns over Christie's weight literally started before she was old enough to remember, and she has had to fight through many setbacks. However, after gastric bypass at age 40, she finally feels as though controlling her weight is within reach. Her highest weight was 312 pounds, and she's now at 219 pounds.

On Being the Overweight Infant and the Dieting, Chubby Nerd

I have had weight issues my entire life. At my check-up when I was six weeks old, my mom got yelled at because I'd gained too much weight. As a kid, I was always chubby and one of the last kids picked for any sports activity. I was always in advanced classes and was in band, so I was that chubby, dorky, band nerd. Luckily, I always had a few good friends, although I was extremely self-conscious and insecure because of my weight. I still have nightmares about mom making me go to aerobics classes with her when I was in 5th and 6th grade.

In ninth grade, I decided that I was tired of being the fat kid, and I pretty much started starving myself. I would skip breakfast, eat 1/2 of a cheese sandwich for lunch, and take a few bites of whatever mom made for dinner and throw the rest away. I bet I didn't eat 600 calories a day for six months or so. I don't know what my starting weight was, but I got down to 170; at 5'6, it was the first time ever I didn't feel like the fat kid! However, we all know you can't live like that, and during my sophomore year in high school, I gained it all back. I started college at 18 years old and 220 pounds.

On Her Attempts to Control Her Weight

I have never been a fad dieter. Every few years I would try to improve my diet and start an exercise program and would lose 30 or 40 pounds but never could stick with it. I was an emotional eater. I'd get stressed out about something or break up with a boyfriend and be back where I started, plus some extra weight. From ages 22 to 29, I bounced around from 240 to 280 pounds. That seemed to be my comfort zone.

At 29, I decided I had had enough. I obviously could not lose weight on my own, and I started looking into bariatric surgery. I was quickly approved and scheduled for RYGB, but a couple weeks before my surgery, my co-worker was fired. My employer revoked my PTO approval for my surgery. Needless to say, I was devastated. I'd finally taken the biggest step of my life, and nearing the finish line, I'd crashed and burned. Soon, I left that employer and pushed thoughts of bariatric surgery to the back of my mind.

On Her Abusive Relationship and Emotional Eating

The following year I met a man, got married, and shortly thereafter got pregnant. My husband turned out to be a con man who lived off of overweight and insecure women. As soon as I became pregnant, he became verbally, emotionally, and, eventually, physically abusive. I was pregnant and broken down, and I felt as though I had lost myself. When I was eight months pregnant, after a particularly atrocious fight, it dawned on me what this man had done to my life. I decided then and there that as soon as my son was born I was leaving my husband (why I didn't walk away that day I do not know, but at least I had a plan!). At my first OB appointment, I weighed 295. I had horrible morning sickness through the entire pregnancy and ended up being a gestational diabetic on insulin. I had to control my weight and diet for my baby – it's funny what you'll do for a child that you won't do for yourself! The day I delivered I weighed 298; meaning I gained three pounds through the entire pregnancy! Better yet, my son was 8 lbs. 11 oz. and perfectly healthy. He had no issues at all from my gestational diabetes.

Five days after the birth of my son, as I pondered how I was getting out of my marriage without either my son or I getting harmed, the county sheriff notified me that there was a warrant out for my husband's arrest and that my son and I were not safe. That was the day we walked away and the last time I saw my ex-husband. As you can imagine, that was a very emotional summer for me. I had a new baby, and I'd lost what I thought was my dream. I turned to food. I hovered around 300 for two years. Then, when my son was two, I again decided that I had to do something about my weight. I was having dull chest pains, and my weight was keeping me from enjoying my son. This was not the life I wanted for either of us. I again decided to get serious about diet and exercise. I joined a gym and was 312 the day I joined. I started eating healthier and eventually got down to 260; however, I was working a fair distance from home and raising an almost three-year-old entirely on my own and eventually, as always, stopped going to the gym. Again I started gaining weight.

On the Lap-Band and Its Challenges

I am a family practice physician assistant and felt like such a hypocrite educating my patients about diet and exercise when I couldn't do it myself. How could I ever expect my patients to take care of themselves when I couldn't? I had mentioned bariatric surgery to my mom on a couple occasions, but she was adamantly opposed that I just didn't need that, and if I really tried, I could do it on my own. In 2009, she saw something on TV about the lap band, and with me at 36 and almost 300 pounds, she actually approached me and suggested it.

In October of 2009, I started checking instance requirements and coverage. I had hypertension, hyperlipidemia, and a fatty liver. My insurance only covered $4,000 toward the surgery, so my mom and dad offered to split the rest of the cost with me as my Christmas present that year. They called it an investment in my future. At the time, the lap band was all the rage; they said it had fewer complications, was reversible, and led to good weight loss. I thought I'd found the Holy Grail. My surgery was in December, after a two-week liquid diet consisting of four to five shakes a day plus clear and sugar-free liquids. Who knew that two weeks could last so long? It was miserable!

Lap band surgery was a piece of cake. I was back at work, although moving slowly, five or six days later. The post-op diet was miserable. About a week post-op, I woke up starving and spent the next two months starving while I was still on liquids and puréed foods. However, I was losing weight, which was the point! I was 295 lbs. before surgery and around 240 by the summer. I had multiple fills in my band to increase restriction, but by summer, I was able to eat almost anything and still always felt hungry, even ravenous.

Then I got sick. In July, my now 6-year-old son gave me a stomach bug. I started throwing up, and then I couldn't get anything down; I was waking up at night choking and throwing up clear liquids. I got to the point that I could barely stand and was so extremely weak I was shaking and ended up getting two liters of IV fluids and an emergency unfill of my band. From that point on things were never right with my band. I kept very little fluid in it, but if I was sick, if my allergies acted up, if I had PMS, or I was stressed, I would be unable to eat. I lived off of hot tea for days at a time. I never got back to the point where I could really eat solid meats, fruits, etc., if I did I got sick. Crackers and cheese saved me.

Eventually I just had everything in the band removed and gave up. My weight went from 220 to 250, and I was getting depressed. I'd had bariatric surgery and failed it, so I gave up. In March of 2012, though, I was still at 250 lbs. on my 39th birthday. I had a very long conversation with myself and decided I'd give my band another shot. I wanted to be less than 200 lbs for my 40th birthday the following year.

I again had a little bit of fluid put in my band and started walking, and I immediately started having band problems. I felt like I was choking all the time, had pain in my chest and left shoulder, and again had issues with solid foods, so I started living off of fluids. About six weeks after the fill I started having horrible reflux, which I had had off and on the entire time I'd had the band. I started waking up at night choking with stomach acid coming out my nose…I went on a completely liquid diet thinking my band just needed a break, but things continued to escalate. When I again got to the point that the only thing I could tolerate was hot tea, I finally admitted I had a problem and saw my surgeon's nurse practitioner. She unfilled my band again and sent me to the hospital straight from the clinic for an upper GI evaluation. The following day we discovered my band had slipped. That was a Friday. They scheduled me for surgery the next Wednesday, and I saw my surgeon on Monday to discuss options.

I had four choices at that point. One was to take the band out and do nothing. The next was to take the band out and get another band. The third was to take the band out and revise to a vertical sleeve gastrectomy, and the fourth was to take the band out and revise to gastric bypass. I had actually decided months before that eventually I wanted my band removed, and after much research, I had decided that RYGB was probably my best bet. I knew I needed something to help me lose weight. Another band was not an option after the miserable 2 1/2 years I'd had with mine. The sleeve was relatively new, and I have a couple of friends and acquaintances that were sleeved but just didn't lose that much weight, so I wasn't comfortable with that option; plus, after the horrendous reflux, I did not want anything that might cause that to return. So I chose RYGB!

To clarify about my insurance, I have a once in a lifetime bariatric surgery exclusion. When I found out about the slipped band, I contacted my insurance to see if they'd cover revision. My BMI was 36 with no comorbidities at that point. Based strictly on their criteria, I would not *qualify for bariatric surgery (BMI > 40 or >35 with two serious comorbidities). I was petrified, but my insurance rep asked me a zillion questions and got records from my surgeon, and by the end of the day that I contacted her, she said that because I'd been compliant and somewhat successful with my lap band, that without some type of assistance, they fully expected me to regain all the weight I'd lost and for my co-morbidities to return. And because I had a mechanical failure (the slip of the band) they would cover revision. In fact, they had revamped their policy, so when I finally had surgery, they paid 80% as opposed to my band surgery, where they only covered $4000. Amazingly, my slipped lap band turned out to be a blessing. And as frustrating as my surgeon can be, I absolutely have full confidence in him and wouldn't have let anyone else do a revision on me. Our personalities don't always mesh, but I absolutely cannot question his skill as a surgeon; he did my band, band removal, and RYGB.*

On Getting the Gastric Bypass

That Wednesday I had urgent band removal and was scheduled for revision to RYGB. I woke up post-op to a very sad mom informing me that the band had done so much damage that my surgeon was unable to complete the revision. He wanted to see me in two weeks but was expecting to be able to do the revision in about a year. A year?! I was band-less and bypass-less, and once the numbness and shock wore off, I was angry. I felt betrayed by my band, by my body, and by everything. I was an emotional mess for about three weeks. I pictured myself back at 300 pounds, although I'd dropped to 225 while sick. After so many years of band life and fearing food, I was once again eating and loving it, and the scales showed it. It was a very emotional month.

At my post-op appointment, my surgeon agreed to do the revision at six months instead of a year. Six months felt doable; I could survive six months. So I counted days, joined BariatricPal. com, read everything, and ate everything. It was the craziest pre-op ever because I'd already done the seminars, met the nutritionist, and been approved by insurance and the surgeon. I had absolutely nothing to do until two weeks pre-op when, I met the surgeon again and started those darn shakes again. I had ballooned back up to 255. Pre-op was easier than before. It was still miserable, but easier. I knew it was a means to an end, and I knew beyond a shadow of a doubt that RYGB was what I wanted. I was dying to get to my surgery on February 11! At about 1 a.m. on February 10 I woke up throwing up with horrid diarrhea. We'd been seeing a ton of patients with a GI bug, and it had finally found me...the day before surgery. I was devastated. I fell asleep on the bathroom floor crying because I knew they'd end up canceling my surgery. After many bouts of nastiness, things finally settled down around noon. I was supposed to be on clear liquids that day anyway, so at least it was the easiest clear liquid day ever! I went to bed that night hopeful, but still nervous. I never did sleep that night, but thankfully the bug had passed.

On February 11, 2013, I finally had my gastric bypass revision surgery. It truly was a breeze. I had some issues with nausea and my surgeon kept me in the hospital an extra night, but I really had no serious issues. The pain was never terrible, walking was slow but it felt good, and it all just kind of fell into place.

On Feeling Hopeful with RYGB

Next week I will be three months post-op. I'm down 40 pounds, which is fairly slow compared to many, but I feel good! I can eat virtually anything, including bread, apples, and meat; none of it bothers my stomach at all. I have to watch simple carbs because I do dump if I eat something with a high carb load and no protein, but otherwise I eat what I want. It just takes tiny amounts to satisfy me. Even if my allergies are flared up, I'm sick, or have PMS, I can still eat normal foods. My gastric bypass and I have already found a peace that my band and I never did. I really do not have food cravings any more either. The foods I want to eat are typically healthy foods. If we have something ridiculously delicious at work and I want a bite or two, I take a bite or two, and I'm satisfied. I never felt satisfied with my band.

I do occasionally, completely randomly get extremely queasy. This happens once every week or two and does not seem to be associated with food. Thank goodness for Zofran when that hits, but even that seems to be occurring less and less the further out I get. Drinking water is also not a problem, although getting the required amount of protein has proven to be a challenge. I no longer enjoy meat as much as I did pre-op. I'd be perfectly happy to live off of vegetables. I have to force myself to drink a protein shake each day to come close to my protein goal. I hate protein shakes. I've bought dozens of different brands with no luck, so it's a daily struggle for me. The scale shows when I've been hitting my required protein or not though; no protein, no weight loss.

I am currently working on a variation of the Couch to 5K, and I'm starting to enjoy it, at least a little. I don't think I'll ever enjoy running, but getting out and being active makes me feel good. As always, finding time is a struggle, so right now I'm averaging 45 minutes three times a week. My son is almost nine and in the "at risk for overweight" category. When we started running; I lost zero, he lost five pounds. Not only is this making me a better and healthier mom, but it's making him healthier as well. What more could I possibly ask for?

One of my biggest concerns pre-op was how I was going to handle family functions post-op. I come from a long line of eaters; we celebrate with food. Much to my amazement, I can still celebrate with food. I eat a small amount, but I eat so slowly and talk so much we all end up finishing close together. I can now order the most expensive appetizer or side and love every second of it. Sometimes my son and I share meals as well.

My family, friends, co-workers, and even patients have all been amazing. I've had one or two give me the "you aren't that big" speech, but for the most part, they've all been nothing shy of fabulous. I'm starting to feel like a girl again for the first time in years. Heck, maybe I'll try that whole dating thing again eventually. I'm no longer exhausted by the end of the day, and I sleep better than I've slept in years. My blood pressure and lipids are excellent. I'm still 65 pounds from my goal but truly feel fabulous.

On Using the BariatricPal.com Discussion Forums

I use the discussion boards because, although everyone in my life is supportive, none of them really understand. They don't realize what it's like to shop in the regular section of the clothing store for the first time ever. They don't know what an amazing milestone that is. They don't understand how frustrating it is to eat 800 calories a day and not lose a pound for three weeks. They just haven't lived in a fat girl's body or mind; while they support me, they have no idea how amazing it is for that fat girl to look in the mirror every day and see changes. I have collar bones! I have a neck! I just realized I have cheekbones, and they're pretty awesome! Having someplace like this where I can come and celebrate the highs or help pull me through the lows has just made this entire journey so much easier. I feel like I have made a couple of true friends, even though I've never met them in person. I'm online almost every day wanting to see others' successes and hopefully encouraging them when they're at their lows. It's a support system I have nowhere else.

My biggest advice to others is to be patient! It took us years to get to this point, so don't expect to lose 30 pounds a month. Some people do, and yea for them, but slow and steady wins the race. I get frustrated on the boards when I read people saying, "I'm eight weeks out, and I've only lost 40 pounds." Holy cow, that's five pounds a week! Celebrate your successes, and be realistic in your expectations!

1   NWCR Facts. The National Weight Control Registry. Web site. Accessed http://www.nwcr.ws/Research/default.htm. Accessed October 31, 2012.

2   National Health Information Center. Get moving calculator: exercise and calories burned. U.S. Department of Health and Human Services. Web site. Retrieved from http://www.healthfinder.gov/docs/doc12322.htm. 2012, July 2. Accessed October 31, 2012.

3   Ainsworth BE, Haskell WL, Herrmann SD, Meckes N. Bassett Jr. DR, Tudor-Locke C, Greer JL, Vezina J, Whitt-Glover MC, Leon AS. Compendium of Physical Activities: a second update of codes and MET values. Medicine and Science in Sports and Exercise. 2011;43:1575-1581.

4   Calorie Control Council. Get moving calculator. Web site. Retrieved from http://www.caloriescount.com/getMoving.aspx. 2012. Accessed October 31, 2012.

5   Physical activity for everyone: physical activity and health. Centers for Disease Control and Prevention Web site. Retrieved from http://www.cdc.gov/physicalactivity/everyone/health/index.html 2011. Updated February 16. Accessed November 1, 2012.

6   Physical activity for everyone: physical activity and health. Centers for Disease Control and Prevention Web site. Retrieved from http://www.cdc.gov/physicalactivity/everyone/health/index.html 2011. Updated February 16. Accessed November 1, 2012.

7   American Cancer Society: Kushi LH, Doyle C, McCullough M, Rock C, Demark-Wahnefried W, Bandera EV, … Gansler T. American Cancer Society guidelines on nutrition and physical activity for cancer prevention. Cancer: A Cancer Journal for Clinicians. 2012;62:30-67.

8   Centers for Disease Control and Prevention, National Institutes of Health, U.S. Department of Health and Human Services. Chapter 4: the effects of physical activity on health and disease. In Physical activity and health: a report of the surgeon general. 1996;Washington, D.C.

9   American Cancer Society: Kushi LH, Doyle C, McCullough M, Rock C, Demark-Wahnefried W, Bandera EV, … Gansler T. American Cancer Society guidelines on nutrition and physical activity for cancer prevention. Cancer: A Cancer Journal for Clinicians. 2012;62:30-67.

10 Vincent, H.K., Ben-David, K., Conrad, B.P., Lamb, K.M., Seay, A.N., & Vincent, K.R. (2012).Rapid changes in gait, musculoskeletal pain and quality of life after bariatric surgery. *Surgery for Obesity and Related Diseases, 8(3)*:346-354.

11 Weak in the knees – the quest for a cure. Exploration Systems Mission Directorate Education Outreach, National Aeronautics and Space Administration. Web site. http://weboflife.nasa.gov/currentResearch/currentResearchGeneralArchives/weakKnees.htm. 2012. Accessed November 2, 2012.

12 About osteoporosis: exercise for healthy bones. National Osteoporosis Foundation. Web site. Retrieved from http://www.nof.org/aboutosteoporosis/prevention/exercise. 2011. Accessed November 2, 2012.

13 Belavy, D.L., Bansmann, P.M., Bohnne, G., Frings-Meuthen, P., Heer, M., Rittweger, J., Zange, J., Felsenberg, D. (2011). Changes in intervertebral disc morphology persist five months after 21-day bed rest. *Journal of Applied Physiology, 111*:1304-1314.

14 Human research program: areas of study: bone health. National Aeronautic and Space Administration. Web site. http://www.nasa.gov/exploration/humanresearch/areas_study/physiology/physiology_bone.html. 2012. Accessed November 2, 2012.

15 Kemper KJ. Complementary and alternative medicine therapies to promote healthy moods. Pediatric Clinics of North America. 2007;54:901.

16 Kline CE, Sui X, et all. Dose-response effects of exercise training on the subjective sleep quality of postmenopausal women: exploratory analyses of a randomized controlled trial. BMJ Open. 2012;2(4).

17 Rosano, C., Venkatraman, V.K., Guralnik, J., Newman, A.B., Glynn, N.W., Launer, L., Taylor, C.A., Williamson, J., Studenski, S., Pahor, M., & Aizenstein, H. (2010). Psychomotor speed and functional brain MRI 2 years after completing a physical activity treatment. *The Journals of Gerontology. Series A, Biological Sciences and Medical Sciences, 65*: 639-47.

18 Kemper KJ. Complementary and alternative medicine therapies to promote healthy moods. Pediatric Clinics of North America. 2007;54:901.

19 Colcombe, S.J., Erickson, K.I., Scalf, P.E., Kim, J.S., Prakash, R., McAuley, E., Elavsky, S., Marquez, D.X., Hu, L., & Kramer, A.F. (2006). Aerobic exercise training increases brain volume in aging humans. *The Journals of Gerontology. Series A, Biological Sciences and Medical Sciences, 61*:166-1170.

20 Boecker, H., Sprenger, T., Spilker, M.E., Henriksen, G., Koppenhoefer, M., Wagner, K.J., Valet, M., Berthele, A., & Tolle, T.R. (2008). The runner's high: opiodergic mechanisms in the human brain. *Cerebral Cortex, 18*, 2523-31.

21 Mechanick JI, Kushner RF, Sugerman HJ, Gonzalez-Campoy M, Collazo-Clavell ML, … Dixon J. American Association of Clinical Endocrinologists, The Obesity Society and American Society for Metabolic and Bariatric Surgery medical guidelines for clinical practice for the perioperative nutritional, metabolic and nonsurgical support of the bariatric surgery patient. Obesity. 2009;17:S1-S70.

22 McVay MA, Friedman KE. The benefits of cognitive behavioral groups for bariatric surgery patients. Bariatric Times. 2012;9(9):22-28.

23 Centers for Disease Control and Prevention. (2011, December 1). Physical activity for everyone: how much physical activity do adults need? Retrieved from http://www.cdc.gov/physicalactivity/everyone/guidelines/adults.html

24 Kaiser Family Foundation. (n.d.) Percent of adults who participated in moderate or vigorous physical activities, 2009. Retrieved from http://statehealthfacts.org/comparemaptable.jsp?ind=92&cat=2

25   Weight-Control Information Network, National Institute of Diabetes and Digestive and Kidney Diseases (NIDDK). (2006, November). Physical activity and weight control. Retrieved from http://www.win.niddk.nih.gov/publications/physical.htm

26   McGuire, M.T., Wing, R.R., Klem, M.L., Seagle, H.M. & Hill, J.O. (1998). Long-term maintenance of weight loss: Do people who lose weight through various weight loss methods use different behaviors to maintain their weight? *International Journal of Obesity*, 22:572-577.

27   Wing, R.R., & Phelan, S. (2005). Long-term weight loss maintenance. *American Journal of Clinical Nutrition*, 82:222S-225S.

28   National Weight Control Registry. (n.d.). NWCR facts. Retrieved from http://www.nwcr.ws/Research/default.htm

29   Shick, S.M., Wing, R.R., Klem, M.L., McGuire, M.T., Hill, J.O. & Seagle, H.M. (1998). Persons successful at long-term weight loss and maintenance continue to consume a low calorie, low fat diet. *Journal of the American Dietetic Association*,98:408-413

30   U.S. Department of Health and Human Services & U.S. Department of Agriculture. (2010). Dietary Guidelines for Americans. (7th edition). U.S. Government Printing Office, Washington, D.C.

31   National Heart, Lung and Blood Institute. (n.d.). Moderate-level physical activities. Retrieved from http://www.nhlbi.nih.gov/hbp/prevent/p_active/m_l_phys.htm

32   Heart rate zone calculator. American Council on Exercise. Web site. http://www.acefitness.org/calculators/heart-rate-zone-calculator.aspx. Accessed November 3, 2012.

33   Monitoring exercise intensity using heart rate. American Council on Exercise. Web site. http://www.acefitness.org/fitfacts/fitfacts_display.aspx?itemid=38. Accessed November 3, 2012.

34   Physical activity: how much physical activity do adults need? Centers for Disease Control and Prevention. Web site. http://www.cdc.gov/physicalactivity/everyone/guidelines/adults.html. Updated 2011, December 16. Accessed November 3, 2012.

35   Get fit facts: strength Training 101. American Council on Exercise. Web site. http://www.acefitness.org/fitfacts/fitfacts_display.aspx?itemid=2661. Accessed November 3, 2012.

36   American Council on Exercise. (n.d.). Get fit facts: strengthen your abdominals with stability balls. Retrieved from http://www.acefitness.org/fitfacts/fitfacts_display.aspx?itemid=2662&category=11

37   American Council on Exercise. (n.d.). Get fit facts: ACE's top ten reasons to stretch. Retrieved from http://www.acefitness.org/updateable/update_display.aspx?CMP=HET_0807&pageID=520

38   Mayo Clinic Staff. (2010, December 18). Exercise: when to check with your doctor first. *Mayo Clinic*. Retrieved from http://www.mayoclinic.com/health/exercise/SM00059/METHOD=print

39   PT careers: role of a physical therapist. American Physical Therapy Association. Web site. Retrieved from http://www.apta.org/PTCareers/RoleofaPT/. 2011, January 15. Accessed November 4, 2012.

40   American Council on Exercise (n.d.). Get fit facts: before you start an exercise program. Retrieved from http://www.acefitness.org/fitfacts/fitfacts_display.aspx?itemid=2612

41   Woods, K., Bishop, P., & Jones, E. (2007). Warm-up and stretching in the prevention of muscular injury. *Sports Medicine*, 37:1089-99. Retrieved from http://www.ncbi.nlm.nih.gov/pubmed/18027995

42   Law, R.Y.W., & Herbert, R.D. (2003). Warm-up reduces delayed-onset muscle soreness but cool-down does not: a randomized controlled trial. *Australian Journal of Physiotherapy*, 53:91-95.

43   Shrier, I. (2012). Should people stretch before exercise? *The Western Journal of Medicine*, 174:282-283.

44   American Council on Exercise. (n.d.). Get fit facts: flexible benefits. Retrieved from http://www.acefitness.org/fitfacts/fitfacts_display.aspx?itemid=2610

45   American Council on Exercise. (n.d.). Get fit facts: cross-training for fun and fitness. Retrieved from http://www.acefitness.org/fitfacts/fitfacts_display.aspx?itemid=2547

46   American Academy of Orthopaedic Surgeons. (2011, October). Cross training. Retrieved from http://www.orthoinfo.aaos.org/topic.cfm?topic=A00339

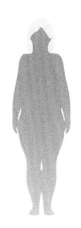

17

The First Year After RYGB Is Filled With Changes

So far in this book, we've covered the benefits and risks of the Roux-en-Y gastric bypass, choosing a surgeon, preparation for and recovery from surgery, and the RYGB diet and exercise program that will help you lose weight and improve your health. Those are the parts of the RYGB experience that probably come to mind first, but your weight loss journey goes beyond this.

The RYGB affects all parts of your life. In this chapter, we will cover some of the changes, beyond the numbers on the scale, to expect during the first year after surgery. Knowing what to expect can help you prepare. Here is what the chapter will cover:

- Physical and emotional changes in the first year
- Common cosmetic surgeries that bariatric surgery patients get after losing a lot of weight
- Other aspects of your life that may change after RYGB surgery

This chapter cannot predict everything that will happen over this exciting year, but knowing even a little bit can be helpful. Something else that will help you get through this year is the knowledge that you are not alone.

The First Year Is Filled with Changes

RYGB is life-changing. While losing weight, you can experience many other changes, both physical and otherwise. Your entire world may change for the better!

Physical Changes – Weight Loss and Other Effects

The first physical change is pretty obvious. You might lose 100 pounds or more in the year after surgery. Your appearance will change quickly, although exactly how quickly depends on your body type, starting weight, and rate of weight loss.

Changes in Weight

*Not everyone will notice your weight loss at the same time…*People who are closest to you, such as your family and close friends, may notice your weight loss soonest. However, some people who see you frequently might not notice your weight loss until you have lost quite a bit of weight. They are not intentionally ignoring your hard work; some people just do not notice others' weights.

Reacting Positively When People Notice Your Weight Loss

You spent so long fighting obesity and defending your weight from other people that you might automatically be defensive when people comment on your weight loss. This is especially likely if you are shy or if the comment comes from someone whom you do not like or who does not know about your surgery. People who do not often see you will be especially shocked by your weight loss. Learn to take each comment as a compliment regardless of how it was meant. You have certainly earned the right to celebrate the new, more attractive, you!

You Will Re-Discover Body Parts That You Had Forgotten You Had

As your fat comes off, you will see new curves and even a few angles that you had not seen or dared to hope think about for years. Your knees and elbows might start to look like joints instead of cushions, and your jaw line — supporting only a single, not triple, chin! — will eventually emerge! With more weight and some exercise, your muscles will begin to show. You will be able to tie your own shoes again, and you will soon be able to see your feet while standing up straight. You will start to sneak looks at yourself in store windows instead of avoiding mirrors and cameras.

Other Physical Effects

You Might Lose Some of Your Hair[1]: Your body's response to rapid weight loss is to conserve energy and nutrients. Hair loss, also known as alopecia, is one effect. Low levels of selenium are linked to a higher risk for alopecia, so you might want to ask your doctor or dietitian about how to get enough of this essential mineral.[2]

Alopecia can make you feel self-conscious, but your thinning hair is probably more noticeable to you than to anyone else. Your hair will grow back as normal when you are at your maintenance weight and you are eating enough calories and nutrients to sustain your weight and support hair growth.

You Might Feel Cold: Feeling cold is another result of your body's conservation efforts. Your body burns energy, or calories, to stay warm. When you cut back on your calorie intake to lose weight, you may feel a little cooler than usual.

> ### Tip
>
> Staying warm is one way your body uses energy and boosts your metabolic rate. **Chapter 1, "Obesity – A Widespread Disease,"** talks about the factors that affect your basal metabolic rate, or BMR, which describes how fast you burn calories throughout the day and night.

Emotional and Social Changes: Your weight loss journey is not only about the number on the scale or even just about your physical health and appearance. The gastric bypass is also about personal emotional growth and improving your interpersonal relationships to improve your life. During this first year of your life-changing experience, you will notice not only physical changes but also emotional ones. Your personal outlook and social relationships can change, and a positive attitude increases the likelihood that these changes will be positive.

Self-Confidence over Self-Doubt: You will probably gain more self-confidence as you lose weight. You are responsible for the decreasing numbers on the scale week after week. Your confidence will increase as you see that you can do what you set your mind to. This belief in your abilities can translate into self-confidence in other parts of your life.

You will have the occasional moment of self-doubt. It might come when you encounter someone who snubs your hard work, when you hit a weight loss plateau, or when you feel excessively hungry and give in to your craving even though you know you should not. The important thing is that you keep it to a moment of self-doubt and do not let it turn into a rut. And once you get used to changing your self-doubt into self-confidence, you will gain even more confidence that even if not everything is perfect, you *can* do this!

Changes in Your Social Life

Many changes will be good. With your weight loss and self-confidence, you will probably have a more positive attitude and energy and be more fun to be around. Spending time with friends and family can be more fun, and meeting people can be easier.

Some people might treat you differently than before:

- Some people who looked down on you because of your obesity might start to treat you with a bit of respect.

- Others might reject the idea of the bariatric surgery. They might treat you like a cheater or act as though you do not deserve to be happy and healthy.

- The people whom you care about and who love you will treat you as you deserve: just as warmly as before surgery but with additional respect for your hard work to lose the weight and get healthy.

In general, people react to the way you tell them about your RYGB. If you are embarrassed about it, they will be embarrassed to talk about it, or they will judge you for getting it. If you are proud and open, they are far more likely to be interested and accepting. You are never obligated to tell people about your surgery.

Changes in Your Quality of Life

Your quality of life, or QOL, basically refers to how good life is for you. Most bariatric surgery patients that lose the amount of weight they had hoped for experience a higher quality of life.[3] This is because of:

- Improved health
- Fewer physical limitations
- More self-confidence
- Better relationships with other people
- Better mood

Changes in Your Relationship with Food

Your relationship with food may change. Many obese patients spend years struggling with food. The RYGB can help you overcome some of these challenges:

- Less hunger: Before surgery, you might have been hungry all the time, leading you to overeat and continue to gain weight. After surgery, you might not be as hungry before meals, and you might get full sooner when you eat.

- Preference for healthy foods: Before surgery, you might have craved salty, sugary, and fatty fast food, comfort foods, sweets, and fried foods. As you get used to the gastric bypass diet, your tastes can change. Cravings for these high-calorie foods can decrease, and you might enjoy more nutritious options, such as lean proteins, vegetables, and whole grains.

- Changes in how you use food: Some obese patients use food as an emotional outlet or as a way to escape their feelings. After Roux-en-Y gastric bypass, you might stop turning to junk food to hide your feelings and instead use healthy foods in a healthier way: to provide essential nutrients.

- Better self-control: You got obese in the first place because you ate too much. A major reason for that might have been lack of self-control. Taking a second helping, finishing the entire package instead of stopping at one serving, and sneaking a bite or two in the kitchen were probably routine for you, and the scale showed it. Self-control with your portions is essential for losing weight and preventing complications.

Changes in Your Health

Obesity caused or aggravated many of your pre-surgery health conditions. High blood pressure and cholesterol, joint pain, asthma, and type 2 diabetes are just a few possibilities. The great news is that you do not have to wait for years after RYGB for your health to improve. Many of your health problems can decrease long before you reach your goal weight. That is right; by the time you lose about five to 10 percent of your initial body weight—that is about 15 to 30 pounds if you started at 300 pounds—you will probably already have improvements in your health.[4] That can happen within weeks or months of surgery!

Improvements in Chronic Conditions

Chronic health conditions can improve if you follow the RYGB diet:

- Lower blood pressure
- Lower total cholesterol and lower "bad" LDL cholesterol levels
- Higher "good" HDL cholesterol (The biggest influence on your HDL cholesterol levels is exercise. So if you start a physical activity program during this time, your HDL cholesterol will go up and your risk of heart disease will go down)
- Lower blood sugar levels[5]
- Decrease in joint pain or arthritis

Your doctor may prescribe lower doses of your medications, such as those to lower blood pressure, cholesterol, and sugar. You might eventually get to stop taking certain medications! Of course, only change your prescription medication use when your doctor tells you to.

More Energy and Feeling Better

Losing weight after RYGB can reduce or cure sleep apnea:[6]

- You will not have to worry about your breathing stopping while you sleep.
- Not waking up during the night leads to better quality sleep and more energy during the day.
- You might not have to sleep with a continuous positive airway pressure, or CPAP, machine.

Another reason for having more energy during the day will be better controlled blood sugar levels. Your energy will be more sustained rather than rising and falling with uncontrolled blood sugar. You will also have more energy because moving around is easier when you weigh less.

Side Effects after Gastric Bypass

Side effects are common. They are not always serious, but they can be unpleasant. Many of them are related to eating too much, eating too quickly, or eating the wrong foods. Before RYGB, you overate and may have eaten fast food or junk food quite often. Now these mistakes cause almost immediate effects. The first few months are usually the most challenging, but a careful diet for life is necessary to minimize consequences.

Gastrointestinal Side Effects Are Likely

- Dumping syndrome: Dumping syndrome can result from eating too much, eating too fast, or eating high-fat or especially high-sugar foods. Symptoms include diarrhea, nausea, vomiting, sweatiness, and shakiness.
- Regurgitation: Regurgitation, or acidic bits of food that rise up in your throat from your stomach pouch, can be a sign of an ulcer. Regurgitation and heartburn are also possible when you eat too much or too fast.
- Vomiting: Vomiting can result from eating too fast, from eating solid foods when you should still be on the liquids or pureed foods diet, or from not chewing your food enough.

First, find out whether the symptoms are serious or not. You might need to call your surgeon or 911 to be sure. When you are sure that you do not need medical attention, try to figure out the cause of your symptoms; usually, the cause is going off of your diet. You may need to return to a liquid or pureed food diet until the symptoms stop.

Avoiding Side Effects Can Motivate You to Stick to the RYGB Diet

The best way to look at these unpleasant side effects is as a blessing in disguise. They are actually the reason why you got the RYGB—these side effects are strong motivation to stick to your diet. They are uncomfortable, but also avoidable and predictable, making them the ideal motivation for sticking to the gastric bypass diet.

You Might Need or Choose Additional Surgical Procedures

Nobody wants to go under the knife twice, but in some cases, you might need or want another surgery. These are some of the possibilities:

- Surgery to correct a serious complication, such as an anastomatic leak, bowel obstruction, or adhesion
- Revisional surgery to a longer-limb RYGB to reduce nutrient absorption
- Placement of an adjustable gastric band (lap-band) around your small stomach pouch to further reduce stomach size and increase restriction
- Plastic surgery, also known as body contouring or cosmetic surgery, to remove excess skin after weight loss

Earlier parts of his book talked about revisional weight loss surgery after disappointing weight loss with the RYGB and serious complications that can require an additional surgery to fix. This chapter will discuss elective surgeries—the ones you choose. You might want elective surgery to improve your appearance and make you more comfortable with your new body. Body contouring surgery is relatively common after successful weight loss following bariatric surgery; one study found that one-third of bariatric surgery patients had had at least one procedure.[7]

Surgeries to Remove Excess Skin

Your body will change a lot as you lose weight. Most of the changes will be great, but you may develop some folds of extra skin. They can be uncomfortable and make you feel unattractive. They can even cause medical problems, such as the following:

- Back pain from the weight of your abdominal skin hanging down in front.
- Inability to keep yourself clean with normal baths and showers because of so much extra skin. Excess skin between the legs can lead to frequent yeast infections in women.
- Risk of regaining the weight because you are too uncomfortable to exercise. When you try, the loose skin flaps and bumps, and you feel very heavy, so you quit.
- Interference with a normal life. Some extra skin, such as around your abdomen, under your arms, or between your legs may be so heavy and bulky that it makes you feel tired and unable to even get through your normal daily routine in comfort.
- Rashes from constant rubbing of skin against skin. Rashes from chafing can be painful and itchy and lead to infections because they are broken skin.

Common Types of Body Contouring or Plastic Surgery after Significant Weight Loss

Many different procedures are available. The best procedure or procedures for you depend on your own problem spots. Following are a few of the more common skin-removal or body contouring procedures for bariatric surgery patients who have lost a lot of weight. In general, successful bariatric surgery patients are most likely to complain about excess skin around the waist and abdomen compared to other areas of the body and most likely to be satisfied with surgery in those areas.[8]

Panniculectomy or Abdominoplasty: You can call it your evil twin, you can call it "Fred," you can call it whatever you want…but the fact remains that your abdominal skin often feels like you are dragging around a second person—who is not on your side! *Panniculectomy* is the term for removing the excess skin and fat of your belly; an *abdominoplasty*, also known as a "tummy tuck," involves removing the excess skin and fat while also tightening up your stomach muscles.

Brachioplasty: This one is more familiar as the removal of your bat wings. It will leave scars under your arms, but your arms will be much lighter and more toned-looking.

Breast Reduction and Breast Reshaping: Some women dream of having bigger breasts, but you may be sick of yours. If you have lost a lot of weight, you may be going through life with heavy, aching breasts, sore shoulders from your bra straps cutting in, and constant back pain from heavy breasts. Daily life can be painful and embarrassing, and do not even mention exercise—the thought of unnecessary bouncing is painful! *Breast reduction* may be for you. *Breast reshaping,* or *mastoplexy*, is cosmetic and probably will not be covered by insurance, but you might choose to get mastoplexy if you are getting breast reduction anyway.

Lower Body Procedures: Walking is a chore when your thighs rub together at every step. Your impressive weight loss will unfortunately leave you with excess skin in your inner thighs and groin area. A *belt lipectomy*, or *lower body lift*, can take care of that so you are not constantly experiencing rubbing, burning, and chafing between your legs. Lower body procedures can also remove extra skin and fat from your buttocks.

The Logistics of Plastic Surgery

Planning for plastic surgery involves deciding on your procedure(s), finding a surgeon, and figuring out the financing.

Find a Qualified Plastic Surgeon

Choose a certified plastic surgeon whose qualifications and credentials inspire your confidence. The American Society of Plastic Surgeons is a private organization that aims to improve plastic surgery care. It includes surgeons from the American Board of Plastic Surgeons and its Canadian counterpart, the Royal College of Physicians and Surgeons of Canada.[9] You can use the Society's search engine to find a certified surgeon in your area. The advanced search function on the Society's website allows you to specify the procedure(s) that you are interested in.[10]

Another option is to go to the American Board of Plastic Surgeons' website and use its search function to find a certified surgeon.[11] The site also has a phone number that you can call to check whether a particular surgeon is certified.

Health Insurance May Cover Plastic Surgery for Medical Reasons

You will not get reimbursed for cosmetic surgery if it is for purely aesthetic reasons, but some health insurance policies cover plastic surgery procedures if you are getting them for health reasons. You and your physician may be able to persuade your health insurance company that your excess skin is a health hazard for which plastic surgery is the best treatment.[12] This can be true if:

- You are at risk for regaining your weight because your extra skin prevents you from exercising.
- You are at risk for infections because of your extra skin.

You will need documentation of your health problems. To assist you in writing a letter requesting reimbursement from your insurance company, the American Society of Plastic Surgeons provides a sample letter, along with medical insurance coding.[13]

Possible Side Effects of Extra Surgeries

All surgeries have risks. However, compared to pre-RYGB, your risk for complications from surgery is lower. That is because you have lost a lot of weight. These are some of the general risks of surgeries that are already familiar to you:

- Infections
- Blood clots
- Excessive bleeding
- Long recovery times with overwhelming nausea and fatigue

Plastic Surgery Has Its Own Risks

These are some risks that are more specific to cosmetic and reconstructive procedures. Your risk of severe complications is lower when your BMI is lower.[14]

- Seromas, or fluid building up near the surgery site under your skin. Your surgeon will need to drain it with a needle.
- Numbness or tingling at the site that your surgeon cuts. It can occur if your surgeon cuts a few nerves and is usually temporary.
- Large scars at the site where the excess skin is removed and your remaining skin is stitched together. These stitches are often in unnoticeable places, such as between your legs or under your arms. Often they are hidden by everyday clothes in most cases.
- Dehiscence—or splitting of the scar site where the stitches are. Reopening of the wound can result from poor stitching techniques or too much stress on the wound. It can lead to bleeding, infections, or even another surgery. You can lower your risk by choosing a good surgeon and by avoiding stretching the wound too much before it is fully healed. Another potential cause of dehiscence is if you regain your weight—yet another reason to treat your RYGB diet as a new lifestyle and not as a temporary fix.

Keep Your Expectations Realistic

Before you get your surgery or multiple procedures done, think carefully about your expectations in the short term and long term. You want to be able to enjoy your new body and feel pride in your hard work. Do not start criticizing your body for smaller and smaller details. Some bariatric surgery patients fall into the trap of wanting more procedures done, after they get the first, in pursuit of perfection.[15] Plastic surgery is not a solution to your self-image problems,[16] http://www.ncbi.nlm.nih.gov/pmc/articles/PMC3443403/but it can help you enjoy your new looks and your healthier body.

What to Expect: Triumphs

This can be a thrilling year! Do you remember all those times over the past five, 10, 20 years, or your entire life, when you felt a sense of failure, disappointment, or shame that was related, in some way, to your weight? As you lose the weight, you are going to relive the *opposites* of those moments—and they will come within the short period of a year or two. Every day or week that you stick to your diet and exercise plan will bring you proud, unforgettable moments on and off of the scale. Making the conscious effort to appreciate each one of your personal triumphs can motivate you to work hard for more triumphs.

Weight Milestones & Non-Scale Victories

These are what will stand out in your mind when you think about your weight loss. The milestones on the scale come at numbers that are important. These might be some of your milestones:

- The day you break 300 pounds and get back into the 200s and the day you break 200 pounds and get into the 100s
- Getting below your pre-pregnancy weight, weighing what you did on your wedding day, or getting back to your weight on the day that you graduated from high school
- Losing a round number of pounds, such as 100 pounds or 200 pounds
- Hitting your goal weight

These might not all come in the first year after surgery, but you will make progress toward them if you stick to the gastric bypass diet.

Non-Scale Victories

A non-scale victory, or NSV, is a triumph that comes during your weight loss journey but is not tied to a number on the scale. The NSVs are as important as your scale victories in making your weight loss experience worthwhile.

NSV: Better Control over Food

Before surgery, food controlled you. You might have thought about food all day: when the next meal is, how soon you can go back for seconds and thirds, whether you can squeeze in a trip to the drive-through on the way to and from work, and so on. After bypass, you might find that you think about food less frequently or that you are able to think about food without giving in to the urge to binge.

One example of a food-related NSV is if you go to a party where in the old, pre-surgery, days, you would have hung out at the food table. The post-surgery NSV comes at the moment you realize that you did not overeat at the party! Instead, you had fun mingling and socializing instead of sneaking over to refill your plate over and over to avoid talking to people, as in the old days.

NSV: Easier Clothes Shopping

Almost every lady dreams of fitting into her "skinny jeans," and quite a few gentlemen have their own dream belts, waist sizes, and other goals for fitting into clothes. Your weight loss journey provides plenty of opportunities for clothes-related NSVs! These are some examples:

- Ordering a 4X dress online and finding that it is too big. You exchange it for a 2X, and by the time it comes…it is already too big because you are down to the 1x size!

- Having fun shopping with your friends because *you* get to shop too. In the pre-surgery days, you were probably good at pretending you were interested in their clothes but did not want anything for yourself, but in reality, there was nothing in the store that fit. Even if there was, you would not have wanted to try it on in public. The NSV comes when you get to browse and have your friends wait for *you* to try things on!

- Clearing out your closet because none of those ridiculously oversized clothes will ever fit you again

- Fitting into your wedding dress

- And for fun? It is an NSV when you drag your old jeans out of the closet and step into them—with both legs in one pants leg!

NSV: More Natural Lifestyle

Until you regained your freedom, you probably did not even realize how much your obesity was holding you back. Sure, you knew that your knees hurt, you got out of breath easily, you felt self-conscious, and you did not fit comfortably into regular chairs and cars. But until your obesity stops being such an obstacle, you might not realize *quite* how hard it was keep up with your grandchildren or friends, how much you avoided eating meals in public, and how often you had to make excuses so that people did not feel bad leaving you behind while you sat and rested. You might not realize the changes all at once, but there may be a few NSVs that will be *ah-ha* moments, as in, "*Ah-ha…This is what the RYGB journey is all about."*

- Your friends will invite you to the movies, and you will say "yes" without worrying whether you will fit into the car with them.

- You will book a flight to your family reunion and choose the cheapest flight instead of scrambling to find the least full flight so that you can use two seats.

- Your daughter will ask you if she can take her tricycle out, and you will go with her on your own bicycle without having to get the car out to accompany her down the block.
- You and your spouse will go to a work party, and you will be able to focus on the people and the scene instead of wondering whether people are staring at you.

The list goes on—all of these new activities will become natural as you lose weight. You will be able to focus on life, not on your weight.

Practice Watching for NSVs

Some will be obvious—who *would not* be delighted with the ability to put her wedding ring on again for the first time in 30 years, for example? And others—you will have to look for them. Not every bypass patient will automatically notice the first time that he was able to let his toddler sit on his lap when his lap appeared from under his belly. With practice, you will be seeing NSVs everywhere and using them as motivation to keep up the good work.

What to Expect: Overcoming Challenges

Many challenges will appear during this year, but you got the RYGB to help you overcome them. You, like many obese individuals, might have gone through life giving up easily. You might have turned away from challenges and turned to food. Now you are going to confront and overcome your challenges because you are a stronger person. Success breeds success, and better self-confidence goes hand in hand with more weight loss.[17]

Common challenges include:

- Trouble sticking to your diet
- Disappointment in your rate of weight loss
- Feeling stress over changes in some of your relationships

Being honest with yourself is important. For example, instead of ignoring behaviors that contribute to weight regain, confront them. Some of these behaviors might be going back to drinking beverages with calories, snacking without recording your food, or going to drive-through outlets. Another risky behavior is having an all-or-nothing attitude, in which you convince yourself that a small mistake makes you a failure, so there is no point in trying any more. A better approach is to recognize a slip-up, think about why it happened, figure out how to prevent it in the future, and go on with your good habits.

Plateaus

Unfortunately, plateaus are to be expected in the first year and beyond. A plateau is when weight loss slows for a while. It might be a couple of weeks or even a month. Plateaus can come on suddenly—you might lose two pounds per week like clockwork for the first four months after surgery and then one week—bam. Nothing. The next week—nothing. You are still following the same diet plan, and your exercise has been consistent. What is going on? It is the dreaded…plateau.

Do Not Let Plateaus Derail Your Diet

Everyone experiences plateaus while trying to lose weight. Plateaus are frustrating enough to drive many dieters off of their diets. Some people throw in the towel during a plateau. They think that trying so hard to lose weight is pointless because of this small setback. You know better than that though! Instead of giving up, persevere, and you will be glad you did.

Weight loss is all about calories in compared to calories out. If you keep up the low-calorie RYGB diet and exercise as recommended, you will eventually break out of the plateau. It may take a couple of weeks or even months. These are two sure things about plateaus:

1. It *will* end if you continue to follow your weight loss surgery diet and burn off more calories than you eat.
2. It *will not* end if you give up and eat too much.

Sticking closely enough to your diet to be able to break through a plateau is something to be proud of. It is another challenge that you have faced successfully, and it is another reason to be confident in yourself.

Only Count Your Weekly Weigh-Ins

Your weight will not go down every day. If you weigh yourself every day, the number will often be the same as the day before. Sometimes it may even go up. These small fluctuations in your weight are normal, and they are not signs that you are gaining body fat. They are usually just from small changes in the amount of water in your body, and there is nothing you can do to prevent them.

That is why it is best to make a deal with yourself to only officially "count" a weekly weigh-in that you will record as part of your weight loss journey. Choose a day of the week to be your weigh-in day, and be consistent with your official weigh-in.

- *Weigh yourself in at the same time of day.* The early morning, right after you go to the bathroom for the first time, is a good time because you have not eaten anything yet so you do not have the extra weight of food or drink inside of you.
- *Weigh yourself naked or wearing just your underwear.* Light clothing is okay, but do not wear shoes.

Daily Weighing for Accountability

Although daily weigh-ins should not be taken as seriously as weekly ones, they can still be important in your weight loss plan. Knowing that you have to face the scale helps you stay accountable. Weighing yourself regularly will likely continue to be a part of your life for years to come. In fact, the National Weight Control Registry, or NWCR, reports that more than three out of every four people who lose at least 30 pounds and keep it off for at least a year weigh themselves regularly.[18]

Depression

Depression is not likely, but it is possible because of the rapid changes in your life. After RYGB, your whole world may seem upside-down. For the first time in years, possibly for the first time in your life, you are losing weight, you are in control of yourself, you are getting compliments about your appearance, and your self-esteem is increasing. Some of your personal relationships may improve while others may fall apart. These changes can be stressful because they are such big, important changes and because they affect all aspects of your life.

These changes can be overwhelming at times and make you thoughtful or moody. Everyone feels a little less energetic sometimes, but these periods should be short and infrequent. You may have mild depression if your feelings of hopelessness or lack of self-worth interfere with your regular activities or your symptoms last for more than two weeks.[19]

The risk for depression is one reason why keeping up your regular appointments with a mental health professional is so important to your postoperative care plan. If you do not have regularly scheduled appointments, you should at least know how to contact a psychologist if necessary. An expert can determine whether you should just wait out your symptoms or whether you should get treated for depression. The sooner you catch depressive disorder, the easier it is to treat.

Depression is not ubiquitous. In fact, losing a lot of weight after your surgery is more likely to improve your mood than make you depressed. This is especially true if you were mildly depressed before surgery because of your obesity and health issues related to your obesity that prevented you from living the life you wanted.[20]

Continued Struggles with Food

The Roux-en-Y gastric bypass is a powerful tool for weight loss, but it is just a tool. It does not instantly erase years of bad habits, get rid of all hunger, or eliminate food cravings. However, some bariatric patients report less hunger and lower cravings for sweets and fast foods.[21]

Unfortunately, not everyone finds the weight loss journey to be so easy. Some patients remain hungry, especially at the beginning. As you progress to pureed, soft, and finally solid foods, the RYGB diet can still be tough because you are not used to eating such small portions and ending the meal before you are stuffed.

Cravings Can Still Hit Hard

Even after surgery, your cravings may remain strong. [22] You may want something that is not on your diet, like a slice of pizza (or, as in the old days, a half of a pizza!) or some fried chicken. These are some options for when a craving strikes:

- *Ignore it until it goes away.* Distract yourself however you can, whether by talking on the phone or going for a walk, until the moment has passed. By the time you are finished with the phone conversation or walk, it will be close to time for your next drink or meal or snack so you can focus on a healthy food or beverage.
- *Reason with yourself.* Weigh the benefits against the disadvantages. A benefit of eating a small amount of the food might be preventing an eventual binge if you try to ignore

your craving. Disadvantages include increasing your calorie intake, feeling guilty, and getting dumping syndrome.

- *Have a very small amount.* Measure a tiny portion, record it in your food journal, and enjoy your serving at your next meal. Be sure to chew it slowly and savor it.

- *Have a healthier, portion-controlled substitute.* For example, instead of one or more slices of meat-lover's pizza, try an English muffin pizza on one-half of a whole-wheat English muffin spread with a quarter-cup of tomato or pizza sauce. Add an ounce of low-fat shredded mozzarella and some diced onions, black olives, and mushrooms. Turkey and vegetarian pepperoni and sausage are low-fat alternatives to beef and pork pepperoni and sausage.

As long as you stay focused on making good decisions, you can get over your craving without doing much damage to your diet. The most important thing to remember is that there is always another chance, so you do not need to slip into a rut. Whenever you feel like you have gone off of your diet, pick yourself up and get right back to work.

Cravings	
Instead of...	**Try...**
Apple pie	Baked apple with cinnamon
Buffalo wings	Chicken breast with barbecue sauce
Fried chicken	Baked chicken breast with high fiber cereal or whole-grain bread breading
Banana split	Half of a banana on a stick dipped in dark chocolate with sweetener; freeze
Brownie or chocolate cake	1 square (1/2 ounce) dark chocolate; 1 cup sugar-free hot cocoa mix
Ice cream	Sugar-free frozen pudding cup; let thaw for 30 minutes
French fries	Oven-baked squash fries/sticks

Table 43: Cravings

Working Hard to Develop New Eating Habits

After surgery, you will need persistence and hard work to break years-old habits and develop new habits. *Examples of habits that you will need to break include*:

- Constantly snacking
- Eating while doing other tasks
- Nibbling while preparing your next meal or snack
- Going to drive-through restaurants
- Choosing food based on taste rather than nutrition

Tip

Chapter 14, "RYGB Diet 101," lists the foods that should and should not be regular parts of your gastric bypass diet. The next chapter goes into more detail about healthy choices.

- Wolfing down your first portion so you can get seconds faster

Good habits to form include:

- Measuring and recording everything you eat and drink
- Focusing on your food, and not on other tasks, while you are eating
- Eating only at the table
- Choosing the most nutritious foods
- Stopping when you are full

Since you spent several pre-surgery years practicing the unhealthy eating behaviors, it will be a while before you naturally weigh out each portion of food, choose proteins and vegetables instead of macaroni and cheese, walk to the store to buy bananas instead of drive to your nearest burger drive-through, and slow down your eating enough to enjoy your food. Your good habits will form slowly but surely if you are consistent. Every time you consciously make a good decision instead of a poor one, your new healthy habits will become easier and more natural, and the old bad habits will seem less tempting.

Side Effects or Complications

You are still at risk for experiencing side effects or developing complications even after you are fully recovered from surgery.[23,24] You could experience the following:[25]

- Stricture
- Vomiting
- Leakage
- Dumping syndrome

You can nearly always prevent or reduce these late complications by following the weight loss surgery diet precisely. Try to figure out the cause of your symptoms. Ask yourself whether your diet changed, whether you chewed your food too fast, or whether you ate too much in one meal. These are common causes of the above side effects.

Remember to call your surgeon if you ever have a situation in which you cannot swallow or drink for more than a few hours or if you are ever concerned for any other reason that your health is in serious danger. It is always better to be safe than sorry.

> **Tip**
>
> Chapter 5, "Roux-En-Y Gastric Bypass: Risks and Considerations," which describes common side effects and complications of surgery. Chapter 13, "Post-Surgery Diet: From Liquid Diet to Solid Foods," and Chapter 14, "RYGB Diet 101," have advice on how to choose safe foods that are not likely to cause problems plus what to do if you start to experience dumping syndrome or other diet-related symptoms.

Smoking

Question: What is the only lifestyle choice that kills more Americans each year than obesity, a poor diet, and not enough exercise?

Answer: Tobacco use!

The Centers for Disease Control and Prevention state that smoking kills one out of every five Americans.[26] Smoking leads to coronary heart disease and peripheral vascular disease; lung cancer; esophageal, throat, pancreatic, and kidney cancer; high blood pressure and stroke; emphysema; chronic obstructive lung disease; and osteoporosis. In fact, smoking harms every organ in your body. What else does smoking do:

- It hurts the people around you because of your second-hand smoke.
- It makes your clothes and breath smell.
- It is expensive. At $5 per pack, a pack a day costs you more than $1,500 per year.
- It makes your teeth yellow.
- It makes your hands shake.
- It is inconvenient. You cannot enjoy anything because all you can think about is getting out for your next smoke and making sure you have another pack handy.

Time to Quit

So where does smoking fit into your post-surgery plans? If you are a smoker, the postoperative period is an ideal opportunity to quit for several reasons:

- *You will still lose weight.* Many people are afraid to quit smoking because they think it will make them gain weight, but that does not have to be true. If you follow your RYGB diet as prescribed, you will still lose weight quickly even if you stop smoking. The gastric bypass journey is a golden opportunity to stop smoking because the effects of a slower metabolism will be so minor compared to the huge calorie deficits you should have.
- *You are taking control of your life.* This period is all about you. You need to focus on yourself and your weight loss goals if you want to lose weight. Now that you are focusing attention on yourself, you can also direct energy to quitting smoking. Your post-surgery care program requires you to work closely with your medical team and attend group support meetings anyway; why not use this time to commit wholeheartedly into your health and go to the extra support groups or doctor's appointments that will help you quit smoking?
- *You are testing your willpower anyway.* You will need to be strong-minded to be able to consistently make the diet and exercise changes necessary for success with the bypass. As you are breaking old eating habits and forming new ones, you might as well break the smoking habit and live a smoke-free life.
- *It is time for a new you.* You have already decided that your body is going to be at the goal weight you have been dreaming of. Why not make it a healthy, smoke-free body?

Some Surgeons Require You to Quit Smoking

Some surgeons might ask you to stop smoking during the weeks leading up to your surgery as a way to prove that you have enough self-discipline to succeed in your weight loss journey. When you schedule the date of your RYGB, you might have to sign a contract stating that you will not smoke again before the surgery. Your surgeon can give you frequent drug tests to make sure that you are sticking to your end of the bargain leading up to surgery. By the time you have your surgery, your cigarette cravings may have diminished.

Replacement Addictions

Replacement addictions, also known as crossover addictions or substitute addictions, threaten a small proportion of bariatric patients. Some obese individuals were literally physically or psychologically addicted to food; you may have actually *felt a need* to use junk food to get you through the day. After surgery, you will not be able to depend on large portions of high-sugar, high-fat foods.

> **Tip**
>
> Chapter I, "Obesity – A Widespread Disease," for information on the addictive power of high-calorie, high-sugar, high-sodium foods.

Replacement Addictions Can Result from Physiological Reasons

Breaking your food addiction helps you lose weight, but it can lead some people to develop replacement addictions to substitute for food. Alcohol is among the most likely addictions to develop because there are actually biological mechanisms that are similar to those of high-sugar foods. Alcohol and sugar are both used to stimulate dopamine, which is a neurotransmitter, or chemical that your brain produces, that gives you a sense of pleasure. When you stop "abusing" sugar as a drug, you might end up replacing your sugar abuse with alcohol abuse.[27]

Replacement Addictions Can Result from Psychological Reasons

Even if you were not chemically addicted to food, you might have been emotionally or psychologically addicted. That is true if you used to eat for comfort or out of boredom or habit. Smoking is an example of a dangerous replacement addiction that might develop if you start to smoke on your lunch hour and short breaks and when you want to take a moment to step outside. In the old days, you might have taken a break to eat; a replacement addiction could develop if you choose to smoke instead.

Choose Healthy Alternatives to Food or Replacement Addictions

If you are concerned that you are developing a crossover addiction, try to figure out why. What role did overeating fill in your life that you are now trying to fill with another unhealthy habit? Then find a healthy alternative to junk food or replacement addictions.

- Your social support system can help if you are lonely or bored: phone a friend, write some emails, or hop onto BariatricPal.com.
- Find a new hobby to fill the gaps between meals, relieve stress, or keep your hands occupied: blogging, sewing, and gardening are examples.
- Crossword puzzles and other mind games can help you distract yourself.
- Go for a short walk or do a few stretches to relieve stress in a healthy way and let the craving pass.

☞ Summary

☞ Losing significant amounts of weight after your surgery will lead to far greater changes than just the number on the scale. You will look different and feel better. Your whole world can change after RYGB. This chapter covered some of these possible changes to help you prepare.

☞ We suggest greeting the changes with confidence, preparing for them as much as possible, and staying aware that you are facing the same challenges and situations as other gastric bypass patients.

Time to Take Action: Looking ahead to the First Year

List three things that you are most looking forward to in your first year after surgery.

Example: I can't wait to go biking with my son for the first time!

1.

2.

3.

List three challenges you expect to have and how you plan to overcome them.

Example: It'll be tough to go to parties and social events and stay on my diet. People are used to me pigging out, and I'm used to me pigging out. I plan to avoid any diet problems by focusing on enjoying the people, not the food, when I go to social events. Also, when it's appropriate, I will bring something healthy to eat so I won't be starving.

1.

2.

3.

1   Faria SL, Faria OP, Lins RD, de Gouvea, HR. Hair loss among bariatric surgery patients. Bariatric Times. 2010;7(11):18-20.

2   E, Riffo A, Papapietro K, Csendes A, Ruz M. Alopecia in women with severe and morbid obesity who undergo bariatric surgery. Nutr Hosp. 2011;26(4)

3   D'Hondt M, Vanneste S, Pottel H, Devriendt D, Van Rooy F, Vasteenkiste F. Laparoscopic sleeve gastrectomy as a single-stage procedure for the treatment of morbid obesity and the resulting quality of life, resolution of comorbidities, food intolerance and 6-year weight loss. 2011. Surg Endosc. 25(8):2498-504.

4   Losing weight: what is healthy weight loss? Centers for Disease Control and Prevention. Web site. http://www.cdc.gov/ healthyweight/losing_weight/index.html. Updated 2011, August 17. Accessed November 24, 2012.

5   Gill RS, Birch DW, Shi X, Sharma AM, Karmali S. Sleeve gastrectomy and type 2 diabetes mellitus: a systematic review. Surg Obes Relat Dis. 2010;6(6):707-713.

6   Edholm D, Svensson F, Naslund I, Karlsson FA, Rask E, Sundborn M. Long-term results 11 years after the primary gastric bypass in 384 patients. Surg Obes Related Dis. 2012.

7   Mitchell JE, Crosby RD, Ertelt TW, Marino JW, Sarwer DB, Thompson JK, Lancaster KL, Simonich H, Howell LM. The desire for body contouring surgery after bariatric surgery. Obesity Surgery. 2008;18:1308-12.

8   Steffen KJ, Sarwer DB, Thompson JK, Mueller A, Baker AW, Mitchell JE. Predictors of satisfaction with excess skin and desire for body contouring following bariatric surgery. Surgery for Obesity and Related Diseases. 2012;8:92-7.

9   American Society of Plastic Surgeons. Active membership process (United States and Canada). Retrieved from http://www. plasticsurgery.org/For-Medical-Professionals/Surgeon-Community/Join-ASPS/Active-Membership-Process.html. 2012. Accessed November 24, 2012.

10 Find a surgeon. American Society of Plastic Surgeons. Web site. http://www1.plasticsurgery.org/find_a_surgeon/. 2012. Accessed November 24, 2012.

11 American Board of Plastic Surgeons. Web site. https://www.abplsurg.org/moddefault.aspx. 2012. Accessed November 24, 2012.

12 Gurungluoglu R. Insurance coverage criteria for panniculectomy and redundant skin surgery after bariatric surgery: why and when to discuss. Obesity Surgery. 2012;517-520.

13 American Society of Plastic Surgeons. ASPS recommended insurance coverage criteria for third-party payers: surgical treatment of skin redundancy for obese and massive weight loss patients. Web site. http://www.plasticsurgery.org/Documents/medical-professionals/health-policy/insurance/Surgical-Treatment-of-Skin-Redundancy-Following.pdf. 2007, January. Accessed November 24, 2012.

14 Langer V, Singh A, Aly AS, Cram AE. Body contouring following massive weight loss. Indian Journal of Plastic Surgery. 2011;44:14-20.

15 Song AY, Rubin JP, Thomas V, Dudas JR, Marra KG, Fernstrom MH. Body image and quality of life in post massive weight loss body contouring patients. Obesity (Silver Spring). 2006;14:1626-1636.

16 Singh D, Zahiri HR, Janes LE, Sabino J, Matthews JA, Bell RL, Thomson JG. Mental and physical impact of body contouring procedures on post-bariatric surgery patients. Eplasty. 2012;12:e47.

17 Batsis JA, Clark MM, Grothe K, Lopez-Jimenez F, Collazo-Clavell ML, Somers VK, Sarr MG. Self-efficacy after bariatric surgery for obesity: a population-based cohort study. Appetite. 2009;52:637-45.

18 NWCR facts. National Weight Control Registry. Web site. http://www.nwcr.ws/Research/default.htm. Accessed November 24, 2012.

19 Depression. National Institutes of Mental Health. Web site. http://www.nimh.nih.gov/health/publications/depression/complete-index.shtml.Revised 2011. Accessed November 24, 2012.

20 Rutledge T, Braden AL, Woods G, Herbst KL, Groesz LM, Savu M. Five-year changes in psychiatric treatment status and weight-related comorbidities following bariatric surgery in a veteran population. Obes Surg. 2012;22(11):1734-41.

21 Leahey TM, Bond DS, Raynor H, Roye D, Vithiananthian S, Ryder BA, Sax SC, Wing RR. Effects of bariatric surgery on food cravings: do food cravings and the consumption of craved foods "normalize" after surgery? Surg Obes Relat Dis. 2012;8(1):84-91.

22 Leahey TM, Bond DS, Raynor H, Roye D, Vithiananthian S, Ryder BA, Sax SC, Wing RR. Effects of bariatric surgery on food cravings: do food cravings and the consumption of craved foods "normalize" after surgery? Surg Obes Relat Dis. 2012;8(1):84-91.

23 Hamdan K, Somers S, Chand M. Management of late postoperative complications of bariatric surgery. Br J Surg. 2011;98(10):1345-1355.

24 Richardson WS, Plaisance AM, Periou L, Buquoi RN, Tillery D. Long-term management of patients after weight loss surgery. Ochsner Journal, 2009;9:154-159.

25 Iannelli A, Dainese R, Piche T, Facchiano E, Gugenheim J. Laparoscopic sleeve gastrectomy for morbid obesity. World J Gastroenterol. 2008;14(6):821-827

26 Health effects of cigarette smoking. Centers for Disease Control and Prevention. Web site. http://www.cdc.gov/tobacco/data_statistics/fact_sheets/health_effects/effects_cig_smoking/. 2012. Accessed November 24, 2012.

27 Common mechanisms of drug abuse and obesity. National Association of Drug Abuse. Web site. http://www.drugabuse.gov/news-events/news-releases/2010/03/common-mechanisms-drug-abuse-obesity. 2012, March 28. Accessed November 24, 2012.

18

The Benefits
of a Strong
Support System

The last chapter discussed some of the changes to expect after your Roux-en-Y gastric bypass surgery. With so many changes in your appearance, health, self-image, and relationships, you will need a lot of support. This chapter will talk about building a fail-proof support system and the sources of support that may be available to you. These include:

- Yourself
- Your family and friends
- Members of your medical team
- Other bariatric surgery patients from your support group meetings and online communities

Building Your Support System

Your support system will be one of the most important factors in your RYGB success story.[1] You cannot prevent struggles, but a support system can help you overcome these struggles through encouragement and advice.

A Strong Support System Is Like a Multi-Level Insurance Policy

Failure is nearly impossible when your support system is solid. It should be a complex organization of people that will hold you up in any situation that you come across. When your support system is in place, you should have encouragement and advice available wherever you are and whatever you face.

The Center of Your Support System: Yourself

This may sound corny, but it is quite true:

- You are your own biggest fan. Nobody wants you to succeed as much as you do.
- You are always there for yourself. There is no denying that fact, so you might as well be a source of support for yourself!
- You are in charge. That means that you have the power to choose the best action.

How You Can Support Yourself

With a bit of effort, you can become a stronger source of support for yourself. These are a few tips:

- *Make yourself proud.* Follow your gastric bypass diet and your exercise routine.
- *Compliment yourself.* Make a conscious effort to recognize your accomplishments. Tell yourself when and why you are proud, just as you would tell your best friends when you are proud of them.
- *Believe in yourself.* You are much more likely to achieve your goals when you are confident that you can. If you let doubts creep in, they can prevent you from trying and succeeding. If you do not succeed the first time, try again. True failure comes when you give up.

- *Prepare to give yourself pep talks.* You will slip up sometimes because you are human, but you prepare for it. If you go off your diet or exercise program, you can pick yourself right back up. Quickly going back to your original plans can become automatic if you practice.
- *Be your own best motivator.* Make a list of reasons why you are losing the weight, and post it where you can see it every day, possibly on the refrigerator or on the wall behind your desk.
- *Make a back-up plan.* When you are feeling down, you might not be thinking as clearly as you normally do. Have a list of your closest support allies with you so that you know whom to call when you need help.

Tracking Your Progress

Tracking your progress keeps you accountable and motivates you:

- *Track your weight.* Write down the numbers or record them on the computer so you can see how well you are doing and be motivated to continue working hard.
- *Maintain a food diary.* Bariatric surgery patients who keep journals are more likely to lose more weight.[2]
- *Keep an exercise log.* The chapter on starting and continuing an exercise program has a sample log and some suggestions for keeping one.
- *Record body measurements.* Measurements that will shrink as you lose weight include the distances around your waist, thigh, bust, chest, calves, hips, and neck. Recording these changes is motivating.

Family and Friends for Support

Some of us are closer to family, while others are closer to our friends. Regardless, nearly all bariatric patients find that some of their closest relationships are supportive of the surgery, while others are not. Often you will not know which are which until you have told them that you are getting gastric bypass or you have already undergone surgery. Friends and family members will likely be in these categories.

Automatic Supporters

They love you unconditionally, and they will automatically support you in anything that you believe is best for yourself without demanding explanations. These are the people who are most likely to be open to learning what they can do to help you on your journey.

Disapproval with an Open Mind

Many people assume that weight loss surgery is weird, cheating, or unhealthy, but they are likely to genuinely listen to your explanation of what the surgery is and what you have to do to make it work. When you explain your reasoning and they see you losing weight, eating healthier, and being happier, they will start to understand your decision and support you.

Even if they never agree with your decision to get the RYGB, people in this category will not look down on you because of your surgery.

Flat-Out Rejection

Some people might be negative about bariatric surgery and refuse to consider changing their minds. Sometimes this happens because they struggle with their own weight and are envious of your dedication and success. Some people decide that weight loss surgery is bad—even if they never bothered to learn the first thing about it. Others may be basing their judgment on a bad experience that a friend of a friend of a coworker's relative had with weight loss surgery. People like this can be frustrating and demeaning, but do not let closed-minded people upset you. Your best option is to ignore them while you keep losing weight and doing your best for yourself.

You will find out soon enough who is supportive, who is neutral, and who is destructive. Do not waste your time and energy worrying about negative people.

Recruit Allies

Specifically ask several of your friends and family members if they are willing to be part of your support system. Different friends and family members each have their own best roles. You can figure out how each of them can help you the best way they can. These are some examples:

- You might need to ask your spouse to avoid eating chocolate chip cookies in front of you, if that is your weak spot.

- You might ask your sister to call you each day on your cell phone at 8:00 p.m. so that she can talk you through your evening walk.

- Your best friend might be your conscience and responsible for asking (politely and with genuine concern) if you are doing okay when he sees that you are down or notices that you have not been telling him proudly about weight loss recently.

- You might ask your children to help you make dinner so that you are not tempted to nibble on food while you are preparing it. Younger children will revel at being the food police and stopping their mom or dad from sneaking forbidden bites.

Here are a few more tips for making the best use of your friends and family member support system:

- Your spouse, friends, children, siblings, and parents all have different roles in other parts of your life. The same is true for your RYGB journey.

- Be specific about what you need them to do. They do not know unless you tell them.

- Understand and clarify the differences between being a shoulder to cry on, someone who gives advice, and someone who is there to give you some tough love or a kick in the pants. Some friends and family members will always be best at one of these. Others can fill multiple roles depending on the situation, but they may need you to tell them what you need in any given moment.

- Do not be afraid to be the weak one. Sometimes you hold your family and friends up; sometimes they hold you up. That is how life works. If you need help in your weight loss journey, ask for it and accept it.

How Can I Prevent Sabotage?

Other people can sabotage your diet if you let them. The sabotage often seems — and may be — intentional. These sneaky people are often the ones who make you feel bad for getting weight loss surgery, for following a diet and exercise plan, or for taking steps to become healthy. Their sabotage may include:

- *Keeping* certain foods in the house that you have specifically asked them not to have around. These might be foods such as fried chicken, ice cream, potato chips, or anything else you cannot control yourself around.

- Inviting you to dinners without serving anything you can eat or pressuring you to eat more than you want.

- Making rude comments or staring at you to make you feel uncomfortable or doubt yourself.

What can you do about these people? Here are a few options:

- *Avoid them*. It is fail-proof but not always possible.

- *Preparing for them*. Psych yourself up: think ahead to what might go wrong when you encounter your saboteur, and prepare to react. What will you say and do? Also, give yourself a pep talk. Remind yourself what a wonderful person you are, how hard you are working to achieve your goals, and how much you deserve your success.

- *Phone a friend or family member* — before and after. When I know that I am going to have an unpleasant encounter with someone who is about to make me feel bad, I ask my sister to be ready with her phone so that I can call her right afterward and she can make me feel better.

- *Be patient*. Believe it or not, some saboteurs actually have the potential to become your friends and allies. Try to be kind, informative, and courteous. Over time and with persistence, you might be able to figure out why they are mean to you and how you can solve the problem. It is possible they are jealous of you or unsure of themselves and need a helping hand that you can provide.

- *Be prepared*. Bring a healthy dish to share if you are going over for dinner; decide ahead of time exactly how many bites you will eat, and remember to take three deep breaths before even considering taking offense at any disparaging comments. You may be taking a lot of deep breaths, but the deep breathing practice will serve you well in the future too.

Everyone faces intentional or unintentional sabotage at some point. You can prevent it from delaying your weight loss as long as you stay cool, collected, and in control of yourself.

A Supportive Work Environment

The average middle-aged working adult spends an average of nearly nine hours per day at work on a typical working day.[3] That is a lot of time. If you want to lose weight, your work environment had better be healthy. Two ways to make your work environment more supportive are to recruit coworkers to help you and to make your own workspace healthier.

People at Work

Everyone's employment situation is different, but if you work outside the home, you probably spend a *lot* of time with your coworkers. Your weight loss journey will be so much easier if you can find one or two supporters. Although everyone's own personal work situation is unique, you can use the following ideas to help you search for your own effective source of encouragement.

A Friend: If you are lucky enough to have one or more close friends at work, by all means take advantage of them! Let them know about your gastric bypass journey and how they can help, if they are willing. Work friends see you each day, so they know how you are feeling day to day. Along with providing listening ears, they can encourage you to keep on track at lunch and break times.

Your Boss: Your weight loss journey will be easier if you are lucky enough to have a sympathetic boss. You need to decide for yourself exactly what and how much you want to tell your boss about your weight loss surgery, if anything. You might not feel comfortable divulging personal information. But if you are pretty sure that your boss will be supportive, go ahead and tell about your weight loss surgery. A boss who is in your corner will enable you to more easily attend surgeon or other appointments in your postoperative care program. It will also help at those times, especially when surgery is still pretty recent, when you want to go home a little early or take it easy at work because you do not feel well.

A Colleague Who Is Also Losing Weight: You are not likely to find someone in your workplace who got weight loss surgery around the same time as you, but you might a coworker who is making a serious effort to lose weight. You two can help each other stay on track and exchange tips and encouragement.

A Colleague Who Is Working toward a Different Goal: A little creativity can go a long way when you are looking for support at work. Support can come from someone who is not trying to lose weight but who is trying to achieve a different life-changing goal. For example, someone who is trying to quit smoking can be a great source of support and inspiration for you. The two of you can go for walks together at lunch so that you can burn calories and your coworker can be distracted from smoking. Inside the office, you can confide in each other with your struggles and remind each other that you are rooting for each other.

If you work a 40-hour work week, you are spending one-third of your weekday life in your work environment. The more support you can get at work, the better off you will be.

A Weight Loss-Friendly Workspace: You can design your workspace to be more encouraging to weight loss. Keep your food environment healthy by following many of the same guidelines as you do at home. For example:

- Keep healthy snacks on hand so you do not need to depend on the vending machine.
- Plan ahead so you know what you will eat for each meal and snack for the entire work day.
- Do not store unhealthy foods in your office or the worksite's refrigerator.
- Keep water on or near your desk at all times.

These are some additional ways that you can promote weight loss at work:

- Keep some sneakers and workout clothes available. You can use them for lunchtime walks or for going to the gym.
- Reduce the temptation of workplace foods, such as chocolates or doughnuts, by trying not to walk by where they are being offered.
- Remind yourself about your goals with post-it notes on your bulletin board or on or in your desk.

Do I Have to Tell People That I Have Gastric Bypass?

Absolutely not! You get to decide:

- Whom to tell: from nobody to everyone
- What to tell: from nothing to everyone
- When to tell: from before RYGB to after hitting your goal weight

Keeping your weight loss surgery a secret is completely normal. Shy and private people are naturally inclined to say nothing as they steadily lose weight and discretely thank people that compliment them on their weight loss. Even outgoing people do not always tell everyone about the bypass. On the other hand, people who share everything about their lives and are super proud of their weight loss are more likely to tell everyone about the RYGB.

To tell or not to tell? That seems to be the question…but the answer can lie somewhere in between! These are some of the decisions we have seen from a variety of weight loss surgery patients:

- Telling everyone because they are proud of their hard work and success
- Telling close friends and family but not saying anything to more casual acquaintances — after all, weight loss can be a personal thing.

- Telling people on an NTK, or need-to-know, basis; that is, tell people who may be able to benefit from hearing about your experience with the gastric bypass.
- Telling people that care. Some people are genuinely interested in you and your life; others are going through the motions. If they ask, and sincerely seem interested in the answer, you might want to tell them.
- Telling almost nobody. If you have heard enough nasty, often uninformed, comments about the gastric bypass, you might not want to open yourself up to more negativity.

By the way, your decision is not necessarily related to your chances of being successful with the Roux-en-Y gastric bypass. Each of the above examples came from people who were losing weight at the rate they had hoped, or who had hit their goal weight and were maintaining their weight.

Support from Your Healthcare Team

Your healthcare team's main goal is for you to succeed, and team members can play a large role in your success by being part of your post-surgery support system. You can take advantage of this support by participating fully in your aftercare program. Weight loss surgery patients who complete their aftercare programs and follow through with their one-year check-in after surgery are more likely to lose the weight they had hoped for by the end of that year than patients who do not take aftercare seriously.[4]

Medical Support: A comprehensive support system includes having support for when you have a medical emergency or just a question. You should have the direct number to your surgeon or someone at the clinic or hospital where you got surgery so that you can get answers to urgent questions. You can call these numbers when you need to know whether the symptoms you are experiencing require medical attention or whether you can treat them at home.

Psychological Support: Your psychologist or mental health professional should be available for routine support.[5] Many weight loss surgery patients actually have regular appointments with their mental health professionals or maintain regular contact when the psychologist leads support group meetings. Psychologists are great for suggesting coping strategies for your situation and ways to stay positive during the tough times. Staying in touch with your psychologist lets you be monitored for signs of depression, which can occur with bariatric surgery patients because of the quick changes in your life.

Dietitian or Nutritionist: Dietitians are not officially responsible for keeping you emotionally grounded, but they can certainly help! Your dietitian is your trusted source for nutrition advice and meal plans. Beyond that, dietitians can be lifesavers, or at least diet-savers, when you are craving something that is not on your diet. Most dietitians understand your situation and are sympathetic; most are willing to accept your calls (or text messages or emails) and offer suggestions when you need help. For example, when you are craving a banana split and you are just about to give in, you can contact your dietitian, who might encourage you instead to stick with a half of a pureed banana topped with some sugar-free vanilla pudding to save hundreds of calories and worlds of guilt. Knowing that your dietitian is there for you no matter what adds an extra layer of support to your system.

Support Group Meetings -- Before agreeing to do the gastric bypass, your surgeon is likely to have you promise to attend support group meetings for at least a year. It is an important part of your post-surgery care program. Support group meetings can help teach you better eating habits, ways to develop better habits, and strategies for getting through the tough times.[6]

In-Person Support Group Meetings -- Research clearly shows that you are more likely to have better weight loss when you attend support group meetings.[7] In one study that followed bariatric surgery patients for a year, the patients who went to their recommended support group meetings lost an average of 42 percent of their original BMI. The patients who did not attend support group meetings lost only 32 percent of their original BMI, even though they had the same surgeon and other aftercare services as the group that attended support group meetings.

> **Tip**
>
> Chapter 7, "Planning for the Gastric Bypass," discusses the process of assembling a strong healthcare team and the role of each member in your success. **Chapter 12, "Aftercare: Your Post-Surgery Care Program,"** talks about taking full advantage of the follow-up appointments with your surgeon and other team members.

Online Support

Support group meetings are great because you learn a lot and meet great people. But they do not always fit into your schedule, and they only meet at certain intervals. Online support groups can fill in the gaps in between your weekly or monthly support group meetings. Online support groups also have an advantage over your own friends and family because members know exactly what you are going through.

Online support resources are there for you at every minute of every day. They can provide encouragement, advice about how to deal with RYGB side effects, and information on diet and exercise. Online support forums include members who are gastric bypass patients— they have been there, done that and can offer advice for any problem that you are experiencing or question that you have. There will also be people who are at the same point of their weight loss journey as you; you can form amazing bonds with these members as you support each other.

There are many weight loss surgery and gastric bypass support groups online. Many are free to join, and they welcome everyone. BariatricPal.com is the largest such group, and it is an independently-run, non-biased board. It is not run by a healthcare company, a bariatric surgeon, or a hospital.

> **Tip**
>
> Chapter 19, "Bariatricpal.Com and Other Online Resources," for information on joining and using BariatricPal.com. The chapter covers the unique features of the site and some of the benefits of membership, which is free for everyone.

✍ **Summary**

☞ You will encounter plenty of challenges with the RYGB, and you will have a head start at overcoming them if you have a strong support system. You are at the center of your system.

☞ Also supporting you will be some of your friends and family members and hopefully a few people at your workplace. Your surgeon, psychologist, and dietitian will also be ready to give you a helping hand as you lose weight after surgery. You can get support from other bariatric patients from your support group meetings and online groups too.

☞ The Internet is likely to play a large role in your success with the bypass, and the next chapter focuses on BariatricPal.com, an online community that is welcoming, free for everyone, and a potentially important component of your social support system.

Time to Take Action: Your Support System

List five sources of social support that you are going to recruit and maintain.

Example: I've already signed up for membership on BariatricPal.com, and I've gotten into some cool conversations with some of the members. I hope they'll continue to be sources of support for me!

1.

2.

3.

4.

5.

1   Positive relationships. Realize. Web site. http://www.realize.com/weight-loss-lifestyle-support.htm. Accessed November 24, 2012.

2   Butryn ML, Phelan S, Hill JO, Wing, RR. Consistent self-monitoring of weight: a key component of successful weight loss maintenance. Obesity (Silver Spring). 2007;15:3091-3096.

3   Bureau of Labor Statistics. Charts from the American Time Use Survey. Department of Labor. Web site. http://www.bls.gov/tus/charts/. Modified 2012, November 16. Accessed November 23, 2012.

4   Harper J, Madan AK, Ternovitis CA, Tichansky DS What happens to patients who do not follow-up after bariatric surgery? The American Surgeon. 2007;73:181-4.

5   Breznikar B, Divneski D. Bariatric surgery for morbid obesity: pre-operative assessment, surgical techniques and post-operative monitoring. J Int Med Res. 2009;37(5):1632-1645.

6   McVay MA, Friedman KE. The benefits of cognitive behavioral groups for bariatric surgery patients. Bariatric Times. 2012;9(9):22-28.

7   Orth WS, Madan AK, Taddecci RJ, Coday M, Tichansky DS. Support group meeting attendance is associated with better weight loss. Obesity Surgery. 2008;18:391-4.

19

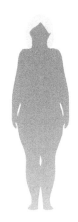

Bariatricpal .Com and Other Online Resources

After reading this far, you are almost an expert on the RYGB journey! Topics in the previous chapters included:

- Learning about the Roux-en-Y gastric bypass procedure and your other options
- Deciding whether to get the RYGB
- Choosing a surgeon and preparing for the procedure
- Having surgery and recovering well
- Your post-surgery diet progression and long-term gastric bypass diet
- Integrating nutrition and exercise into your new lifestyle
- Life changes to expect as you lose weight

You already know a lot about RYGB, but there is always more to learn. This chapter gives you pointers on where to go when you have questions throughout your weight loss journey. It provides advice on making the most out of online resources so you know what to believe. In particular, this chapter focuses on BariatricPal.com. This social network and comprehensive weight loss surgery resource center has already been mentioned in this book.

Online Resources Are Nearly Indispensable

Nowadays the Internet is essential for staying in touch, finding locations, researching products and services, and keeping up with the news. We are connected at home and away on computers and mobile devices. You can take advantage of technology and online information and communication to help you in your RYGB journey. This section suggests ways to use the Internet more effectively.

Online Social Communities

You already know that your support system is fundamental to successful weight loss after gastric bypass. In-person members of your support system likely include your family, friends, support group members, and medical team. Virtual buddies can be just as important. Online social networks let you meet far more weight loss surgery patients online than you can in person.

Some general sites, such as Facebook and Twitter, enable you find and communicate with other gastric bypass patients. Other sites are designed to facilitate meetings with people in your area. BariatricPal.com has these features as well but has the major advantage of being dedicated to the weight loss surgery community, with hundreds of thousands of members.

Benefits of Online Resources

Online resources are unlimited sources of information, and they are always available. You can get your questions answered after business hours and on weekends. You can meet and communicate with friends around the world and in different time zones. Online resources can be as private as you want them to be so you can feel free to ask questions that you think are silly. For example, maybe you are lying awake wondering whether you can eat non-fat cottage cheese for breakfast on your soft foods diet, but you would feel silly letting people know that you are worried. You can ask anonymously online, get your answer, and sleep peacefully knowing that yes, cottage cheese is allowed.

Being Cautious with Online Resources

Online resources can be credible and complete, but they are not always. Anyone can post materials online without being accurate. Blogs, company or personal web pages, and all other resources can be accurate or inaccurate. Often you have to use your own judgment to decide whether a site is accurate. These are some warning signs of sites that probably are not trustworthy:

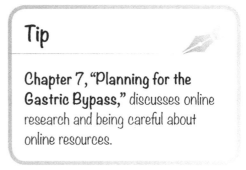

Tip

Chapter 7, "Planning for the Gastric Bypass," discusses online research and being careful about online resources.

- Distracting ads that direct you away from the site
- Contains at least some information that you know is wrong, so you can assume that other information on the site might be inaccurate too.
- Includes a noticeably high number of posts or contributions that are redundant and by a single person. That person might be trying to get you to buy something.
- Has tons of links to an external (different) site. That is a sign that someone is just trying to get you to visit the other site and the owner of the original site may receive a payment each time a visitor goes to the other site.

A lot of resources look authentic at first glance, but as you dig deeper, you might start to notice some of the above red flags. You can develop your own set of trusted sites as you continue to search for information on the gastric bypass online. Information from your surgeon and informal advice from social networking sites where you have developed close friendships can be dependable sources.

Online Communities

Thousands of weight loss discussion boards can be found online. They may be dedicated to weight loss, to bariatric surgery patients in general, or to gastric bypass patients in particular. They may be sponsored by companies, by hospitals, or by individuals.

There is no single "best" board for everyone. If no single board meets all of your needs, you might join and regularly visit multiple communities. These are some of the criteria to consider when you are test-driving to find one or more good communities:

- Friendly
- Option to provide as much or little personal information as you want
- Offers mobile apps
- Policy against selling your information to advertisers
- Additional features, such as live chat rooms and instant messaging

Introduction to BariatricPal.com

BariatricPal.com is the largest online social network dedicated to the weight loss surgery community. It is for bariatric surgery patients, people that are considering surgery, and any of their supporters.

BariatricPal.com Weight Loss Surgery Support

Originally, WLSBoards.com included four separate Weight Loss Surgery (WLS) boards, or discussion forums, with hundreds of thousands of members. Each board was dedicated to a specific type of weight loss surgery:

- LapBandTalk.com, the original WLSBoards community dating back to July of 2003, was for the laparoscopic adjustable gastric band, or lap-band.
- VerticalSleeveTalk.com, started in February of 2009, was for the vertical sleeve gastrectomy.
- SleevePlicationTalk.com, started in May of 2011, was for the sleeve plication procedure.
- RNYTalk.com, started in July of 2011, was for the Roux-en-Y gastric bypass.

Now the four boards are all housed within BariatricPal.com, which is a comprehensive online resource for the weight loss surgery community. You are welcome to hang out with other RYGB patients in the gastric bypass board, to hop on over to the other weight loss surgery forums, or to chat in a general section for all weight loss surgery procedures. Together, the boards have more than two million posts per month.

The Story of BariatricPal.com

A unique feature of BariatricPal.com is that it is independent and not affiliated with a major company or medical care group. Its founder, Alex Brecher, is himself a bariatric surgery patient—and one of the authors of this book. At 5 feet 7 inches tall and 255 pounds, Alex got the lap-band in July of 2003. When he got home from the hospital and looked online for sources of information and support, he was disappointed that he could not find a comprehensive source of trustworthy information and friendly encouragement. That is when he started LapBandTalk.com.

Alex did not forget the trials of obesity and the gift that bariatric surgery was for him. When he saw that patients of other types of weight loss surgery needed information, he started the other communities within BariatricPal, or what was then known as the (weight loss surgery) WLS Boards network.

With over 200,000 members, BariatricPal is the largest online social network dedicated exclusively to bariatric surgery. Thousands of RYGB patients regularly use the discussion forums, track their progress, blog, and post their photos on BariatricPal. Alex and his team work daily to keep the boards up and running, to update the news items, and to monitor the discussions to make sure that they are friendly and never rude. BariatricPal.com continues to serve anyone who is part of the RYGB community by providing free membership to everyone. Alex truly hopes and believes that the boards can play a role in your own RYGB success.

And how does Alex's own bariatric story end up? He is doing great! Since hitting his goal weight of 155 pounds, Alex has maintained his 100-pound weight loss for over seven years now. When Alex is not working on BariatricPal or related projects to help weight loss surgery patients, he loves to run and spend time with his family.

A Brief Tour of BariatricPal.com

The boards are user-friendly. You can see links to the discussion forums on the home page. You can navigate to other parts of the site, such as your profile, your message center, or the surgeon directory, from the home page or any other page. The board rules of courtesy and friendliness are very strictly enforced; negative posts are taken down, and posters can be banned for violating the terms of use.

There is a lot to discover at BariatricPal.com, from discussion forums to the informational library. Our advice is to start with the basics, such as creating your profile when you sign up and learning how to read and reply to posts. You will discover new features as you spend more time on the boards. You can get help by posting a question in the general forum, clicking on the "Help" link on each page, or by contacting Alex or another administrator by clicking on "The Moderating Team" from the home page.

Discussion Forums

The discussion forums are the foundation of BariatricPal.com. The nearly two million posts include nearly any bypass-related, somewhat weight-related, and not at all weight-related topic that you can think of. BariatricPal.com gastric bypass forums are divided into different categories, each with their own focus. Here are some examples:

- *Introductions:* This is where you will find out how welcoming the community is. As soon as you post your introduction here, you will probably get a warm welcome from one or more established members.

- *Pre-Surgery Questions*: In this forum, you can read about and ask questions about preparing for the surgery and what to expect.

- *Post-Surgery Questions:* This forum is geared toward helping you after surgery. Topics might include pain medications, your post-surgery diet progression, and how to treat possible side effects.

- *The "Main Forums":* Here you will find discussions on nutrition, exercise, cosmetic surgery, complications, and everything else that can help you throughout your entire journey.

- *Support Groups:* Whatever your situation is, there is a support group for you. (And if there is not, you can start your own.) There are groups based on your location, personal interests, when you got the bypass (or are scheduled to have your surgery), age, religion, special health conditions, and more.

- *The "Community Center":* This is where you can find the most recent news articles on the gastric bypass, on bariatric surgery, and on obesity; a forum for board suggestions; and feedback and archived newsletters. You can discuss off-topic topics in the Lounge.

BariatricPal.com Grows with You

BariatricPal.com adapts to your changing needs as your gastric bypass journey progresses. Your first visits to the boards, for example, might be to learn about others' experiences and ask your own questions as you decide whether to get RYGB. The site's surgeon directory and reviews can help you find a surgeon. BariatricPal.com members can help you through the surgery and recovery process as they answer your questions about diet and recovery. Later, as your own weight loss is well underway, you will probably find yourself shifting from always asking for help to occasionally providing advice for others. Throughout the process, BariatricPal.com may become one of your favorite online social hangouts where you can kick back and relax.

BariatricPal.com Library

BariatricPal.com's wealth of information about bariatric surgery is particularly convenient if you are already spending time using the site's social features. Topics go from before surgery to afterward. In addition to tips on choosing a surgeon and reducing side effects of surgery, you can find food lists and meal plans, among other topics.

Other Features on BariatricPal.com

BariatricPal.com is not just about the boards and library. It has a variety of other features that make it unique and attractive. These are a few of them:

- *Newsletters:* You receive an electronic newsletter each month. Newsletters include various features such as site updates, detailed profiles of BariatricPal.com members, weight loss tips, and news on weight loss surgery.
- *Surgeon directory*: The surgeon directory lets you search for surgeons in your area. Surgeons are rated and reviewed by BariatricPal.com members so you can be confident that they are trustworthy.
- *Private messaging*: The private messaging system lets you directly contact a specific member or group of members without posting publicly on the boards.
- *Chat rooms*: Live chat rooms let you "talk" in real-time with anyone else who happens to be hanging out in the room.
- *WLS magazine:* Each WLS ("Weight Loss Surgery") magazine, available from the main page of the forums, contains articles on information that can be very valuable in your journey. Topics might include diet, social support, plateaus, and family issues that come up as the result of your weight loss. Authors include bariatric patients, dietitians, psychologists, and other professionals with expertise in bariatric surgery and weight loss.

Mobile Features

BariatricPal.com has been mobile since 2012, when the site celebrated the launch of its new apps for the Apple iPod, iPad, and iPhone, as well as for the Android and the Kindle. The apps are free and fully functional, so you can carry BariatricPal.com with you anywhere. You can read and post to discussion forum topics, send private messages to your friends, post status updates and photos, and do anything else that you can do from a computer on BariatricPal.com.

These apps are great because they let you stay connected with the board at all times. Let's say that you need to know what to order at a restaurant or which foods at a luncheon are allowed on your diet or that you are feeling down and need some encouragement to go out for a walk. BariatricPal has so many members that you are almost sure to be able to connect with people whenever you need them.

You can also use smartphone apps and the app for the Kindle to get answers to burning questions that come up when you are on the go. For example, you might find yourself at a fast food restaurant with friends and you want to find out what to order that is best for your meal plan. You can probably find some suggestions on previously posted discussion on BariatricPal.com. The smartphone app makes it possible for you to find the best choice even when you did not plan ahead.

Your Profile and Options – Making BariatricPal.com Your Own

In this section, we will talk about getting started on BariatricPal.com and some options for personalizing your experience and making it your own.

Getting Started and Setting Up Your Account

Only members can post on the boards, so the first step is to sign up and create an account. Again, your full-featured account is free. These are the basic steps of creating an account:

- Click on "Register Now" toward the upper right corner of the page and follow the prompts.
  - *Step 1: "Your Account."* Choose a username and password, enter your email address, select your gender, and check the box that states that you agree to the terms of use.
  - *Step 2: "Your Surgery."* Answer the questions in as much detail as you want. You can always come back later and fill in blank answers.
  - *Step 3: "Confirmation."* A confirmation email will come to your inbox.
- Activate your account by following the prompts in the confirmation email that you receive.
- When you are ready, you can set up your account preferences for which notifications you would like to receive, such as friends' status updates, personal messages, and general messages to the community from BariatricPal.com administrators.
- You can always edit your profile information and account settings later.

Profile

You do not have to complete a full profile, but it helps everyone else know who you are. There is space for you to write your RYGB story; for your beginning, current, and goal weight and BMI; and for identifying your surgeon. You can also put in personal information, such as your location, age, hobbies, and occupation. You have the option of linking your BariatricPal.com account to your Facebook and Twitter accounts.

Everyone loves before and after photos, and there is a place for them on your profile page.

You can post additional photos in the "Photo Gallery," which is like a photo album that you get to share with the entire community if you choose.

Stay on Track with Trackers

Lose weight and stay on track when you log and record everything, including your progress. BariatricPal.com *trackers* are basically online mini-logs—you get to track your measurements and see how far you have progressed toward your goals. You can put in your weight and your body measurements. You can also keep a food log using your tracker so that you always have a place to record what you ate.

Mark Your Progress with Tickers

The *tickers* are what you will see under some members' signatures when they post in the forums. You can set yours to show your BMI, your percent body fat, your body weight, or, if you have not had surgery yet, a countdown of the number of days until your surgery is scheduled. The ticker is sort of a ruler; on the left of the ruler is your starting BMI, percent fat, body weight, or number of days when you started counting down to surgery. At the far right is your goal value or surgery date. A ticker marker moves from left to right as you make progress toward your goal. You get to customize your ticker by choosing from a variety of designs for the ruler and for the ticker marker. If you choose, your ticker marker will be displayed under your post every time you post in the forums.

You do not have to share your tracker if you do not want. You can set yours to be private so that only you can see it or set it so that only your approved friends on BariatricPal.com can see it. If you like to be held accountable by a lot of people, you can keep your tracker public so that everyone who looks at your profile can see it.

Automatic Updates Are Optional

You can set your account to send updates to your email address or smartphone. Some people like to get emails and push notifications from BariatricPal.com every time there is an update. Some members, on the other extreme, prefer to only rarely receive emails or push notifications; they would rather only see board updates when they log in.

Most people like the occasional email or phone notification from the boards. These reminders can also provide additional inspiration to keep working at your RYGB diet. These are examples of some of the email or smartphone notifications that you can choose to receive if you want. You can always change your settings from your profile page if you change your mind about what email or smartphone updates you want to receive.

- Updates on any discussion thread of your choice so you know when someone has replied to a conversation that you are in or you think is interesting
- Delivery of the board's regular newsletter
- Communications from Alex Brecher, the board's founder, or any of the staff at the boards. These kinds of messages come only a few times a year when there is big news, so we recommend signing up for these.

- Delivery of private messages from other board members
- Alerts on your friends' status updates and members' replies to your own status updates

If you choose not to receive a notification via email, you can still find the information on BariatricPal.com the next time you log in. You will see a little icon near your name at the corner of the screen when you log in. It tells you that you have notifications to check out.

Keeping Your Profile Current and Customized

There are plenty of ways to keep your BariatricPal.com information current so that everyone is up to date on your latest news. As with all of your information on BariatricPal.com, you can set your profile information to be as private or public as you choose. Many members choose an intermediate option by allowing only their approved BariatricPal "friends" to see their information.

You can update your profile at any time. This includes features such as tickers, trackers, your gastric bypass story, and your photo gallery. These are some of the options that BariatricPal.com offers to keep your profile and information personal and current.

Member Blog

BariatricPal.com hosts members' blogs. The blog is automatically linked to your account, and you access it from your profile. You can use it just like any other blog, where you post entries about your life or whatever you want. Some members keep their blogs strictly focused on the gastric bypass and weight loss, while others include pretty much everything else about their lives—almost as a regular diary or journal.

Personal News Feed

The news feed feature on BariatricPal.com is similar to those on other online social networking sites. The feed shows your social activity on BariatricPal.com. Members can see when you update your profile photo, when you add new friends, and when you make new posts on the discussion boards. The profile feed is a feature that allows you to post short sentences about what you are doing so everyone knows.

Photo Ops

BariatricPal.com has space for your photos. Besides posting before and after photos on your member profile page, you can choose a photo—or any image you want—as your profile picture. That is what everyone will see when they read your posts or get private messages from you. You can also take advantage of the photo gallery to post as many photos as you want and let everyone see them!

The Social Side of BariatricPal.com

Come for the information; stay for the friends! You might start going to the boards to gather information about the gastric bypass. Even if this book does not inspire you to look for the site, you will probably find it when you do online searches. When you make your way to BariatricPal.com, you will probably find not only the answers you needed but more encouragement and positive support than you expected.

In fact, do not be surprised if you come back to the boards because you like the atmosphere and start to meet some people that you really care about—and that really care about you. You might even start to count some members as some of your best friends. Just as you can on other social media sites, you can become board "friends" with other members by inviting them to be your friends or accepting their invitations to be theirs. This lets you see each others' updates faster and send private messages straight from your profile.

Special "Groups" Let You Make Closer Friends

As mentioned above, the group forums are for members with common characteristics or interests. The groups provide ideal opportunities to share experiences with members who may be going through the same struggles and triumphs as you. Just like in the real world, where you are more likely to make close friends with people who have a lot in common with you, you might feel a closer bond with BariatricPal.com members who have more in common with you than just the bypass. They might be your age, have children of the same age, live near you, or share the same religious beliefs or hobbies, for example.

Using BariatricPal.com Daily

Some gastric bypass members check out the boards daily or even more frequently as they start to depend on it for instant advice, sympathetic listeners, and, finally, close friends. The site gives you a sense of belonging and accountability.

Giving Back to the Bariatric Community and BariatricPal.com

Membership to BariatricPal.com, including each of its services and features, is free for everyone. You can set up your account and get instant access to the boards, including to the smartphone and Kindle apps. Alex Brecher, the founder of BariatricPal.com, is committed to helping you throughout your weight loss journey. His mission is to make the community accessible to everyone who needs this resource for their success. A lot of people depend on this free service. Opportunities are available if you are interested in giving back just a little. These are some of the ways you can help out.

Review and Rate Your Surgeon

The Surgeon Directory is invaluable for patients who are looking for a surgeon. You can help keep the Surgeon Directory complete by writing a review of your own surgeon and rating him or her. You might be more motivated to write an honest, detailed review when you remember how difficult it was for you to find a surgeon and how much you appreciated each bit of information that helped you make your decision confidently.

Post Fliers in Your Clinic

BariatricPal.com depends on growth and is always eager to welcome new members. You can help spread the word and attract new members by posting promotional BariatricPal.com fliers in your surgeon's office or waiting room, where your bariatric surgery group support meetings are held or anywhere else that bariatric surgery patients are likely to gather and see the posters. The fliers are already prepared and are available from BariatricPal.com, so you just have to print them out and post them.

Be a Good Community Member

You can also help simply by being proactive on the boards. The BariatricPal.com community is based on a foundation of positive energy and member participation. One of the ways you can help out is to keep an eye out for inappropriate posts, such as negative posts, off-topic posts, or spam posters that are obviously there to promote their own interests. Alex and his team work daily to prevent these situations, but extra eyes can always help.

Another way that you help out the community is to provide support for other members. In the beginning, your support might be more geared toward encouragement. You can also play a role in welcoming new members. As you lose weight, you will be gaining more knowledge. You will soon be an expert at knowing what works and what does not with the RYGB. This experience enables you to provide more advice and answers to specific questions.

Other Online Resources

BariatricPal.com is the biggest discussion forum and support system on the web, but it is not your only possible source of support and information. Additional sources include other online discussion forums and social networks, bariatric surgery clinic sites, and government-provided information.

Sources of Information

Government resources, such as Medline Plus and the Weight Information Network, are considered trustworthy sources of information. They are both provided and maintained by the National Institutes of Health within the Department of Health and Human Services. Many bariatric centers at large hospitals and universities have relatively extensive sites. They often provide a good deal of practical information about the bypass, such as how the procedure goes, how to prepare for surgery, and how to progress with your post-surgery diet.

Select the Resources That You Prefer

Which resources you use are completely up to you. You might be the type of person who trusts only what your doctor says and stays far away from online information and social networking. That is okay, as long as you are sure to get the information and support you need from real-life sources, such as family, close friends, coworkers, and members of your support group. If you are an Internet junkie, you will probably be online constantly, looking at every possible resource. You will probably end up using a few different sites regularly. You might, for example, have a favorite hospital site for when you need to look up basic rules on your diet, plus one or two social networking sites to connect with your new friends.

✍ Summary

- Preparation, without a doubt, increases your chances of success after bariatric surgery, but you cannot possibly know the answer to every question ahead of time. Luckily, finding answers and support is easier with the Internet. This chapter encouraged you to explore the Internet as a valuable resource and provided advice on making the most out of what you find.

- Reading this book puts you far ahead of most other bariatric surgery patients in terms of knowledge, preparation, and what to expect. You have learned about every step of the way, from the possible risks of obesity, to whether RYGB is for you, to how to get through surgery, to what kind of lifestyle you will be or are leading. You are more prepared than someone that jumps in blindly, and this gives you a better chance of success.

- You should have confidence in your ability to track down the information you need to stay on track and make the right decisions when you are not sure what to do. Just as the gastric bypass is a tool to help you lose weight, this book is a tool to help you learn what you need to know to lose weight with gastric bypass. It is a good starting point.

Time to Take Action: How Can the Internet Help You?

This book covers a wide range of topics, but there's no way it could cover everything you need to know. What is something that you still need to find out?

Example: I still don't know which cuts of beef are healthiest.

1.

2.

3.

What questions do you think will come up later as you make progress toward your weight loss goal and eventually hit your goal?

Example: I'll probably start to wonder how I can meet new exercise buddies as I get in better shape.

1.

2.

3.

The Internet is almost certain to play at least a small part in your weight loss success. Resources are unlimited, free, and instantly available. What roles do you see the Internet playing in your vertical sleeve journey?

Example: I'll probably be looking up recipes to find out how to make my diet more interesting!

1.

2.

3.

BariatricPal.com is the world's largest online social network dedicated to the bariatric community. List three of BariatricPal.com's features discussed in the chapter and explain how you think they might help you.

Example: gallery for before and after photos. I think I'm going to be very excited to show the world the differences. It'll keep me motivated to keep losing weight so that I can keep changing my after photo!

1.

2.

3.

Epilogue

This is the end of *The BIG Book on the Gastric Bypass: Everything You Need to Know to Lose Weight and Live Well with Roux-en-Y Gastric Bypass*. We have taken you from the beginning of your weight loss journey, through surgery, to your new everyday lifestyle after gastric bypass. The book was designed to be a complete guide to enable you to take control of your weight, health, and life.

The book covered the effects and challenges of obesity, how RYGB is a tool to help you lose weight for the long term, and what kind of weight loss to expect after the procedure. You've learned about the side effects and possible complications from RYGB and what you can do to lower your risk. You now know how to choose a surgeon, get ready for surgery, and recover more quickly. The book discusses the importance of exercise and gives some tips and tricks to get you started and turn an active lifestyle into a long-term habit. And you have worked on building your support system to keep you motivated.

Your diet is among the most important factors in your weight loss success. From the post-surgery dietary progression to your weight loss diet, you are practically an expert on nutrition and the gastric bypass diet. You know which foods to choose, which foods to avoid and what to do if you have a reaction to a food. You even know how to create a daily menu that has the nutrients you need and which nutritional supplements may be necessary to stay healthy.

We know that your weight loss journey does not stop here. You will continue to have new questions, try new recipes, overcome, and share happy moments with your friends and family that might not have happened if you had not gotten weight loss surgery.

We sincerely hope that this book has been and will continue to be an excellent resource for you. We suggest that you keep it handy as one of your valuable references so you can look things up when you have questions. You can use it to look up facts about the bypass, refresh your memory on basic nutrition, and design a meal plan based on the food phase you are in. Chapter 15 is always there for you too, for whenever you feel ready to get started with an exercise program or you need some strategies to motivate yourself to continue your program.

We also recommend, if you have not already, signing up for BariatricPal.com, the world's premier online social network dedicated to the weight loss community. It is a source of information and support, and it will grow with you. No matter where you are in your weight loss journey or how many new questions and experiences you have, you will be able to find someone to sympathize with you, offer you advice, or point you in the right direction. You will probably also make a few very close friends on BariatricPal.com. Your account is free and takes only minutes to set up, so there is no reason not to try it out. We think you will be glad you did!

We would like to thank you for letting this book be a part of your Roux-en-Y gastric bypass journey. Regardless of where you are in your weight loss journey, whether or not you choose to get the surgery or whether you read the book so that you could offer support to a loved one who is a RYGB patient, we hope that this book has met your needs. Our goal was to provide honest and complete information to allow you to make the best decisions for yourself, and we truly hope we have succeeded.

We wish you the best of luck in your bypass future.

Alex Brecher and Natalie Stein

Glossary of Terms

Abdominoplasty (also panniculectomy) – This is also known as a "tummy tuck." It is when your cosmetic surgeon removes the excess skin and fat that are left in your stomach after you lose a lot of weight, such as hitting your goal weight after getting the Roux-en-Y gastric bypass. The surgeon might also tighten up the abdominal muscles too.

Adjustable gastric band (AGB) – Also known as the lap-band or the band, it is a band that goes around the upper part of your stomach to create a smaller upper pouch, called a stoma. The larger part of your stomach remains below the band, which slows the flow of food from the stoma to the lower part of the stomach. The gastric band restricts your food intake to help you lose weight because your stoma fills up quickly and you feel full. The tightness of the gastric band can be adjusted by filling it with saline solution to make it more restrictive. An unfill, or removing saline solution, loosens the band and makes it less restrictive.

Adverse events – These are harmful side effects or complications that are associated with a specific medication or medical procedure, such as the gastric bypass. A low rate of mild adverse events means that the procedure is pretty safe, while a high rate of severe adverse events means that the procedure is pretty risky.

Bariatric surgery (weight loss surgery) – This is any surgery that is designed to help you lose weight. The more common types in the United States are the gastric sleeve, or vertical gastrectomy, the roux-en-Y gastric bypass, the adjustable laparoscopic gastric band, or lap-band, and the sleeve plication surgery. Bariatric surgery itself does not cause weight loss. Instead, it is a tool that helps you eat less and/or absorb fewer nutrients so that you can lose weight.

Biliopancreatic Diversion with Duodenal Switch (BPD-DS) – This bariatric procedure is restrictive because it removes most of the stomach, and it is malabsorptive because it redirects some digestive juices and food to the large intestine for elimination from the body. The BPD-DS is a two-step process and is used most often in morbidly obese patients.

BMI (body mass index) – This is a calculation that is used to indicate whether you are at a healthy weight or whether you should lose weight. The formula to calculate BMI considers your height and weight. Chapter 1 shows you how you can calculate your BMI and determine whether you are at a normal weight or if you are overweight, obese, or morbidly obese.

BMR (basal metabolic rate) – This is also known as your metabolism. It is the number of calories you burn per day just to stay alive. Your body uses calories, even while resting and sleeping, for things like keeping your heart beating, your blood flowing, and your lungs breathing. Your BMR is higher if you are a man, you are a younger rather than an older adult, and if you are heavier.

Brachioplasty – This procedure, also known as an arm lift, is cosmetic surgery to get rid of your "bat wings," or the skin that hangs down from your arms after you lose a lot of weight.

Calorie balance – Also known as "energy balance," this is a comparison of the calories you consume, or take in, versus the calories you burn off, or expend. You consume calories by eating; you expend calories with your basal metabolic rate (see "BMR"), from digesting food and from physical activity. You are in calorie balance when you are eating the same number of calories that you are expending. Your weight will not change when you are in energy balance.

Calorie deficit – Also known as a "negative calorie balance," this is when you are expending, or using, more calories than you are consuming. A calorie deficit leads to weight loss. A deficit of 3,500 calories leads to one pound of weight loss, so you need to average a deficit of 500 calories per day if you want to lose one pound per week. You can create a deficit by eating fewer calories or increasing your physical activity.

Calorie surplus – This is also known as a "positive calorie balance." It happens when you consume more calories than you expend. Basically, if you eat more than you burn off, you will gain weight.

Cholesterol, total – Your total cholesterol is measured with a simple blood test, usually as part of a lipid panel. Your doctor or the laboratory can let you know whether you need to be fasting. High cholesterol is a risk factor for heart disease. A normal cholesterol level is under 200 milligrams per deciliter (200 mg/dL or 5.2 mmol/L); borderline high cholesterol is 200 to 239 mg/dL (5.2 to 6.2 mmol/L); high cholesterol is 240 mg/dL (6.2 mmol/L) or above. You can lower your cholesterol by losing extra body weight and eating more fiber, which is in fruits, vegetables, beans, nuts, and whole grains products. (See Chapter 15, "*The RYGB Diet & Nutrition,*" for more information).

Cholesterol, HDL – High-density lipoprotein cholesterol, or HDL cholesterol, is known as the "good" cholesterol. Like total cholesterol, you will get your HDL measured in a blood test as part of a lipid panel. A high value of HDL cholesterol means that you have a lower risk for heart disease. Women naturally have higher HDL cholesterol than men. A desirable value for HDL cholesterol is above 60 milligrams per dL (60 mg/dL; over 1.5 mmol/L). HDL cholesterol under 40 mg/dL (1 mmol/L) for men and below 50 mg/dl (1.3 mmol/L) for women is a risk factor for heart disease. Increasing your physical activity increases your HDL cholesterol levels.

Cholesterol, LDL – Low-density lipoprotein cholesterol, or LDL cholesterol, is known as the "bad" cholesterol because a high value increases your risk of heart disease. Your doctor might recommend keeping your LDL under 70 milligrams per deciliter (70 mg/dL, or 1.8 mmol/L) if you have a high risk for heart disease; otherwise, the general goal for your LDL cholesterol is under 100 mg/dL. LDL cholesterol from 160 to 189 mg/dL (4.1 to 4.9 mmol/L) is high, and over 190 mg/dL is considered very high. You can lower your LDL cholesterol by losing excess weight and reducing your intake of saturated fat, such as from fatty meats, dark-meat poultry, butter, dairy products, and palm oil.

Comorbidity – A disorder related to the primary disease; in this case, the primary disease is obesity, and common comorbidities include obesity-related diseases, such as type 2 diabetes, hypertension, and osteoarthritis.

Contraindications – These are reasons to refuse to provide a certain medical service or procedure. Some of the contraindications for the gastric bypass, or reasons why you would not be a good candidate for the RYGB, are congestive heart failure, drug or alcohol addiction, and lack of understanding of how the sleeve works.

Copay – This is a flat fee, rather than a percentage, that your insurance company makes you pay each time you see a healthcare provider. In most cases, your copay amount is not affected by the services you end up getting at the appointment. An example of a copayment might be $30 each time you see a physician within your health coverage plan.

Deductible – This is the amount you need to pay, usually annually, before your insurance plan actually starts to cover your expenses. The "better" your insurance plan is, the lower your deductible rate; that is, your insurance plan pays for services before you have paid very much out of your own pocket. Let's take an example. Let's say that your insurance plan covers 80 percent of your expense and that your deductible is $1,000 annually. You, yourself, are responsible for paying the first $1,000 in medical bills in each year. Your insurance will only start to pay 80 percent of your bills for the rest of the year after you have already gotten—and paid for by yourself—$1,000-worth of services.

Dehiscence – This is a complication of surgery that is the splitting of the scar site where the stitches are. It can happen after RYGB along the line where your surgeon stitched your stomach. Dehiscence is more likely if you do not follow your surgeon's instructions for taking care of yourself after surgery.

Diabetes (type 2 diabetes) – This is the type of diabetes that is often known as adult-onset diabetes. It is most commonly linked to obesity, unlike type 1 diabetes, which usually occurs in childhood or adolescence. Diabetes occurs when your blood sugar levels are out of control. Complications include kidney disease, blindness, amputations, infections, and heart disease. (See also gestational diabetes.) RYGB can help reduce diabetes.

Dietitian – A dietitian, or registered dietitian, has taken a variety of nutrition classes, practiced clinical skills in an internship, and passed the national dietetics examination. Dietitians help you plan meals, work through food challenges, choose healthier foods, and improve your recipes. You can recognize a dietitian by the "RD" credential. A nutritionist is not necessarily a dietitian, although many nutritionists are just as highly qualified. They might have an "MS" or "PhD" in nutrition.

Dumping Syndrome – A side effect of malabsorptive procedures that leads to diarrhea, nausea, weakness, and fatigue after you eat. It happens when undigested food gets into your large intestine and is worse for high-sugar and high-fat foods. Dumping syndrome is less common with VSG than with gastric bypass or BPD-DS.

Dyslipidemia – This is a condition when your blood lipids, or total cholesterol, LDL cholesterol, HDL cholesterol, and/or triglycerides, are not at normal levels. Dyslipidemia is a risk factor for heart disease, and it is often caused by obesity.

Empty calories – These are calories or high-calorie foods that do not provide many essential nutrients, such as vitamins and minerals. Examples include sugar, sweets, French fries, doughnuts, and bacon.

Excess Weight Lost (EWL) – This is usually expressed in a percentage as the amount of weight lost divided by the amount of excess weight that you started with. To calculate your starting excess weight, take your starting body weight and subtract your ideal body weight.

Fully-insured plan – This is a health insurance plan that you or your employer pays for.

Gastric band – This is the key weight loss tool in the lap-band procedure. The gastric band is literally a band that goes around your stomach (the gastric tissue) to create a smaller stoma above and the larger stomach portion below. The gastric band is cushioned and has room for saline solution. A fuller gastric band makes you feel more restriction to lose weight faster; a less full band makes you feel less restriction.

Gastric bypass – This is a type of weight loss surgery that divides your stomach into a smaller upper pouch and smaller lower pouch. The intestine connects to both. The procedure is restrictive, like the lap-band, but unlike the lap-band, gastric bypass is also malabsorptive so the amount of nutrients that you absorb decreases. The most common kind of gastric bypass is Roux-en-Y.

Gastric sleeve (see vertical sleeve gastrectomy)

Gestational diabetes (GDM) – This is a type of glucose intolerance, or lack of blood sugar control, that occurs during pregnancy. It often goes away after you give birth, but you are at higher risk of developing type 2 diabetes if you had GDM during one or more pregnancies. Obesity increases your risk of developing GDM.

Ghrelin – Sometimes called the hunger hormone, it is produced by your stomach and pancreas, and it makes you feel hungry. You have higher levels before meals and lower levels after meals. Gastric sleeve patients have lower levels of ghrelin after surgery than before, so this hormonal change may play a role in helping you lose weight.

Glucagon-like peptide-1 (GLP-1) – This is a gut hormone whose levels are lower between meals and higher after meals. It tends to make you eat less. Obese individuals have lower levels of GLP-1 than normal-weight individuals. The RYGB leads to higher GLP-1 levels, which might help you lose weight by making you feel more satisfied after meals.

Glucose – This is the type of sugar that is in your blood. It provides energy to most of the cells in your body, but very high or uncontrolled levels of blood glucose cause pre-diabetes or type 2 diabetes. Your glucose levels go up as you start to develop insulin resistance.

Glucose tolerance test (or oral glucose tolerance test—OGTT) – This is a test of how well you are able to control your blood glucose levels. You drink a very sweet sugar solution, and the laboratory technician draws your blood periodically for a couple of hours after that to monitor the changes in your blood sugar levels. You may have diabetes if a glucose tolerance test causes your blood glucose levels to spike high and fast.

Health maintenance organization (HMO) – This is a type of health insurance plan that helps cover expenses for doctor visits, medical services, and prescription drugs. Your HMO might cover a certain percentage of most services.

Hypertension (high blood pressure) – This is when the force of your blood beating against your blood vessels is higher than it should be. You get your blood measured, probably at most doctor's visits, when a nurse puts a cuff around your upper arm, inflates the cuff, and slowly lets the air out. Hypertension means your heart is working harder than it should, and it also puts a strain on your kidneys. High blood pressure increases your risk for heart disease, kidney disease, and stroke. If you are obese, losing weight can probably lower high blood pressure.

Ideal body weight – This is a theoretical value that is considered to be the healthiest body weight at your height. It is often set at a BMI of 22.

Ileal brake – Combined effect of peptide-YY and glucagon-like peptide-1 to make you feel full when food reaches the far end of your small intestine—the ileum.

Indications – These are characteristics that make you a potential candidate for a medical treatment. Some indications for getting Roux-en-Y gastric bypass, for example, are having morbid obesity or having a BMI of at least 35 and a comorbidity, such as type 2 diabetes.

Inpatient – This is often defined as an overnight hospital stay or a stay that lasts at least 24 hours.

Insulin – This is a hormone that is necessary for regulating your blood sugar levels. It is produced by a kind of cell, called beta cells, that are in your pancreas. Type 2 diabetes occurs when you develop insulin resistance and your body can no longer control your blood glucose levels.

Insulin resistance – This describes what happens when the cells in your body are no longer as responsive (or as sensitive) to the effects of insulin. The result is that high levels of glucose stay in your blood. Severe insulin resistance leads to pre-diabetes and then type 2 diabetes.

LAP-BAND® or adjustable gastric banding system (AGBS) – This is the brand name for the adjustable laparoscopic band made by the company Allergan, Inc. It consists of a gastric band, thin connection tubing, and an access port. The system comes in two sizes and is designed to be adjustable and reversible so that you can reduce your risk of health complications with the surgery and afterward.

Laparoscopic surgery – This is also known as minimally invasive surgery, or MIS. Laparoscopic surgery requires smaller incisions than regular surgery. Instead of actually opening up your body and controlling the instruments with his or her hands, the surgeon uses a camera to visualize the patient's interior and controls the instruments with robotic systems.

Laparotomy – This is an open surgery that your surgeon might choose to do if unable to perform the laparoscopic surgery on you. The laparotomy involves a single deep cut in your abdomen to give the surgeon access to your abdomen. Recovery time is longer after the laparotomy and you have a higher risk for infections, but you might need it if your heart and lungs cannot handle the pneumoperitoneum required in laparoscopic surgery.

Leak – A leak is a complication of RYGB in which the staple line of your stomach pouch is no longer tight. Food and bacteria from your gastrointestinal tract can get into your abdominal cavity and lead to peritonitis. A leak may require a stent or another surgery to fix the leak.

Leptin – A hormone that is involved in appetite control. Leptin may reduce appetite, but obese individuals have higher leptin levels than normal weight individuals. That may mean that obese individuals respond differently to leptin. The gastric bypass can improve the effects of leptin on your appetite, but the research results are not yet clear.

Lipid panel – Also known as a lipid profile, this is a standard set of tests that your doctor uses to help determine your risk for heart disease. It includes your total cholesterol, LDL cholesterol, HDL cholesterol, and triglycerides. It is a simple blood test, and you will often get your blood glucose, which is a test for diabetes, tested at the same time. You will need to fast for a complete lipid panel.

Managed care – This is a general term for health care programs that are designed to reduce total costs to you and the system. Private examples include HMOs and PPOs; public examples of managed care programs include Medicare for older adults and Medicaid for low-income children and disabled adults.

Magenstrasse and Mill – This is an early version of the vertical sleeve gastrectomy developed in the United Kingdom. The surgeon removes the majority of the stomach and makes a long tube out of the lesser curvature of the stomach that goes from the esophagus to the antral mill, where food grinding occurs. The procedure is simple, does not require foreign implants, and retains regular digestion of food to prevent dumping syndrome.

Malabsorptive procedure – A bariatric surgery procedure that interferes with regular nutrient absorption. This helps with weight loss because you absorb fewer calories from your food, but it puts you at higher risk for nutrient deficiencies because you are not absorbing all of the vitamins and minerals that you eat. Another side effect is dumping syndrome. Gastric bypass and biliopancreatic diversion with duodenal switch (BPD-DS) are examples of malabsorptive procedures; the sleeve is not malabsorptive.

Maximum out-of-pocket – This is the highest total amount of money that you yourself will need to pay in a specific time period, such as a year, before your insurance company will pay for absolutely all the rest of your medical costs. Having a maximum out-of-pocket protects you against catastrophic financial results in case you end up needing unexpected and expensive emergency care or a long hospital stay.

Medicaid – This is the government-run health insurance program for low-income individuals. It is run partly by the federal government and partly by the state government, so there are lots of variations between states in their Medicaid programs. You might have to do a bit of quick research to find the specific name of the Medicaid program in your state.

Medical tourism – This is when you go to a foreign nation to get your medical procedure done. Mexico is a popular destination country for bariatric surgeries. Some Americans go to Canada, India, or other nations to get their surgeries. Medical tourism can be cheaper than staying in the U.S. for patients whose insurance will not cover it, and you can usually get package deals with transportation, accommodations, and medical care included.

Medicare – This is the national health care insurance program for adults over age 65 years. It is a managed care program. Hospital services are covered in Part A of Medicare, and outpatient services are covered in Part B.

Metabolism (see BMR)

Morbid obesity – This is when your BMI is 40 or above. It is a level of obesity that is associated with a very high risk of chronic diseases, such as heart disease, stroke, and type 2 diabetes. If you have morbid obesity, you may qualify for the Roux-en-Y even if you do not have any other health conditions because you are at such a high risk for developing them soon.

Non-Steroidal Anti-Inflammatory Drug (NSAID) – These are common painkillers that also fight inflammation. Many, such as ibuprofen and aspirin, are over-the-counter and familiar. Ketorolac is a prescription NSAID that is common after the VSG. Using NSAIDs can reduce the amount of narcotic painkillers that you need.

Nutrient-dense – These kinds of foods provide a lot of essential and beneficial nutrients, such as dietary fiber, healthy fats, vitamins, or minerals. Examples include fat-free yogurt, tuna, skinless chicken breast, fruit, vegetables, and beans. Most nutrient-dense foods are fairly low in calories, but some, such as nuts and avocados, are high in calories because they are full of healthy fats.

Obese – You are considered obese if your BMI is at least 30. Obesity is considered a risk factor for a variety of chronic conditions, including heart disease, stroke, high blood pressure, some cancers, sleep apnea, asthma, and osteoarthritis. You may be eligible to get gastric bypass if your BMI is greater than 35 and you have a chronic condition that puts your health at risk.

Osteoporosis – This is a chronic condition with low bone mineral density, so you are at high risk for bone fractures. The disease takes years to develop, and you may not know you have it until you break a bone. RYGB patients need to be sure to get enough calcium and vitamin D to avoid a higher risk for osteoporosis; this can be challenging with the limited food intake on the sleeve diet.

Outpatient – This refers to any procedure that does not require an overnight stay in the clinic or hospital. Sometimes "outpatient" is defined as any hospital visit that takes less than 24 hours. The Roux-en-Y is often an outpatient procedure, but many insurance plans require an overnight stay before you get reimbursed for the surgery. You will have to check your plan and discuss the requirements with your surgeon.

Overweight – You are considered overweight if your BMI is between 25 and 30. You may not have visible health effects from being overweight (but you might), but you are at higher risk for becoming obese than if you were at a normal weight.

Panniculectomy (see abdominoplasty)

Peptide YY (PYY) – This gut hormone forms part of the "ileal brake" with glucagon-like peptide-1. PYY increases your feelings of fullness after a meal. Levels are higher in obese individuals than normal-weight, and they sometimes, but not always, decrease after RYGB— which may contribute to your weight loss.

Pneumoperitoneum – Inflation of the wall of your abdominal cavity, created by pumping in carbon dioxide gas, that allows your surgeon access to your stomach to be able to perform a laparoscopic surgery. It is a strain for your heart and lungs and may cause shoulder or neck pain after your surgery.

Post-anesthesia care unit (PACU) – This is where you are likely to wake up after your RYGB surgery. It is a room where patients that just had surgery and are still under the effects of anesthesia can recover. The benefit of having a single PACU, instead of sending you off to an isolated hospital room, is that the PACU nurses continually check on you to make sure that everything is going smoothly. Smaller clinics might not have a PACU, but the staff there will still take care of you.

Preferred provider organization (PPO) – This is a type of health insurance plan that charges based on a fee-for-service. That means that you pay for each service that you receive, but the amounts that you are charged are lower than for someone who is not in the PPO.

Pre-diabetes (impaired fasting glucose; IFT) – This is when your blood glucose levels are higher than normal but not high enough to put you in the category of being diabetic. Your doctor can diagnose pre-diabetes using a fasting blood glucose test, which you can get in any medical laboratory. Pre-diabetes puts you at very high risk of developing diabetes. If you are overweight or obese, losing weight can often put your blood glucose levels back to normal so that you are no longer pre-diabetic.

Quality of life – Also known as QoL, this is an overall indicator of how good your life is. It considers your physical health plus other factors, such as your social connections, how happy you are, and how well you are able to move around and do the things you want to do. A variety of different tests are available to measure QoL. The RYGB can help improve QoL.

Restrictive procedure – A bariatric procedure that limits the amount of food you are able to eat and therefore helps you lose weight, the Roux-en-Y gastric bypass is a restrictive procedure. The smaller stomach pouch helps you feel full sooner so you eat less.

Roux-en-Y gastric bypass – A gastric bypass weight loss surgery procedure in which the upper part of the small intestine is divided to connect to a smaller upper stomach pouch and a larger lower stomach remnant. It is reversible, but only through a difficult procedure. RYGB works through malabsorption and restriction.

Self-insured plan – This is a plan that your employer purchases; it may have specific benefits or exclusions that your employer has chosen as part of an individualized package.

Sleeve gastrectomy (see vertical sleeve gastrectomy)

Stent – A small tube that is often used to treat leaks in the sleeve, it may contain a sticky substance designed to slowly seal up the leak.

Stomach stapling (see vertical banded gastroplasty)

Summary of benefits (SOB) or certificate of coverage – This is a critical piece of paper (or online document) that tells you your insurance policy if you are in a fully-insured plan. It tells you which services are covered under your plan. You might have to call the insurance company to have them send you the summary of benefits if you cannot locate it yourself.

Summary Plan Description (SPD) – This is a critical piece of paper (or online document) that tells you your insurance policy if you are in a self-insured plan. It tells you which services are covered under your plan. You might have to call your employer's human resources department or the insurance company to have them send you the summary of benefits if you cannot locate it yourself.

Triglycerides – These are a specific kind of fat that float around in your blood stream. Very high levels increase your risk for heart disease. Normal triglyceride levels are under 150 milligrams per deciliter (150 mg/dL, or 1.7 mmol/L). Your triglycerides are high if they are between 200 and 500 mg/dL (2.3 to 5.6 mmol/L) and very high if they are over 500 mg/dL (more than 5.6 mmol/L). You can lower high triglycerides by losing excess weight, exercising regularly, and reducing your intake of sugar and saturated fat.

Type 2 diabetes (see diabetes)

Vertical banded gastroplasty (VBG) – Also known as stomach stapling, this bariatric procedure involves partitioning the stomach with staples and a band to block off the majority of the stomach. The VBG has a similar principle as the VSG, but the stomach is only folded away, not removed, in the VBG. Because of the high rate of weight regain and complications, such as staples coming loose and gastroesophageal reflux (GERD), the VBG is rare in the U.S. today.

Vertical sleeve gastrectomy – This is also known as the gastric sleeve, gastrectomy, greater curvature gastrectomy, and simply the sleeve. It is an irreversible procedure that can help you lose weight because it helps to restrict your food intake. The surgeon removes approximately 85 percent of your stomach, leaving only the upper 15 percent. The smaller stomach pouch is then attached to the small intestine.

Weight loss surgery (see bariatric surgery)

New Terms

There are always more words to learn about the Roux-en-Y gastric bypass. For easy reference, just add them to the glossary. Use this table to add new terms and their definitions. Also make note of where you came across the term so you can go back and look it up if necessary.

Term	Where You Found It	Definition

Made in the USA
Monee, IL
07 October 2023

44137364R00260